FOWLERS AND WELLS'

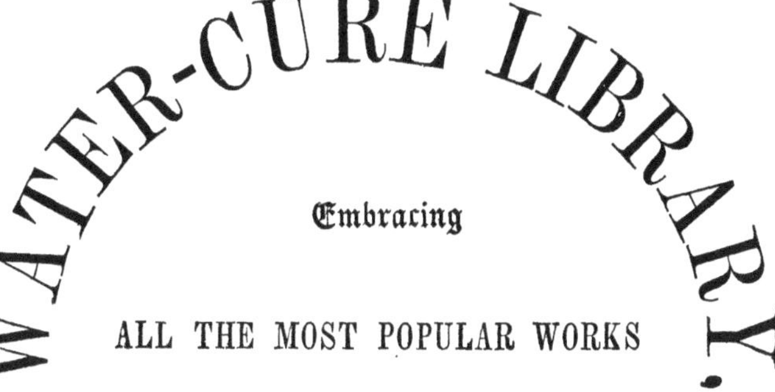

ALL THE MOST POPULAR WORKS

ON THE SUBJECT:

INCLUDING

INTRODUCTION TO THE WATER-CURE;
HYDROPATHY, OR THE WATER-CURE;
EXPERIENCE IN THE WATER-CURE;
THE CHOLERA, AND BOWEL DISEASES;
WATER AND VEGETABLE DIET;
THE PARENTS' GUIDE;
TOBACCO: ITS NATURE AND EFFECTS;
CURIOSITIES OF COMMON WATER;
WATER-CURE MANUAL;
WATER-CURE IN EVERY DISEASE;
WATER-CURE IN PREGNANCY;
HYDROPATHY FOR THE PEOPLE;
ERRORS IN THE WATER-CURE;
WATER-CURE IN CONSUMPTION.

IN SEVEN VOLUMES.

VOL. II.

INTRODUCTION TO THE WATER-CURE;
EXPERIENCE IN THE WATER-CURE;
THE PARENTS' GUIDE.

NEW YORK:
FOWLERS AND WELLS, PUBLISHERS,
CLINTON HALL, 129 AND 131 NASSAU STREET.
SOLD BY BOOKSELLERS GENERALLY.

AN

INTRODUCTION

TO

THE WATER-CURE:

A CONCISE EXPOSITION OF THE HUMAN CONSTITUTION; THE CONDITIONS OF HEALTH; THE NATURE AND CAUSES OF DISEASE; THE LEADING SYSTEMS OF MEDICINE; AND THE PRINCIPLES, PRACTICE, ADAPTATIONS, AND RESULTS OF HYDROPATHY OR THE WATER-CURE; SHOWING IT TO BE A SCIENTIFIC AND COMPREHENSIVE SYSTEM FOR THE PRESERVATION AND RESTORATION OF HEALTH;

FOUNDED IN NATURE, AND ADAPTED TO THE WANTS OF MAN.

BY THOMAS L. NICHOLS, M.D.

NEW YORK:
FOWLERS AND WELLS, PUBLISHERS.
NOS. 129 AND 131 NASSAU STREET.
1850.

BANER AND PALMER, STEREOTYPERS,
201 William street, corner of Frankfort.

INTRODUCTION

TO

WATER-CURE.

OF THE SUBJECT AND THE AUTHOR.

THE TITLE of this work expresses its intention. There are many able treatises on WATER-CURE or HYDROPATHY, but it can not be expected that people will read them, until they have, in some way, become interested in the subject. To be interested in any person or thing, we must form some degree of acquaintance; and the usual way of making an acquaintance is by having an introduction. I have, therefore, taken it upon myself to introduce the reader to a knowledge of the nature, principles, and results of that system of curing diseases, and acquiring and preserving health, which is, from its chief agent, properly designated—the WATER-CURE.

But an introduction, to be well received, supposes some knowledge of the introducer; and where he is not already known, and has no one to introduce him, there comes the evident, though awkward necessity, that he should introduce himself. It seems proper, in this case, that I should give such an account of myself, as may enable the reader, to whom I am not in any way known already, to form an idea of my qualifications for the important task I have assumed. I say *important*—for his health, his happiness, his very existence may depend upon the impression which he may get from these pages. Feeling this, I earnestly entreat a candid perusal of what I am about to write. I wish to make it acceptable; but I write with the feeling that style, and taste, and literary merit, are all of trifling importance, compared with the great truths to which I would call the attention of intelligent minds.

I was born in the state of New Hampshire, where I commenced my medical education, under the instruction of Dr. M. R. Woodbury, about the year 1832. After the usual preparatory studies, I attended a course of medical lectures at Dartmouth College, in 1834, when the medical department of that ancient institution boasted at least two professors of some eminence; I mean the late Professor Oliver and Professor Muzzy, now of Cincinnati. With my preceptor, Dr. Woodbury, I saw, and to some extent assisted in something better than the usual routine of country practice; but, pleasant as I had found the study of medicine, its practice had no charms for me; and though I did not wholly abandon the desire to complete my course of study, I was never attracted to the "art of healing," as taught in the schools. I gave lectures on various subjects, particularly on Phrenology and Physiology; I wrote for the press; and finally, for more than twelve years, worked steadily as editor and author. In all this period I found my medical knowledge of great use to me. I preserved my own health, I gave advice to others, I wrote much upon sanitary reforms. These writings, generally unconnected with my name, have had a very wide circulation, and, as I believe, considerable influence.*

My attention was first called to the Water-Cure, by the celebrated letter of Bulwer, which was an earnest and enthusiastic, but in some respects mistaken advocacy of the system. From that time, I read such works upon the subject as came in my way, but was too much absorbed in my editorial duties to give it much attention. In 1848, I became acquainted with Mrs. Mary S. Gove, whom I had known by reputation as an eminent lecturer and writer. Her "Lectures to Ladies on Anatomy and Physiology," published by the Harpers in 1846, established her scientific reputation; while her novels, tales, and poems, would have given her a wide literary celebrity, had they not been published either anonymously or under a *nomme de plume*. I found her, not only a lady of high literary and scientific attainments, respected and beloved by all who knew her, but the most scientific and successful of Water-Cure physi-

Among my later writings are my editorial articles during two years, in the New York "Dispatch," and the "Universe;" a historical work, entitled "Woman in all Ages and Nations;" the "Religions of the World;" and "The World's Reformers," in the same papers, not yet published in book form; a series of articles on "The Science of Life," in the "Monthly Bulletin;" a series on "Sanitary Laws," and another on "The Curiosities of Medical Science," in the "Sunday Times;" and various others.

cians. A new light broke upon my career—the mingled rays of love and wisdom. My destiny was joined to hers, in the holiest of bonds; and our studies and work, as well as our lives, lay hence forth in the same track.

Every day I saw, and heard of, the triumphs of Water-Cure. Taking charge of the male patients of our establishment, I saw the practice, while I diligently read the theory in the works of the best writers; I also gained no little knowledge in assisting to prepare for the press the "Experience in Water-Cure," written by Mrs. Nichols, and lately published. And, as if Providence had determined to take every stumbling-block out of my way, at this period, my two partners conspired to plunder me of my share in the proprietorship of a newspaper, of which I had been for two years an editor; and I was left, with a loss of some thousands of dollars, by this piece of unimaginable rascality, to enter without hindrance upon the professional career so strangely marked out for me, and into which I was at once attracted and driven.

As a first step to success in that career, I resolved to complete my regular education as prescribed by law; and for that purpose I attended my second course of lectures in the Medical Department of the University of New York, where, after some five hundred lectures and cliniques, by Professors Mott, Pattison, Payne, Dickson, Bedford, and Draper, I presented my credentials, passed the required examination, and received the diploma of my degree of Doctor of Medicine.

Nor did I think even this full and legal course of regular education in medicine and surgery sufficient. With a competent knowledge of the allopathic system of practice, as certified by the highest authorities, I have carefully examined the systems of Hahnemann and Dickson—Homœopathy and Chrono-Thermalism—and have seen some practice in the former. In an earnest love for TRUTH as the greatest good, with a strong desire for usefulness, I have attentively considered these leading systems and doctrines of medicine, and have deliberately adopted that which I believe to be not only the best, but the only system founded in nature and adapted to the wants of man.

With this conviction, my duty is clear. With knowledge that can benefit my fellow creatures, I am impelled to use it. Knowing the truth, I have no right to conceal it. Thousands around me are ignorantly sacrificing health and life—thousands are suffering from disease and pain—thousands are cut off in the flower and prime of existence; and I should stand condemned of my own conscience, and accursed of God, if, knowing the means of preserving health, of curing disease, and saving life, I neglected to use them.*

These means are all comprised in what is called Hydropathy, but which I prefer to term the WATER-CURE. The name must not be received in any narrow sense. It means more than giving sick people plunge baths, wet sheet packs, and douches. It comprehends, in the sense in which I shall use it, a knowledge of the relations of man to the universe. It is a central science; a pivotal system; the desideratum of progress, and the basis of reforms.

OF HEALTH AND DISEASE.

HEALTH is the natural condition of every organized being. It is that condition in which all animals enjoy the highest development, beauty, vigor, and happiness. It is a state of harmony with nature, and a fulfillment of the ends of creation.

The same laws of life apply to all organized beings. Their natural condition is one of health during all their progress up to maturity; their only natural disease is the slow decay which precedes dissolution. Vegetables, animals, and men, are governed by the same organic laws.

Let a plant spring from a perfect seed, in a well adapted soil, with the proper moisture, temperature, and electrical conditions, and it will be healthy, well developed, and beautiful. Change any of these conditions, and it will be diseased, stunted, and short-lived.

The animals, in their natural state, are full of health and vigor. Confined, pampered, and abused by man, they grow sick and short-lived. Our horses, oxen, sheep, and swine are the prey of diseases arising from the unnatural lives to which we subject them, and which they never know in a state of nature. The wild horse needs no veterinary surgeon, the buffalo needs no cow doctor.

Man is an animal, with the same tissues and organs as the whole class of mammalia to which he belongs. Like them he has bones, muscles, blood-vessels, and nerves. Like them he has senses, powers of locomotion, organs of nutrition, of reproduction, and of thought. He is, like them, hungry and thirsty; subject to heat and cold. Like them he has his origin, his gradual development, his maturity, his gradual decay, and finally he dies when his race

* To withhold from society facts regarding health, is a sort of felony against the common rights of human nature.—*Dr. Lambe.*

is accomplished. Such is the law of nature; but very different, in some of these things, is the sad reality of fact.

Every plant and every animal has a certain period of existence assigned to it by nature. There are plants and animals whose entire existence lasts but a few hours. The oak endures for centuries. The antediluvian life of man is said to have been as long as that of the oak, and it is predicted that in some future period "his life shall be as the life of a tree." What is the present term of man's existence? Three score years and ten is set down as its ordinary limit; but there is no law which confines it to that, for we have all around us persons of eighty, ninety, and a hundred. We have rare cases, indeed, in which men live to one hundred and fifty, and, it is said, even two hundred years, at the present day.

The natural life of man, then, may be from seventy to a hundred years; and those who go over or fall short of these periods, must be set down as exceptions to a general law. Every plant, every animal, enjoying proper conditions, ought, accidents excepted, to reach the period of existence it is fitted by nature to attain. We should think that a bad field of corn in which not one stalk in a hundred came to maturity; we should think that a bad breed of animals of which one half should die in infancy, and nineteen-twentieths before old age. In one case, we should suspect that the seed was bad, the soil inadapted, the climate insalubrious, or the cultivation poor; in the other, we should think we had been imposed upon by a worthless breed, or that our animals were placed in unnatural conditions.

The natural condition of the human animal is a healthy birth, a robust and happy infancy, a joyous youth, a vigorous maturity, a calm old age, and a painless death. This is nature; and it is the instinctive desire of every human being. It is what man is fitted for in his anatomy and physiology. It is in harmony with all nature around him. It is his proper destiny; and every other life than this is a violation of the will of God, as revealed in His own universe.

Men are subject to disease and premature death, the same as all organized beings are, and in no other way. The plant may be crushed, or a drouth may wither it. The worm may be trodden upon, or the lamb become the prey of the tiger. Men, like all other animals, may be burned with fire, drowned with water, or frozen with cold. All animals may be diseased with poisons, and men may, if they choose, shorten their lives in many ways; but these are all violations of the great laws of life.

The natural state of man, as of all plants and animals, is one of uninterrupted health. The only natural death is the gradual and painless decay of old age. Such a life and death are in happy harmony with nature; pain, and disease, and premature mortality are the results of violated laws. I can not insist upon this too strongly. Every pain we feel, every distress we suffer, is but the sign that some law of our being has been outraged. All sickness is a discord with nature—health is harmony.

Health, moreover, is the condition of beauty and happiness. Every organized being is beautiful in its perfect development, and health is the sole condition of such development. We have, from similar causes, dwarfed, stunted, and miserable trees, animals, men, and women. All animals are happy in the free exercise of their faculties, and there can be no such exercise without health. In health, every period of life and every phase of existence is full of happiness.

OF THE CONDITIONS OF HEALTH.

If it be admitted that health is the natural state of man, and it must be, unless we can conceive that nature has made a woful blunder in his organization, what are the conditions in which all his functions are harmoniously performed? In other words, what are the conditions of health?

A plant requires a good seed or germ, a good soil, a suitable degree of moisture, free access to air, light, and a proper temperature. An animal requires, also, a sound germ, healthy food, light, air, a proper temperature, and the exercise of its faculties and passions. The plant draws its food from the soil; the animals draw theirs directly or indirectly from vegetables. The stomach of the animal answers to the soil of the plant. The plant extends its absorbent vessels after food in the earth—we bring food within reach of our absorbents, by conveying it into the stomach. Plants and animals alike need light, air, and moisture, and can not be developed without them.

Man, the head of the animal kingdom, demands, then, for his proper development, or for health—first, that he be well born, the child of healthy parents; second, that he be well fed with nutriment adapted to his digestive organs, in kind and quantity; third, that he breathe pure air; fourth, that he live in the light; fifth, that he gratify the instinct of cleanliness, and so keep his skin in proper condition; sixth, that his muscular powers have due and pleasant exercise; seventh, that his intellectual faculties and social affections are developed in harmony with the ends of his existence.

The conditions of health are few and simple. They are in accordance with our own unperverted instincts, and may be learned of our near relations, the beasts of the field and the birds of the air. The life of a bird or beast, in its natural state, is one of simple conformity to nature, and health and fullness of days are the consequences. Let man be as true to his nature as are the unperverted beings around him, and he would be as healthy and proportionally as long-lived.

What! would you have us live in a state of nature? Assuredly. Would you violate nature? God made us as He made all nature, and His works should be in harmony. But, by a state of nature, I do not mean a savage or barbarous state. There are other vices than those of civilization, and other perversions of nature than its so-called refinements. What man really wants, for health, may be comprised in a few words. A good constitution, simple food, cleanliness, a pure air, proper shelter and clothing, exercise, freedom from care, refining pursuits and recreations, and happy domestic relations.

HEALTH, being the result of the regular performance of all the functions of life, any variation from such regularity is disease. Health gives full and beautiful development; the want of such development is a symptom of disease or disordered function. Health is characterized by vigor; weakness and indolence are the effects of disease. In health we have "strength of body, serenity of mind, and a keen enjoyment of all the blessings of life." In disease we have weakness of body, perturbation of mind, and so much pain and distress that life often becomes a burden.

As the natural condition of all living things is one of health—as health may itself be defined as the *fullness of life*—so are they all subject to disease. A plant in a barren soil has but a sickly growth; deprived of moisture, it withers; kept from the air, it suffocates; in darkness, it has neither color nor strength. Take away the conditions of health, and it is subject to disease and death. It is the same with animals, the same with man.

All organized beings are endowed with a principle of vitality or life. It is in vain that we try to understand this principle. All we know of it, is learned from observing its effects. It has intimate relations with light, oxygen, and electricity, or galvanism. This principle of life, contained in the germ of the plant or animal, presides over its development to maturity; and when this principle is exhausted, the result is death; when it is weakened or obstructed, the result is disease. Disease, then, may be considered the struggle of the principle of life against morbific agencies.

The constitutions of organized beings are adapted to the relations of this life principle with the elements of nature. In temperatures varying from twenty degrees below zero to one hundred or more above, the life principle keeps the temperature of the human body at ninety-eight degrees, with slight variations. Deprive the human body of life, and it would quickly broil or freeze in such temperatures. This is one of many examples of the influence of the life principle. The force of our vitality marks the measure of our health; its continuance makes the duration of our lives. The secret of health and long life, then, is the preservation of the energy of this vital principle.

Strictly speaking, there is but one disease; or, we may say that all the forms of disease, arising from a multitude of causes, come from one central source—a weakening of the nervous energy or principle of life; as all the varied forms of death may be resolved into the destruction of this principle. An acute disease, as a fever, is a quick, sharp struggle of a vigorous vitality to overcome or cast out some diseasing influence. A chronic disease is a weaker and more protracted effort for the same purpose. Pain is, at once, the friendly monitor, to warn us of evil influences, and the chastisement of nature for some violation of her laws. A headache or toothache, the gout or rheumatism, is just as natural and inevitable, and just as much a sign that we have violated some law of our being, as the pain which comes from our putting our hands in the fire, or screwing them in a vice.

OF THE HUMAN SYSTEM.

I HAVE little room for the details of anatomy and physiology; but all that is necessary may be given in a few words. The human system, complete, harmonious, admirable in its adaptations, wonderful in its displays of creative wisdom, though each part is inseparably connected with and necessarily dependent upon every other, may yet be divided into three parts—the NUTRITIVE SYSTEM, the ACTIVE, and the REPRODUCTIVE. Under the nutritive system, I comprehend all the organs which build up, support, and strengthen the body; as the stomach and intestinal canal, the lacteals and absorbents, the heart, arteries, and veins, the liver, lungs, skin, glands, lymphatics, etc. The system of action comprehends the apparatus of thought, passion, and motion, including the brain, spinal chord, nerves, and muscles. The reproductive system has its own peculiar organs, the proper development and healthy condition of which are of the highest importance to the individual and the race. Over all these presides the principle of life, which seems to reside in a nervous system of its own, which pervades the entire system.

The health and energy of the whole nutritive system, it will be seen, is absolutely necessary to the growth, development, and vigor of every organ of the body, its own included; for as the heart supplies itself with blood, as the arteries and veins have their own vessels, so all the organs of nutrition are obliged to supply continually the waste of their own action. All action is accompanied by waste. The steam-engine can no more be propelled without a loss of steam—the water-mill can no more move without an expenditure of water—than any thought or action of our bodies can take place without an actual loss, both of vital power, and of the matter of which the various tissues of our system is composed. This is why thought fatigues our brains, and exercise, our muscles. This is why we need repose and sleep. It is the office of the function of nutrition to continually supply this waste matter of the system. This is why we require food every day and air every moment.

Not only must new matter be constantly supplied to the entire system, bones, muscles, nerves, etc., but the waste matter must be constantly carried away. Once used up, it is foreign matter in the system, clogging and poisoning it. It passes off through the lungs, the kidneys, the intestinal canal, and especially through the skin. It is easy to see that a vigorous and active state of every organ connected with the function of nutrition, is of the last necessity to a healthy condition.

It is of absolute necessity to health that the brain and muscular system should have proper exercise. With too little, the mind grows dull, and the muscles weak and flabby. Tasked too much, the head is wearied and the strength of the muscular system overtasked. We must have activity and enjoyment; we must avoid indolence on the one hand, and on the other, all excess of labor or pleasure.

The importance of the reproductive system is scarcely enough dwelt upon. It gives us flowers and fruit in the vegetable world, it prolongs the races of animals, and greatly influences the character of individuals of the human race. It is connected, in some mysterious way, with all that is *manly* in man and all that is *womanly* in woman. Deprived of this function men are effeminate and women coarse. Its disorder affects the whole system, its abuses sap the fountains of life.

OF THE CAUSES OF DISEASE.

As HEALTH requires that all these functions be maintained in vigor and harmony of development, disease must inevitably arise from the want of such a condition; and we can now go understandingly into a consideration of the causes of the various forms of disease.

The first cause of disease is hereditary transmission or predis position. A child may be born actually diseased, as with syphilis, scrofula, salt-rheum, tubercles in the lungs, etc., derived from the father or mother, or with such a weakened vitality that it can not resist the common diseasing influences. A diseased father can not beget, a diseased mother can not bring forth, a healthy child. A child, the very germ of whose existence is depraved, who partakes, for the nine months of its fœtal life, of the weakness, pain, and suffering of a sick mother, whose very life-blood is made of bad food and impure air, narcotics and medicinal poisons, and who continues to live for some months longer on the same unhealthy nutriment, drawn from her breast, has a poor chance for life, and none at all for a healthy existence.

The period of infancy past, impure, insufficient, or excessive nutrition is one of the great causes of disease. All vegetables feed upon gasses or their combinations, certain chemical principles found in air, water, and the soil in which they grow. All animals live upon the substances thus elaborated by vegetables. Some animals live directly upon vegetables, others get the same materials indirectly, by eating other animals. The order of animals to which man belongs is naturally frugivorous, or fruit eating; hence our best sustenance is derived from fruits, grains, roots, nuts, etc. To these we add milk, eggs, fishes, the flesh of animals, etc. A large portion of the human race lives entirely upon vegetables; a very small portion lives almost entirely upon animal food. We can live far better on vegetable food without animal, than we can on animal, without vegetable. The more the vegetable preponderates over the animal, the purer is our diet, and the better adapted to health—and health is vigor of body and mind. The best flesh contains about twenty-five per cent. of nutritive matter—the best vegetables, such as wheat, corn, and rice, contain eighty or ninety per cent. Vegetable food is the purest, as it is the cheapest, human nutriment.

An impure diet conveys morbid matter into the system. Unhealthy vegetables and animals are alike unfit for food. Animals, fattened for the market, are often full of scrofula and other diseasing matter, and those who eat their flesh can not avoid their diseases. This is especially the case with pork, and generally with animal fat, which should always be avoided.

An insufficient diet, not properly sustaining the organs of life, leads to disease, decay, and death. Want of food causes typhus fever, consumption, and a general weakness and breaking up of the system.

But excess is a far more frequent cause of disease. Gluttony kills hundreds where one dies of starvation. A single ounce more of food than we need for our proper nutrition, tasks the vital powers and weakens the system. Eating too fast and eating too much, are our greatest vices; and these are caused, in a great degree, by an artificial cookery and the use of condiments and spices.

The only drink is pure water. All that we join to it is one of two things—it is either food or poison. Milk and sugar are food, coffee, tea, and alcohol, in all its forms, are poisons. They excite, weaken, and deprave. They belong to the same class of substances as opium and tobacco, and none of them can be used in any quantity without an exactly corresponding amount of mischief. This is a hard saying, but it is God's own truth. All science proclaims it, and all experience confirms it. Let each one take it to his own conscience, remembering that every violation of nature is a sin that inevitably brings its punishment. Such are the laws of the universe.

Breathing an air deprived of its proper proportion of oxygen, by being breathed over, or by other processes of combustion, or loaded with foul gasses and emanations, is another common source of disease. At every beating of the heart, blood is sent into the lungs, where it receives oxygen from the air we breathe, and there can be no healthy blood unless this is supplied in its fullness and purity. Any diminution is a cause of disease—privation is death. Morbid matter contained in the air, enters the lungs and poisons the vast surface of millions of air vessels. Can we wonder at the terrible effects of miasma and the crowd poison, as the air of crowded and unventilated ships, jails, and hospitals? Our churches, theaters, and concert rooms are often as bad, only we do not breathe in them so long. Few of our dwellings, and especially our sleeping rooms, are sufficiently ventilated, and the whole atmosphere of large cities is poisoned by a thousand nuisances, made by cupidity and permitted by ignorance.

Exercise without fatigue, thought without care, enjoyment without excess, are all conditions of health, and the deprivation or violation of any of these conditions, may be the cause of disease. In all these things, in all that belongs to the active functions of life, we require pleasant labor, variety, and cheerful excitement. Our social instincts must, also, be gratified. Solitude, disappointed love, or ambition, and unhappy associations, may be causes of disease. The mind and body act reciprocally on each other. Both must be healthy or both will be diseased.

The reproductive system has its own special diseases, and any irregularity in its functions affects the whole body. This is more markedly the case in the female than the male. Four fifths of all the diseases of women are connected with derangements of the reproductive system. The excesses and abuses of this function, in both sexes, cause an untold amount of disease and suffering.

The want of personal cleanliness is a common cause of disease. In a general sense, this has already been mentioned, for eating impure food, or breathing impure air, filled with fetid and disgusting emanations is, surely, a great lack of cleanliness; but, in its special sense, the want of personal cleanliness weakens that great cleansing organ, the skin, clogs its myriads of pores, through which the effete matter of the system should be constantly thrown off, and by this means the whole system becomes filled with a rank poison, which deranges its whole action, and in the struggle which ensues, often overpowers the vital energy. Health and purity are synonimous terms. An impure system must be a diseased one. The whole skin requires its daily bath of cold water, as the eye wants light, the lungs, pure air, and the stomach, healthy food. How many thousands wash their faces and hands every day, without thinking that every square inch of their skin needs ablution as much, and would be as much refreshed by it!

There are other causes of disease, connected with clothing, sleep, and other artificial habits, such as tight lacing, living in darkness, and turning night into day, exhausting excitements, unhealthy employments, etc., but they are generally comprehended in the preceding observations; there is, however, one cause of disease, which, though it will be treated of hereafter, I can not pass over here without notice. I mean the administration of drugs for medicinal purposes. Under the common or allopathic system of medicine, we are poisoned from before our birth, through our whole existence, and very often ignorantly and heedlessly poisoned to death. Poisons, of the most horrible kind, are sent to the unborn babe in the blood of its mother; poisons are commonly sucked in with the mother's milk, even such as opium, antimony, arsenic, calomel, and corrosive sublimate. Children are poisoned with paregoric or laudanum, and made to swallow filthy, nauseous, and poisoning drugs, through all the diseases of infancy; and in this way are laid up in their bodies the causes of future aches, pains, depressions, dyspepsies, epilepsies, and a whole train of disorders. It is a matter of grave doubt with the most eminent members of the medical profession, whether they do not kill more than they cure, and whether the general effect of medicine is not to shorten life.* I have long been past all doubt on that point, and every day's observation satisfies me that the drug medication of the present day is a potent cause of disease and premature death. I am well satisfied that mankind would not only be far better off were the whole medical profession, and all knowledge of the use of drugs, swept out of existence, but that many diseases would disappear, and the average period of human life be greatly lengthened.

There are diseases which are the result of virus, as of a rattlesnake, or the bite of a rabid animal, and the virus of syphilis. These may be classed with those produced by mercury, quinine, antimony, opium, and the other violent poisons of the materia medica. There is also a class of contagious diseases, as measles, small-pox, and some would add yellow fever, plague, and cholera. These all appear to be the offspring of those artificial habits of life

* "A monarch, who could free his state from this pestilent set of physicians and apothecaries, and entirely interdict the practice of medicine, would deserve to be placed among the most illustrious characters who have ever conferred benefits on mankind. There is scarcely a more dishonest trade imaginable than medicine in its present state."—Dr. Forth.

It is a curious fact that the two poisons, opium and murcury, were introduced into the medicine of Europe by "a malignant quack and drunken vagabond, who rejoiced in the resounding name of Aurelius Phillipus Hohenheim Theophrastus Bombastus Paracelsus." Yet no two medicines are now so often given, and no other two have produced such lamentable results.

which we call civilization. Some are of comparatively recent date, and all belong to unhealthy conditions. To those who obey the laws of life, they have no terrors. The victims of all these diseases are those who violate, or in whom are violated, the conditions of health. They are severe and fatal just in proportion as vitality is weak and loaded down with the causes of disease. It is doubtful whether any truly healthy person can take one of this class of diseases.

OF SICKNESS AND MORTALITY.

LET us see to what extent these causes of disease produce their appropriate effects. In any proper conformity to natural laws, health and long life would be the rule ; and disease and premature death the exception. Human ignorance and perversity have reversed the rules of life, and those greatest of blessings, health and longevity, are the rare exceptions in human history.

The statistics of human mortality have a melancholy completeness. About one fourth of all the children born in all civilized countries, die within the first eleven months of their existence. One half die before they reach their eighth year. Two thirds die before the thirty-ninth year. Three fourths before the fifty-first. According to Buffon, only one in nine, of all that are born, reaches the age of seventy-three, and only one in thirty lives to eighty; one in twelve thousand lives to a hundred.

In large cities, where people are crowded together in poverty and filth, where none of the conditions of health exist, and where the causes of disease are multiplied, the mortality is far greater. In London, according to the tables of Dr. Price, half the number born, die under three years of age; in Vienna and Stockholm, under two. The proportion of those who die annually in the great towns of Europe, is one nineteenth or twentieth of the whole population. In all these cities, improved conditions, such as widened streets, sewerage, and greater attention to cleanliness, have improved the public health. In New York the annual mortality is about one in thirty-seven.

There are some good people who believe that God sends our diseases, and appoints the hour of our death, though our diseases are caused by our own gluttony and intemperance, and our deaths are hastened by the bleeding and drugs of the doctors. But how is it that in one quiet place in the country, one in every eleven or twelve reaches the age of eighty, while in London not more than one in sixty attains to the same age? Is there one Providence for the town and another for the country, or do disease and death obey certain laws of God's appointment?

In the city of New York, in 1847, there were 15,788 deaths, of which 7,373 were of children under five years of age. In 1848 the deaths were 15,919, of which 8,899 were children!

In the single month of March, 1850, there died in New York 1,107 persons, of whom 518 were under five years of age.

We have no record of the amount of sickness, but we may suppose twenty cases of sickness to one of death, or an average mortality of five per cent. in all diseases. This would make three hundred thousand cases of disease annually in the city of New York, and this would correspond pretty nearly to the number of medical men and the amount of their professional business.

Taking the month of March, 1850, as an example, we have the following statistics of the various diseases which proved mortal. Of the 1,107 deaths, 308, or nearly one third, were from diseases of the lungs; 77, diseases of the bowels; 124, of fevers, and so on. Taking our former estimate, there were in the month of March, over twenty-two thousand cases of sickness in the city of New York.*

Where shall we lay the blame of this disease and death? Shall we charge it upon a mysterious Providence, when abundant causes exist in our violations of the laws of life? Shall we blame the Almighty for the consequences of our disobedience of His laws? No: let us not add this blasphemy to our other sins. In our ignorance and recklessness we bring upon ourselves all this misery, disease, and death; and the sin of ignorance, in the disregard of natural law, never goes unpunished. Fire burns, water drowns, bad food, bad air, uncleanly habits, and the use of poisons, either as stimulants or medicines, shorten our lives and render them wretched. These are sins that can not be forgiven. The true record of the sins of a people may be found in the bills of mortality!

The varied forms of disease seem to be determined by age and circumstances, rather than by the causes that produce them. In infancy we have marasmus, cholera infantum, and convulsions, all diseases of a weak vitality struggling with morbific agencies. Then

* Out of the whole population of New York, how many persons are there who ever enjoy full and uninterrupted health for a year, or for six months together? What people call "pretty well, I thank you," and "well, middling," and "so as to be crawling," is not what we call HEALTH.

come measels, hooping cough, scarlet fever, and dysentery; stronger efforts of the vital energy to cast out the matter of disease. Then come other fevers, inflammations, apoplexy, consumption, and the long train of chronic diseases that gradually wear out our lives. All diseases, according to the chrono-thermal doctrine, belong to the single type of intermittent fever, varying in local lesions, according to the weakness of particular organs. The great mass of diseases, according to Hahnemann, is caused by morbid matter in the system. According to one school of allopathists, the humors are depraved; the solids are affected, according to another; a third class makes all disease depend upon a loss of nervous power. They are all right; for a loss of nervous energy must deprave both fluids and solids, and allow of the accumulation of morbid matter in the system.

OF THE ART OF HEALING.

Before speaking of the Water-Cure as a medical system, let us take a brief glance at the present condition of the art of healing, as practiced by some of the leading sects of our medical faculty. The common qualifications of a physician, are a knowledge of anatomy and physiology, surgery, and the theory and practice of medicine and midwifery. The anatomy is useful in performing surgical operations and making post-mortem examinations. Physiology is seldom understood, and in some of our highest medical colleges makes no part of the regular course of education. We come, then, to the practice of medicine, surgery, and obstetrics.

The common medical treatment, in allopathic practice, consists of bleeding, vomiting, purging, counter-irritation, stimulation, palliation, and the administration of alteratives and tonics. Blood-letting, by the lancet, the cupping-glass, or by leeches, is continually resorted to, and the healths of thousands are undermined, and thousands of lives sacrificed by this barbarous practice. The circulation becomes disordered in the struggle of nature, which we call disease, and our doctors know no better method than to let out the vital fluid, and subtract so much from the strength and life of the patient, a practice never necessary, always dangerous, and often fatal. It has been well said, that the lancet has slaughtered more men than the sword. The homeopathists, the chrono-thermalists, all the reformed schools of medicine, renounce and denounce blood-letting. In Water-Cure, the most violent inflammations are controlled without it, with perfect ease; and our recoveries are proportionally rapid and complete. The physician who bleeds now, belongs to the dark ages; yet, with few exceptions, all allopathic doctors still bleed, and their patients die accordingly, or linger miserably through a long convalescence, and never fully recover.

Vomiting and purging are produced by the most violent poisons of the materia medica, such as antimony and mercury, poisons which can never be introduced into the human system without great and irreparable mischief. Men, drugged in their childhood, carry the effects of their poisonings to their graves, often pining through years of pain, and dying prematurely and miserably. In Water-Cure we relieve the stomach and bowels with simple water, and do away with all necessity for other emetics or cathartics; for water answers every useful purpose of both.

Counter-irritation is a way of relieving some internal pain or disease, by producing a greater one upon the surface. It is done by blisters, mustard plasters, moxas, antimonial ointment, croton oil, or some other way of burning or poisoning. It is a miserable system of torture, which we entirely dispense with, having much better and more effectual means of relieving pain and congestion. In Water-Cure, we excite a vigorous action of the whole surface of the body, instead of burning and destroying any portion of it. Our wet-sheet packing is worth a hundred blisters, even were we to allow that the latter were ever useful. If they ever were, they are now fortunately superceeded by a process at once pleasant and efficacious.

Stimulants are medicines given to excite the whole system or some particular organ. They are uniformly poisons, which the energy of the whole system is roused to expel, and exhaustion is the necessary consequence of this unnatural stimulation. It is the strength of the drunkard, which soon gives place to prostration. The poisons given to produce it are always liable to be retained in the system, aggravating all the causes of disease. In Water-Cure, we rely solely upon the vigor and recuperative energy of nature, with her natural stimulants of water, air, exercise, and a pure diet. All the strength gained is real, and there is no going backward in the cure. Tonics are a kind of stimulants, acting more slowly but upon the same principles, and they are liable to the same objections.

The palliatives of allopathy, consist chiefly of the vegetable narcotics, at the head of which are opium, and, according to Professor

Dickson, quinine. They are medicines that allay pain, and control diseased action, by their deadening influence. They change disease, but never cure it. These are the favorite remedies of the profession, but they are never given but to purchase present ease at the expense of future misery. All medicines of this class are violent poisons, and can not be taken with impunity. One who takes them, has as much need to be cured of his medicines as he had of his disease.

The alteratives consist chiefly of the most deadly poisons, given in small doses, so as to have a gradual effect in changing the action of the system, and the seat of disease. They consist chiefly of calomel, arsenic, antimony, corrosive sublimate, iodine, etc., articles whose natural action is to destroy life, which they never fail to do, more or less rapidly, according to the extent to which they are administered. Water-Cure produces all the effects which are vainly hoped from these medicines, simply, and in beautiful harmony with the laws of nature and the constitution of man.

The whole system of allopathy is one of weakening and poisoning. Every good it gains, is by the infliction of some mischief. Its evils are acknowledged by its ablest teachers; but they are taught as necesary evils. Water-Cure has demonstrated the contrary. We have shown, by thousands of cures, of the most hopeless cases, and in all manner of diseases, that this whole system of bleeding, torturing, nauseating, and poisoning, is as unnecessary as it is destructive.*

But shall we not respect the accumulated wisdom of three thousand years? ask the upholders of this system. Where, I ask, is the wisdom for us to respect? I see nothing but an accumulation of absurdities and barbarities. I must respect, in medicine, that which saves life, and not that which destroys it. "The accumulated wisdom of three thousand years!" Look at the diseased

* Among the allopathic medicines in common use, we have the *paralysers*, aconite and hemlock, and the *convulsives*, strychnia and prussic acid, and the *delirifacients*, henbane, stramonium, and deadly night-shade; seven poisons, the most virulent and sudden in the whole kingdom of nature. Using these, we can only wonder that the virus of the rattlesnake, or the saliva of hydrophobia was not added to the list, and dealt out to suffering invalids on the authority of formal recipes. Next to these we have the less active, but still powerful poisons, opium, cinchona, digitalis, scammony, gamboge, hellebore (correctly characterized by its first and very mildly by its last syllable), croton oil, colocynth, and a long list of vegetable poisons; as if the whole vegetable kingdom had been ransacked, and when any substance was found, fetid to the smell, nauseous to the taste, and deadly in its action, it follows that men must take it for medicine—for health.—*Democratic Review.*

humanity around us; look at the bills of mortality; look at generation after generation, cut off in the very spring-time of life, and then talk of wisdom or science!

The practice of surgery, in its mechanical or operative department, has made respectable progress, and achieved some brilliant triumphs; but in the saving of life and limb; in preventing the necessity of operations and mutilations, by the cure of disease, it has miserably failed. Resorting to the same system of depletion and poisoning, it has had the same want of success. The Water-Cure is destined to effect a great and happy revolution in this department. With its power of absolutely controlling inflammation, and imparting the highest vigor and activity to the powers of life, thousands of limbs will be saved, that are now sacrificed, and diseases cured which baffle all the resources of an art in which, hitherto, failure has been the rule, success the exception. In such diseases as cancer, hip-disease, white-swelling, and other scrofulous affections, the Water-Cure is successful beyond all expectation—I need not say beyond all example.

The other systems of medical practice in vogue require a brief notice. Homeopathia is a great improvement on allopathia, if we neither admit its principles, nor credit the potency of its medicines. It prescribes an excellent dietetic system, which of itself is sufficient, with time and nature, to cure many diseases. Its medicines are given in too minute doses, to have the poisonous effects of allopathic drugging, and it uses neither bleeding, blisters, nor emetics. All these are great negative improvements, and quite sufficient of themselves, to account for the superior success claimed by homeopathic physicians.

The leading principle of homeopathy is given in the Latin phrase, *similia similibus curantur;* which means that medicines cure a disease or a symptom, in virtue of their power of producing a similar one in a healthy person. So, to cure any morbid affection, the homeopathists give some poison which would produce one of a similar character. To cure headache, they give some drug which would cause it—and so of affections of the stomach, lungs, etc. In cholera, they give copper and white hellebore; in inflammation of the stomach, arsenic, or corrosive sublimate, and so on. But these poisons are not given in appreciable doses; not in grains, or twentieths of grains, not ordinarily even in thousandths. The usual doses range from the ten millionth to the decillionth of a grain. In Hahnemann's Organon of Medicine, which is the highest homeopathic authority, it is said :

"If *two drops* of a mixture of equal parts of alcohol and the recent juice of any medicinal plant, be diluted with *ninety-eight drops* of alcohol, in a phial, capable of containing one hundred and thirty drops, and the whole *shaken twice* together, the medicine becomes exalted in energy to the first development of power, or, as it may be denominated, the first potence. The process is to be continued through *twenty-nine* additional phials, each of equal capacity with the first, and each containing *ninety-nine drops* of spirits of wine; so that every successive phial, after the first, being furnished with *one drop* from the phial or dilution immediately preceding (which had just been twice shaken), is, in its turn, to be shaken *twice*, remembering to number the dilution of each phial upon the cork, as the operation proceeds. These manipulations are to be conducted thus through all the phials, from the first up to the thirtieth or decillionth development of power, which is the one in most general use."

In a note to this section, a caution is given against shaking the phials more than twice, as a larger number of shakes would increase the potency to a dangerous degree. Medicines which can not be dissolved in alcohol are comminuted to the same degree, by being triturated in a mortar, with sugar of milk. Prepared in this manner, even such commonly inert or harmless substances as salt, charcoal, cuttle-fish, bones, chalk, etc., by these triturations are said to acquire high medicinal potencies.

It is difficult to give an idea of the extent of these dilutions. If a single drop or grain of any medicine were dropped in the reservoir of the Croton aqueduct, a tumbler full from a hydrant would medicate the whole population of New York. The first dilution gives the one-hundredth part of a drop or grain; the second, the ten-thousandth; the third, the one-millionth; the fourth, the one hundred millionth; the fifth, the ten thousand millionth of a grain or drop. This is to be carried up to the thirtieth dilution, but my pages will scarcely contain the figures necessary to express this quantity, which, as it is inconceivably minute, is well called infinitesimal.

But great care must be taken that even these medicines are not given in too large doses, or too frequently repeated, a common mistake with homeopathic practitioners. Hahnemann's favorite dose was to take one globule of sugar of milk, as large as a pin head or mustard seed, moisten it with the thirtieth dilution or decillionth of a drop, put it in a phial and let the patient smell of it once, or at most twice, "every fourteen, twelve, ten, eight, and seven days;" and these subtile doses, he assures us (Organon, §247) are given "with the best and frequently almost incredible effects."

The operation of these medicines is liable to be interfered with or prevented by tasting or smelling of any substance that can neutralize their virtues, such as the flavors of spices, odors of flowers, tobacco, etc. It is especially necessary that the patient should not be exposed to the smell of an apothecary shop, even at a distance.*

I have but little to say in regard to this system. I have spoken of its evident advantages over the monstrous bleedings and poisonings of allopathy, but I have neither seen nor heard from any reliable authority, any evidence of the power of these medicines, or any effects accompanying their administration, which could not be accounted for by the influence of diet, regimen, faith, hope, perhaps the magnetic influence of a kind physician, and the recuperative powers of nature. I have no idea that the decillionth of a grain of charcoal can do any harm; but if an infinitesimal dose of arsenic or strychnia has any potency, it must be an evil one, and should be avoided.

The influence of faith, in the cure of disease, is well illustrated by a historical account of a circumstance that took place at the siege of Breda, in 1625, as related in Ives's Journal.

"That city, from a long siege, suffered all the miseries that fatigue, bad provisions, and distress of mind could bring upon the inhabitants. Among other misfortunes, the scurvy made its appearance and carried off great numbers. This, added to other calamities, induced the garrison to incline toward a surrender of the place, when the Prince of Orange, anxious to prevent its loss, and unable to relieve the garrison, contrived, however, to introduce letters to the men, promising them the most speedy assistance. These were accompanied with medicines against the scurvy, *said to be of great price*, but of still greater efficacy; many more were to be sent them. The effects of the deceit were truly astonishing. Three small phials of medicine were given to each physician. It was publicly given out that three or four drops were sufficient to impart a healing

* Yet we see the professed followers of Hahnemann allowing their patients to use tobacco, drink coffee, and live upon a diet at entire variance with the homeopathic system. In fact, Hahnemann's own example, in respect to tobacco, was inconsistent with his doctrines, for, according to an authorized account of him before me, he fumigated his own patients, and of course neutralized his medicines, by smoking at his consultations.

virtue to a gallon of water. We now displayed our wonder-working balsams. Not even were the commanders let into the secret of the cheat upon the soldiers. They flocked in crowds about us, every one soliciting that part may be reserved for his use. Cheerfulness again appears in every countenance, and a universal faith prevails in the sovereign virtues of the remedies. The effect of this delusion was truly astonishing, for many were truly and perfectly recovered. Such as had not moved their limbs for a month before, were seen walking the streets, with their limbs straight, sound, and whole! They boasted of their cure by the prince's remedy."

All medical history is full of such examples; and there is no doubt that faith, hope, confidence, and enthusiasm, have not only given effect to things quite inert, but that they have also done much to counteract the bad effects of medicinal poisons. But such a plan as this can not be urged to intelligent minds, in favor of any system of drug medication.

The chrono-thermal system, promulgated in London by Dr. Dickson, has been advocated here with great zeal, by Dr. Turner. His book, entitled "The Fallacies of the Faculty," may be read with much advantage. Dr. Dickson's theory is, that all disease is resolvable into a single type, the intermittent, and that it consists essentially of a periodical derangement of temperature, or alternations of fever and ague, heat and cold. Hence the name chrono-thermal, meaning time and heat, or periodicity and temperature. The practice is to cool in the hot stage by emetics and baths, to warm in the cold stage by stimulants and plasters; and to endeavor to break up the recurrence of the fits, by giving such drugs as quinine, opium, arsenic, prussic acid, strychnia, colchicum, nitrate of silver, preparations of mercury, copper, zinc, bismuth, and iron, turpentine, musk, etc. The great value of Dr. Dickson's book is, that it proves the uselessness and terrible murderousness of the lancet, and the common allopathic systems of medication. The use of the cold plunge, shower bath, and douche, will account for much of the success of the system; but its medication is infernal. Its short list of medicines comprises the most frightful poisons of the allopathic materia medica.

The Thomsonian, and other vegetable systems, have their positive and negative virtues; but do not demand any special attention. It is a great mistake to suppose that a vegetable poison may not be as bad as a mineral. On the contrary, several of them are worse than any known mineral preparation

But why, it is asked, did God make all these poisons, if we are not to take them? They were, doubtless, made for some wise purpose, as were all things, but the very fact that they are nauseous poisons, is proof that they were not intended to be put into our mouths or stomachs. When a thing is nauseous, disgusting, and poisonous, we ought to be satisfied that it was not intended for us to swallow. Because we do not know what a thing was made for that is surely no reason that we should eat it.

OF THE WATER-CURE.

I COME now to the history, principles, practice, and results, of the Water-Cure, which I have defined to be the application of the principles of nature in the preservation of health and the cure of disease. It comprehends the maintenance of all the conditions of health, the removal of all the causes of disease, and a thorough and scientific application of proper agents, in assisting the recuperative powers of the vital energy, or principle of life, sometimes termed *vis medicatrix naturæ*.

The agents, constituting the materia medica of Water-Cure, are diet, exercise, recreation, heat, cold, electricity, air, and water in its various uses. These are the positive remedies; the negative consist in the removal of the causes of disease, physical and moral. The proper application of such a system, it will be seen, requires no common degree of wisdom and knowledge.

To a greater or less extent, the Water-Cure has been known from the earliest ages of the world. Wherever men have lived in simple conformity to nature, and in the observance of the rules of cleanliness, they have so far practiced the Water-Cure. It is the system instinctively practiced by the lower animals for the preservation of health and the cure of disease. The birds bathe themselves daily; cattle plunge in the water to cool the fever occasioned by intense summer heats; wounded animals resort to the first stream or pool to bathe the part affected; a horse turned out to die, by his ignorant master, has been known, day after day, to hold his wounded neck under an artificial spout until it was healed, without any other teaching than his own instinct or God-inspired wisdom.

Ancient philosophers, sages, and priests, taught temperance and cleanliness. Moses taught it to the Jews, and Mohammed to the Arabs. Cleanliness is akin to godliness. Purity is one of the doctrines of our religion. The Greeks and Romans knew the effects of exercise and bathing, and spared no pains to preserve the public health by building costly and magnificent Water-Cure establishments for the people. Pindar says, "the best thing is water, the next gold." Water was recommended by Pythagoras to fortify body and mind. The Macedonian women knew enough of the Water-Cure, in obstetrics, to wash themselves in cold water after childbirth, as the females of the North American Indians do at this day. The hardy inhabitants of ancient Italy immersed their newly-born children in the rivers, and accustomed them to bathe in cold water. Charlemagne encouraged cold bathing throughout his empire, and made swimming one of the amusements of his court. Hippocrates and Galen cured fevers and numerous diseases with water. Dr. Hoyer published a work on the medicinal use of water, in 1702. Dr. Hancock advocated its use in fevers, in 1772. The celebrated John Wesley wrote a valuable work on water treatment, and the work of Dr. Currie, in 1797, is one of the best Water-Cure books extant. I might quote from Richerand, Cullen, Gregory, Rush, Oliver, Johnson, Greville, Zimmerman, Hoffman, Hufeland, and scores more of eminent physiologists and physicians, to prove that, to some extent, the principles of Water-Cure have been recognized by men of science in all times; but this point needs no elucidation.

The world owes the present system of Water-Cure to the genius of Vincent Priessnitz, a peasant of Austrian Silesia. His first cure was of a severe injury upon his own person; a cure so remarkable that it attracted the attention of his neighbors, and he was sought for to give relief to others. In a few years he had a large practice, and was obliged to accommodate patients from a distance. In this simple way began the world-renowned establishment of Grafenberg, which has since numbered thousands of patients, among whom were princes and nobles from all parts of Europe. The astonishing success of the treatment of Preissnitz, chiefly in cases where all other means had failed, not only attracted to him patients from all quarters of the world, but caused similar establishments to be opened in various parts of the continent of Europe, in England, and America.*

A knowledge of the system is now spreading among the people,

* In a Water-Cure periodical before us, we find the advertisements of eleven Water-Cure establishments, most of which are in different sections of the state of New York, not including those in this city.

and it bids fair to take the place of all other systems of medical practice.

But this change is not to be effected without a corresponding effort and struggle. The interests involved are too great not to excite violent opposition. General health, attained by a knowledge of the Water-Cure, will do away in a great measure, with the necessity for a medical profession. The sick will be cured, the cured will keep well, and the well will remain so. A little knowledge will enable people to get well and keep well. Now, in this city alone, more than a million of dollars is paid yearly in doctors' bills, and probably a still larger sum for medicines. It is directly for the interest of our thousand doctors and apothecaries that there should be a great deal of sickness, and very much against their interest that people should take the Water-Cure. They can neither wish nor pray for the blessing of public health, since it would bring ruin and starvation to themselves and their families. With a thousand doctors and druggists; paying two millions of dollars yearly for advice and medicines; with a community full of disease and suffering; a mortality of fifteen thousand a year, half of the victims of which are children, and nearly all in the prime of life, and applying such statistics to all civilized countries, we may well hail the progress of medical reform, and thank Heaven for Preissnitz and the Water-Cure.

As usually happens with great discoveries, this was the result of seeming accident, and was made by the last man, perhaps, that the world would have selected for that purpose. But Providence orders these things well; and a more scientific man would have made a less thorough reformer. A doctor would have brought the prejudices of education into play, and have spoiled his water treatment, by mixing with it poisonous drug medication.*

Preissnitz, in the simple earnestness of his character, has kept clear of all this. A strong common sense, whose results were like intuitions, has been his guide, and when he has committed errors,

* Now that the Water-Cure is becoming fashionable and popular, bidding fair to become universal at no distant period; now that it is the system resorted to and believed in by the most intelligent persons in the community, our doctors, of various schools, who, a short time ago, denounced it, are beginning to say, "Oh! yes, the water; yes, I believe in the water. I have found it very useful in many cases. In fact, we have always known about the use of water. It is an excellent thing in many cases, but it won't answer in yours." And some even go so far as to prescribe a shower bath, to go with their cod liver oil and calomel—almost the only kind of bath that is never used by a Water-Cure physician, and one which few invalids could take without injury.

his experience has corrected them. The system, once established, has doubtless been improved by the science and thought of more cultivated minds.

The Water-Cure consists, as I have said, in the removal of the causes of disease, and in substituting the conditions of health; but it has another work to perform, and in this rests chiefly its claim as a system of medicine. It is not enough to remove the causes of disease; it is not enough to surround a man with the conditions of health. Those causes of disease have produced their legitimate effect, and there exists a condition of pain and suffering, a morbid habit, and deranged functions. A weakened vitality, and a wrecked constitution ask the aid of science to enable nature to do her work.

Disease is a terrible reality; pain must be relieved; obstructions must be removed; the forces of nature must be guided in their action. Nature can maintain health if her laws are not violated; nature can do much to restore, but she is not sufficient without the aid of art. It is the office of Water-Cure to remedy the wrongs done her by false and perverse habits. When a man, by breathing bad air, by eating improper food, by the use of narcotics, and by inattention to cleanliness, has filled his body with disease, and it breaks out in the form of fever, or consumption, or scrofula, or rheumatism, whether it effects the whole system or some particu-organ, we must indeed take him out of his bad conditions, and place him in good ones, but we must do much more. We must do something to rouse his vital energy, and strengthen and invigorate his whole system. We must cleanse every pore of his body, and excite his skin to vigorous action, that it may carry on its great work of purification. There is a stomach to be cleansed, and invigorated to perform a healthy digestion, so as to furnish fresh matter to build up the depraved tissues. There is a liver to be waked from its torpidity, and made to perform its office of purifying the venous blood of the portal system; there are kidneys, whose strainers must separate from the vital fluid those effete substances that have been once used, and are now poisons to the animal economy. The whole track of the alimentary canal must be brought into action, by its sympathy with the skin, and all the healthy processes of nature quickened into new life.*

* The extent to which Water-Cure expedites the operations of nature, in the renovation of the system, has been well expressed by the great chemist, Liebig, in his letter to Sir Charles Scudamore. He says: "By means of the Water-Cure treatment a change of matter is effected in a greater degree in six weeks, than would happen in the ordinary course of nature in three years."

This is the work of Water-Cure; and to do this, to find agents to accomplish these results, all the kingdoms of nature have been ransacked, for her most violent and subtile poisons; we have seen with what deplorable effects. Yet all this is done with the Water-Cure. Is there fever? it can be cooled to any desirable point, and the pulse regulated in an inflammatory disease, from hour to hour, with certainty and safety, and without taking a drop of blood, by the various applications of water. Is there local congestion, as of the brain, lungs, liver, etc.? it can be relieved, and the equilibrium of the circulation established. Is there pain? the cold bath, and the wet sheet pack are more rapid and efficient than opium in relieving it. Is there inflammation? * it can be absolutely controlled with water. Is the stomach oppressed? water is the best of all cleansing emetics. Are there obstructions or constipation of the bowels? they can be removed quickly, and without pain or danger, by water enemas, and permanently relieved by the sitz bath, and the bandage. Have we debility, a loss of nervous energy, and muscular power? cold water, in the pack, the plunge bath, and the douche, is the best of tonics. Is the blood filled with impurities? water is the great cleansing agent of universal nature. Are our solids depraved and loaded with morbid matter? water, the only solvent in nature, can penetrate through every tissue and wash them from all corruption. Are the nerves loaded with poisons, as of scrofula, psora, or syphilis? water, taken into the stomach, coursing through every blood-vessel, and passing off by the skin, the lungs, the kidneys, and the intestines, can give them purity and health.

OF THE CONSTITUTION AND PROPERTIES OF WATER.

Yes, all this, and much more, can be done by water, in its thoroughly scientific application.

"What! water? simple water? common water?

How few have ever rightly considered what this *common water* is!

When oxygen, the vital part of the air, unites with hydrogen, the lightest of known substances, and the first of electro-positive agents, supposed by chemists to be in reality a metal, there is a flash of flame, intense heat, a blaze of light, and the result of this union of these two of the most glorious elements of nature is

* It was formerly thought that a certain amount of inflammatory action was necessary to the reparative processes of nature, but it has been ascertained that they go on much more rapidly and effectually without it. The more healthy the constitution, the less disturbance is occasioned by any injury, and the more quickly is it repaired.

WATER. All the water contained in the vast oceans, the lakes and rivers of the world, all that lies hidden in the bowels of the earth or suspended in the atmosphere, must have been formed by this union of oxygen and hydrogen gasses with the evolution of light and heat, which always accompanies this combustion. This process is continually going on around us. Wherever we see the flame of combustion, from the burning of a taper, to the conflagration of a forest, it is always accompanied with the production of this most wonderful of all the forms of the material world. It exists in invisible vapor in the atmosphere, in clouds, in its liquid state, and in its solid form of ice; each form depending chiefly on its temperature.

Water, wherever we see it, is full of use, and beauty, and glory. From the dew that distils upon the rose leaf, to the ocean that heaves its vast tides around the world, it is a perpetual wonder and delight. In the dawn of creation the spirit of God moved upon the face of the waters. Water makes the beauty of our silvery clouds and golden sunsets, it spans the heavens with the hues of the rainbow, it dances to the earth in April showers, it murmurs in brooks, and thunders in cataracts; it waters the earth in rivers, and bears our navies on the rolling seas.

Look at the relations of water to organic life. Without it, the earth would have for ever remained one mass of barren rock. It was the water that dissolved and disintegrated the primitive granite, and from which were deposited all the subsequent geological formations. Water has given the earth its covering of soil.* Without the presence and action of water, no seed could ever have germinated, and no plant ever have been nourished. It is only by being dissolved in water that the elements of vegetable matter ever take on their beautiful forms. Deprived of water they all droop and wither. And as the whole animal creation lives, directly or indirectly, upon the vegetable, all life is dependent upon water.†

* "That vast expanse of water, the ocean—what recollections, what thoughts it recalls! A poet can never look at it without rapture, nor speak of it without enthusiasm; for it is the breath of God condensed on what were otherwise a cold and barren mass of rock; a breath which has communicated fertility, and beauty, and life."—PROF. DRAPER.

† "No living thing can exist except it contains WATER as one of the leading constituents of the various parts of its system. The distribution of organized beings all over the world, is, to a very great extent, regulated by its abundance or scarcity. It seems as if the properties of this substance mark out the plan of animated nature. From man, the head of all, to the meanest vegetable that can grow on a bare rock, through all the various orders and tribes, this ingredient is absolutely required."—PROF. DRAPER.

But let us look at the relations of water to the human system. The germ of fœtal life is little more than a drop of pure water. The new-born infant consists, in all its tissues, of about ninety per cent. of water. Take away water, and all that remains is a few ounces of dust. The adult body is about eighty per cent. water. Water forms about ninety parts in a hundred of the blood, the living fluid which supplies every part with its vitality. Nearly the whole mass of the brain and nerves is pure water. Observe the eye, the most perfect and beautiful of human organs; it is little more than a collection of sacks of transparent water. Evaporate the water from a full grown human body, and its dry solid matter will weigh from thirty pounds to not more than twelve.

But water not only enters thus largely into the composition of the tissues of the human body, but is the grand agent in all its vital functions. Not a particle of nutriment can enter into the composition of the blood, and thence into the various organs, until it is first dissolved in water; and the whole process of digestion is simply a breaking down and comminution to favor that process. It is by water that the system continually receives its new matter, and it is water that continually carries away the old. It passes with the vapor of water from the lungs, with the insensible perspiration from the skin, with the urine from the bladder. Water is the very element of our life. Food is of secondary importance.*

And now, gentle reader, after reflecting upon these truths, and all they must suggest to you, what do you think of "common water?" Is there any drug in the materia medica to compare with it? Will you place beside it all the nauseous, poisonous prescriptions of the pharmacopœas? Might we not reasonably expect the living waters, which are to all organic nature the fountain of life, to be also the fountain of health to diseased humanity?

And that they are such, the Water-Cure has proved. Well has water been deemed, in all ages, a sacred element. It is not strange that the Hindoos pay divine honors to the river Ganges; that the Egyptians worship the Nile; that the fountains of Greece were chosen for the sites of temples; that water was the symbol of purification among the Jews, and the element of Christian baptism. We read of the waters of salvation, and the waters of the river of life in paradise. Water is the symbol, throughout the sacred

* "A man of average size requires half a ton weight of water a year; and when he has reached the meridian of life, he has consumed nearly three hundred times his own weight of this liquid."—Prof. Draper.

writings, of life, and health, and purity, and holiness. It is the express correspondence of the divine truth, as it is every where the medium of creative power.

OF AIR, DIET, AND EXERCISE.

WATER is the chief, but by no means the sole agent relied upon in the Water-Cure, for the eradication of disease, and the restoration of health. Pure air is of vital necesssity; air free from noxious emanations, foul gases, and diseasing influences, and having its full proportion of oxygen, which, being the chief component of water, is also the vital ingredient of the air. The blood requires, every instant of our lives, to be supplied with a certain proportion of this element. By its union with oxygen, the blood takes on its ruddy, arterial hue. As the ogygen is consumed in the body, the blood becomes dark, as we see it in the veins. Deprive the blood of its supply of oxygen and it ceases to flow, as in drowning or other strangulation. The combustion in this union of oxygen with carbon and hydrogen in the body is the source of vital heat. Pure air, then, is necessary to the vitality of the blood, to the proper nutrition of all the organs of the body, and to the evolution of animal heat. Air, deprived of its due proportion of oxygen, performs this work insufficiently; air, loaded with poison, carries it into the lungs and depraves the whole system. Consequently an attention to ventiliation, especially of sleeping apartments, is an essential part of the Water-Cure treatment.*

Some pathologists contend that there is no such thing as a local disease, except in case of injuries. All disease, they say, is first general, and then local, by showing itself in some organ weaker than the rest. Others, who contend that diseases are both general and local, also admit that in any local affection all the functions are disordered. It is not a question of any practical moment. The central powers of life are those engaged in the function of nutrition, including digestion, circulation, respiration, the deposition of new matter, and the absorption and removal of the old. This function is always deranged in disease, or, as some contend, it is the de-

* Many facts indicate that we breathe, so to speak, by all the million pores of the skin, as well as by the million air cells of the lungs. The contact of fresh air with the skin warms and invigorates, especially if the skin is kept pure and active by bathing. Deprive the skin of access to air, and death is the consequence. In a French spectacle, a little boy was covered with gold leaf, and the result was fatal. Subsequent experiments on animals showed the cause. There is no organ more vital than the skin, and none on which health and disease more closely depend.

rangement of this function which causes all disease. A healthy digestion and pure nutrition are at the foundation of health.

Diet, therefore, is a matter of prime importance in the Water-Cure. As a large proportion of our diseases originate in errors of diet, and are kept up by bad habits of living, its careful regulation is one of the first steps toward a cure. In many diseases, abstinence from food does much toward effecting a cure, but there are others which demand all the nutrition consistent with the strength of the organs.*

I do not propose, in this introduction, to fully discuss the matter of diet. Beyond all question, however, the purest food, and that best adapted to all the wants of man, is furnished by the farinacea, as wheat, rice, barley, Indian corn, rye, oats, etc. Modern chemistry has shown that some of these grains contain exactly the materials required to make the best blood and to nourish every tissue of the body, and in the exact proportions in which they are required. Bread is the staff of life. Then come the fruits, agreeable to the palate and refreshing to the system. Then we have a a great variety of roots and edible plants, as potatoes, beets, turnips, carrots, squashes, cabbages, asparagus, etc., and pulse, as beans, peas, and lentils—a variety, from which we may cull and combine the most nutricious, delicate, and healthy dishes. Next in order, come the slightly animalized substances, milk, butter, cheese, and eggs, with shell and scale fish, and then the flesh of birds and the warm-blooded animals. But as the flesh of oxen, sheep, etc., is made from vegetables, we are merely eating grass and grain at second hand, and often, especially if the animal is diseased, with added impurities. Chyle and blood made directly from vegetables resist putrefaction many days longer than that made from a diet of flesh.

The articles prohibited in a Water-Cure diet, either for the preservation of health, or the cure of disease, are all substances absolutely poisonous, as the narcotics, tobacco, coffee, tea, and alcoholic mixtures; all stimulants and condiments, such as pepper, mustard, most of the various spices. Salt, vinegar, and some of the aromatics, are used in moderation. Among the common articles of food, we absolutely prohibit all pork, believing that the laws of Moses and

* A Water-Cure physician of some notoriety has made what is called the hunger-cure so much a hobby, that he neglects some of the most powerful and efficacious of the Water-Cure processes; but judgment and true science avoid the errors of such extremes.

Mohammed, in this respect, were based upon a sound physiology; all fat meat, blood, and intestines, as the liver, kidneys, etc., believing in the wisdom of the Divine command to the Israelites (Lev. iii. 17). "It shall be a perpetual statute for your generations, throughout all your dwellings, that ye eat neither fat nor blood." This perpetual statute, being founded in the principles of nature, can not be repealed. We prohibit, also, smoked and manufactured meats, mince-pies, head-cheese and sausages, veal, ducks, geese, and other oily water-fowl, oily fish, all grease and gravies, except butter, or vegetable oil of undoubted purity, and in general all things impure in quality and difficult of digestion; and in some cases it is necessary to entirely prohibit the use of flesh. The quantity is regulated to the condition and wants of the system.

Exercise is an essential requisite to the cure. Some cases require walking, some riding, and others a course of the most active gymnastics. In distortions of the body, curvatures of the spine, and cases of muscular debility, properly directed exercises have much to do with the cure.

OF PROCESSES, ADAPTATIONS, AND DISEASES.

THE processes of Water-Cure, in the various applications of water, are of considerable number, and require to be greatly varied, and, in some cases of acute disease, adapted, hour by hour, to the condition of the patient. Every variety of disease, general and local, and every variety of constitution and temperament, requires a careful adaptation of the treatment. The same applications that would be of the greatest benefit to a robust man, would not answer at all for a delicate woman or child. The degree of vitality and the reactive powers of each patient, must be estimated with great care, and often tested by repeated experiments. Mistakes have been made in this respect, and mischiefs done, by prescribing the same heroic treatment to patients with all degrees of reactive power. Such practice as this is no better, save in the medicines, than the common routine of allopathy.

The water is used at all temperatures, from the freezing point, and even below it, to as hot as the skin can bear. The temperature is always adapted to the nature of the case, and the constitution of the patient. We use hot fomentations to relieve violent pain or congestion, tepid rubbing baths in fever, and ice-cold applications in uterine hemorrhage. We have plunge baths, pouring baths, sponge baths, dripping-sheet baths, half baths, rubbing baths, and sitz baths. We have vapor baths and dry blanket packs for profuse sweating, wet-sheet packs, alterative, derivative, and tonic; partial packs for local diseases and low reactive power; and heating and cooling wet compresses and bandages, cold affusion, and that most powerful of all applications, the douche; injections at different temperatures and for various purposes, water emetics, water cathartics, water diuretics, water sudorifics, water rubifacients; yes, and if we ever needed them, water epispastics!

Such is a brief and imperfect view of the materia medica of hydropathy.

One of the chief objects of this work is, to endeavor to remove the common errors and misapprehensions respecting the adaptation of the Water-Cure to different constitutions and forms of disease. It has been thought that this practice, though adapted to the robust, could not be borne by the delicate; others have thought that, though suited to the delicate, it was not active enough in its operations for the robust. Some have supposed that, while it is well adapted to fevers and other acute forms of disease, it could have little efficacy in chronic and nervous disorders, while a still more general impression has been that though admirably suited to the renovation of worn-out constitutions and the cure of diseases of long standing, it could not be depended upon in sudden emergencies, and in the violent and rapid forms of disease.

One side of all these impressions is true. The Water-Cure, founded in nature, has a wide adaptation to the human system, in all its multiplied forms of disease.* Its processes are greatly varied, and easily adapted to all circumstances. Let me give a few examples. One of the most sudden and terrible of diseases is apoplexy, and the lancet and the most powerful drugs are commonly resorted to for its relief. In many cases, a stroke of apoplexy is a stroke of death. No treatment can relieve it. But whenever it is curable, the most rapid, the most effectual, and every way the best treatment is the Water-Cure. This fact is now recognized by many of the most eminent practitioners of other schools. Pouring

* "You claim too much for Water-Cure," it is sometimes said by those who imperfectly understand it. "You claim that it will cure every thing." No. We claim that it is adapted to the human constitution in every condition of sickness and health; that it will promote the cure of all curable diseases; that it gives relief in all cases, if rightly applied. It not only relieves symptoms, but removes the causes upon which all disease depends. It is useless to give a list of diseases which can be cured by water as all are cured in proportion to their curability. Patients must understand the system, and then they can judge of the universality of its application.

cold water upon the head, says Professor Dickson, will often give relief while the physician is tying up the arm to bleed. It has been demonstrated that, in cases of apoplexy, bleeding is often fatal. The most violent forms of congestive fever I have ever seen, have proved perfectly manageable, and have never lasted beyond a single week, with the Water-Cure. With its use, the inflammatory and exanthematous diseases, as measles, scarlet fever, croup, lung fever, etc., have absolutely lost their terrors. Cases which seemed hopeless, and which have been given up under other systems, have speedily recovered under the applications of Water-Cure. Its success in the cholera is a striking proof of its adaptation to the most violent and commonly fatal diseases.

When the tone of the system is low, when vitality is exhausted, when the nerves are oppressed with morbid matter and drug poisons, as in dyspepsia, and other chronic disorders, the Water-Cure imparts new energy to the vital forces, excites the skin and other depurating organs to cleanse the system of its "perilous stuff," stimulates to a healthy nutrition, and renovates the entire economy. The change is wonderful, and rapid beyond belief. All the processes of life are quickened. Sometimes quinine, mercury, opium, or other drugs, taken years before, are brought out through the pores of the skin, or made to pass off in some salutary crisis. Strange as this may appear, it has been proved times without number, and without the possibility of mistake. There seems to be an entire making over of the system. Freshness comes to the cheek, brightness to the eye, strength to the limbs, and elasticity to the motions. There is appetite for food, vigor for exercise, and keen enjoyment of life. I can refer to such cases in this city, where persons had suffered miserably, for from two to twelve years, under continual medication, and have been restored to sound and vigorous health by Water-Cure. In the "Experience in Water-Cure," elsewhere referred to, several such cases are given.*

The Water-Cure is peculiarly adapted to the cure or eradication of scrofula, in all its forms. We may dispute about the nature and causes of this morbid condition; but there it is. It is hereditary, and almost universal. Its effects are all around us. We see them in eruptions, abscesses, white swelling of the joints, hip-dis-

* It is no uncommon thing for patients who have been bed-ridden for weeks and months, and even years, to be walking about, after a few days of Water-Cure treatment. Few patients think of lying in bed, unless in certain diseases, where absolute rest, for a brief period, is deemed necessary to a cure.

ease, ulceration of the bowels, and consumption. Allopathy treats this disease, or parent of diseases, with its most virulent poisons, arsenic and corrosive sublimate. Its cure, thorough and permanent, is one of the triumphs of hydropathy. Under its genial action the morbid matter is thrown out of the system, by the quiet action of the skin, by eruptions, sometimes by boils, and large abscesses; but the result is purification, and with purity comes health. The consumption is thus often prevented; it is frequently checked in its early stages; I do not wish to task the reader's credulity, but there are many cases in which it has been cured, after giving the most unmistakable signs of its progress. The cough has ceased; the ulcerated lungs have cicatriced; the terrible night-sweats have been checked; the flush of hectic fever has given place to the rosy hue of health; skeleton forms have been clothed with healthy muscles and adipose matter, and persons given up despairingly to die, have enjoyed long years of health and happiness.

Observe, I do not say that this has occurred in a multitude of cases, but I know it has in some. I do not say that the water-treatment, however well managed, will cure every case of well-seated, tubercular consumption; but I do say that there is no case in which it will not afford relief, and where death is inevitable, it undoubtedly prolongs life, assuages pain, promotes the comfort of the patient, and, more than any other mode of treatment, smooths the pathway to the tomb. In the work just referred to, the causes and treatment of consumption have been thoroughly explained by one whose own life has been saved by the treatment, and who has been instrumental in saving the lives of many others.

The facility with which the diseases of the digestive system, whether in the form of dyspepsia, constipation, diarrhea or dysentery, can be controlled and cured by the water-treatment, lies at the foundation of its success in all diseases of the function of nutrition, comprehending by far the greater number of all forms of disease. The intelligent reader will have little difficulty in applying to the treatment of these affections, the general principles of the system.

Not to go over a list of diseases or symptoms to which Water-Cure is adapted, it may be well to show its applicability to a few extreme cases, which may be considered as examples of classes of similar affections. Of diseases of the nervous system, then, take the two cases of delirium tremens and paralysis. The first is an intense and morbid excitement of the nervous system, the latter an extreme prostration. For the former disease our routine doctors give immense quantities of the terrible poison, opium; for the latter, potent doses of the equally or more terrible poison, strychnia. The opium is given to overpower the disordered brain, induce sleep, and give the system a chance to recover from the effects of disease and medicine; the strychnia, to cure paralysis, by producing convulsions; but generally with a poor effect. In the Water-Cure treatment of delirium tremens, the cold wet-sheet pack coming in contact with the millions of nervous fibers, distributed to the whole surface of the body, soothes the whole nervous system in the most beautiful manner. The pores are opened and the body relieved of its poison by transpiration; a cold bath invigorates the frame, and quickly and surely the cure is accomplished. In paralysis, the shock of the doucho sends a tingling thrill to every nerve, and wakes the dormant powers to action. The system is excited, toned, invigorated, and cleansed of its impurities. The wheels of life are set in motion, and gradually quickened to their normal speed, and gradually, little by little, the paralytic recovers the action of his nerves and the command of his muscles. Epilepsy, St. Vitus' dance, and insanity are all, in many cases, successfully treated.

In one disease, sometimes the punishment of vice but too often the misfortune of innocence, for which mercury has been by many supposed to be a specific, the Water-Cure manifests its cleansing and curative power in an extraordinary degree. I have found that, in the cure of nearly all diseases, the water treatment brings out much foul matter through the pores of the skin. It is manifest to the senses of sight and smell, and its peculiar character can often be distinguished. The odors of typhus fever, of rheumatism, and of gout are all peculiar; so are the medicinal substances, which for years, perhaps, have been lurking in the system. But whatever may be thought of other diseases, in syphilis, whether a recent affection, one of long standing, or a hereditary taint, no one can doubt that there is an absolute poison, a real virus, which nature often tries to cast out of the system by ulcers, cutaneous eruptions, and other tendencies to the surface. Mercury was once thought to be an antidote to this poison. That idea is now abandoned; but it is supposed that by poisoning the patient with mercury, a great effort will be made, and that in casting out one poison the other will go with it. This sometimes *seems* to be the actual effect produced; but in many cases, the poison of the mercury is added to that of the syphilis, and both remain in the system. It is hard to say which is worse, but both together are truly horrible. Now, if there is any thing in the whole range of nature that will wash both these poisons completely out of the human body, it is the Water-Cure. Wherever there is vitality enough remaining to act upon, both syphilitic and mercurial diseases can be cured fully and completely by this method.

The Water-Cure is said to have succeeded, in Germany, in the cure of hydrophobia. If so, it is the only treatment that has ever cured, and if I had a case, I should certainly resort to it. I see no good reason to doubt its efficacy. Indeed, I can not conceive of any diseased condition of the human system, where the Water-Cure would not be better than any other known system of medication. I except, of course, cases of poisining, where chemical reagents can be used to neutralize the poison, as albumen for corrosive sublimate, or the hydrated peroxide of iron for arsenic; and, also, injuries, aneurisms, etc., requiring surgical operations.

And here let me say, that in saving parts from violent inflammations and consequent mortification; in saving limbs from the necessity of mutilation; in discussing tumors, and eradicating various surgical diseases; in the prevention and cure of those terrors of surgery, tetanus and erysipelas; in preparing patients to endure operations, and in the after treatment, the Water-Cure is destined to win even greater honors than even in the cure of diseases falling under medical treatment. Our surgeons have yet to find the uses of water, and to know that all their lotions, poultices, and embrocations are good only as water makes a part of them, and that they are very mean and poor compared with the scientific application of the pure element.*

The use of the Water-Cure in the cure of neuralgia, tic-doloreux, rheumatism, gout, sick headache, and other painful nervous disorders, need not be dwelt upon. The cases of relief are so numerous, that there can be very few who have not had some within the sphere of their own personal observations.

* It must be expected that Water-Cure, like any other system, is liable to suffer from the errors of its practitioners. The ignorance of some, the prejudices others, timidity on the one hand and rashness on the other, may prevent the proper effects of this mode of treatment, and even lead to serious mischief. When a Water-Cure physician has no more judgment than to apply the same heroic treatment to a delicate woman, or a child just sinking from exhaustion, that would be just the thing for a strong man in a high fever, what can we expect? Even injudicious and routine water-treatment is doubtless better than drug medication, but true science, judgment, and skill, are needed, to do justice to the system and those who seek its aid.

OF FEMALE DISEASES, GESTATION, AND CHILDBIRTH.

But there is one class of diseases to which the adaptation of the Water-Cure ought every where to be known, and no false delicacy will atone to my conscience for not giving them the prominence they deserve. I allude to the diseases of women. Women are sadly subject to all the diseasing influences of civilization. Especially do they suffer from want of out-door exercise, bad air, enervating indulgences, and errors in dress. With great nervous susceptibility, their reproductive systems are highly developed, and here, in most cases, when disease exists, will it be found established. In consequence, physicians are called to prescribe for menstrual irregularities, morbid discharges, displacements of the uterus, and many painful affections. For all these, medicines and all the usual modes of treatment fail, or worse than fail; but, as the reader will have anticipated, if he has understood the principles I have advanced, these diseases are such as yield readily and certainly to the Water-Cure. Women, if no others, have cause to bless the genius of Preissnitz! Medicines mock the patient with a temporary palliation of symptoms, but in the end the disease is aggravated. The Water-Cure gives complete relief.

I have left to the last what is to me the most interesting and, perhaps, the most important of all the results of Water-Cure; I mean its use in gestation and childbirth; and were I not supported by an abundance of facts and experience I should feel that I put my reputation in peril by the statements I am about to make. Childbirth is the terror of the female sex, in civilized countries, from its pain and danger. It is not so with the simple children of nature, with whom it is attended by neither pain nor peril. Under the blessings of the Water-Cure, by a judicious course of treatment, woman may be so prepared and strengthened, and so assisted in the progress of labor, and at its termination, as to make the process almost or entirely painless, and almost wholly free from dangerous consequences. This is done by giving tone to the nervous system, and making the reproductive organs perfectly healthy. When this is done, the contractions of the uterus have no more pain than those of a healthy stomach or bladder. Mrs. Gove Nichols states in her "Experience" that the duration of labors, under her care, has been from twenty minutes to four hours and a half. Ladies who had formerly suffered inconceivably forty-eight hours, have been delivered under her care in one hour, and in several cases in a few minutes; often with pain so slight as to be scarcely noticed. But in these cases there must be preparatory treatment. The children, born under these circumstances, are remarkably robust and healthy. In her tract, "The Water-Cure," Mrs. Nichols says:

> "The writer has had a large obstetric practice for several years, and has never had a patient who was not able to take an entire cold bath, and sit up and walk, the day after the birth of a child. I need not say, that life would often be the forfeit of even rising from the bed at an early period after delivery, where patients are treated after the old methods. The water-treatment strengthens the mother, so that she obtains a great immunity from suffering during the period of labor, and enables her to sit up and walk about during the first days after delivery. In all the writer's practice, and in the practice of other Water-Cure physicians, she has never known an instance of the least evil resulting from this treatment."

This subject is of such momentous interest, and so new withal; women are so incredulous of what seems to them miraculous, though it is perfectly natural, and in conformity with all the principles of true science, that I will give another brief extract, from the same writer, in the April number of the WATER-CURE JOURNAL.

> "I have been very much gratified with several births that have recently come under my care. One young lady, who was really far from being strong, but who had been living very carefully on Water-Cure principles through her pregnancy, encouraged and supported by a strong, earnest husband, suffered slightly one quarter of an hour. Another, with a first child, and whose friends frightened her all in their power, took the cure under my care, and when she was delivered she could hardly be said to suffer at all. I was uncertain whether the expulsive efforts were accompanied by pain. I said, after the birth, 'were these efforts painful?' She hesitated, and then said, '*slightly*.' The same day she sat up and held her babe, and said she felt *well*.
>
> "Another, the last case I had. The babe was born with three expulsive efforts, each of which was somewhat painful. *This was all.* The lady was up the day after the birth, and about house, as usual, in a week."

And these, I can assure the reader, are but samples of many cases of a similar character. Have I not properly described the Water-Cure as a comprehensive system, extending through the whole domain of human disease and suffering? I have done so conscientiously; the reader must judge with what capacity of forming a correct judgment.*

OF THE MEANS OF TREATMENT.

How shall the patient reap the greatest advantage from the Water-Cure? Doubtless, by going to some Water-Cure establishment, in whose physician he has confidence, and giving all his time and attention to the cure. In this course there are several advantages. There is change of scene, relief from customary labors and anxieties, the encouragement of companionship, etc. But some of these establishments are distant; others are expensive. Invalids dislike to be separated from their relatives and friends, and to be deprived of the kindness and care which no money can purchase.

In this city, and wherever there are Water-Cure establishments, persons are taken as day patients; who, residing at their own houses, come regularly to the Water-Cure house for advice, packs, douches, and such of the applications as can not be conveniently made elsewhere. They have in this way the advantage of riding or walking, and the excitement of a visit, with all desirable treatment; without leaving home, and in many cases, with but little interruption to their customary employments.

But there is no reason why people should not take the Water-Cure at home, when desirable, as well as submit to any other medical treatment. All our best houses are furnished with baths, and it will not be long before no house will be considered tenantable without one. Even in the country, it will take but a little expense or trouble to fit up a Water-Cure apparatus that will answer all necessary purposes. A tub or trough, which any carpenter can make, will answer for a plunge bath, and one or two pails will form a pouring one. A douche is simply a stream of water falling from the height of a few feet; and a sitz bath, is a half filled wash-tub. Wherever there is pure cold water, I would engage to give the

* This, it must be remembered, is intended as an *introduction* to Water-Cure, and by no means a full account of it. Those who are interested in the subject, will find further information in the works of Gully, Wilson, Johnson, Francke or Rousse, Horsel, Munde, Houghton, Shew, and others. Ladies will find the published lectures of Mrs. M. S. Gove Nichols, and her "Experience in Water-Cure," of great advantage. The latter has been pronounced by very competent judges the best work yet written on the subject, and it is unquestionably the one best adapted to the wants of females.

Water-Cure. A pouring bath, a dripping sheet, a sponge or towel bath, a sitz bath, a wet sheet or blanket pack, can be taken any where. It is certainly best to have all the conveniences of a Water-Cure establishment, but no one should go without the treatment for the lack of these. Water is everywhere; and there are no insurmountable difficulties in its application.

I trust that the time is not distant when we shall have Water-Cure hospitals and dispensaries, where the poor can be treated at prices within their means, or where they are not able to pay at all, gratuitously.

A WORD OF CAUTION.

I HAVE more than once intimated, in the preceding pages, that the practice of Water-Cure is liable to errors and abuses. When a new system becomes popular, it is liable to be taken up by the unqualified and incompetent, as "fools rush in where angels fear to tread." In all schools of medicine people intrust the care of health and life to men to whom they would not intrust their property. Water-Cure is no more likely to be exempt from ignorance and a mercenary spirit than any other system, and from these no system is free. With every day's increasing popularity of this mode of treatment, will increase this danger. It is inevitable that Water-Cure must sometimes fall into the hands of empirics and quacks; as it is notorious that what is called the regular profession is full of such.

I have endeavored to show briefly, indeed, but I trust not the less clearly, that the proper application of the Water-Cure demands of the practitioner a profound knowledge of the human system, its diseases, the causes which produce them, the process of cure, and the means by which that process may be brought about. A diseased human system is not a thing to be trifled with, or treated with blind ignorance. The powerful processes of the Water-Cure demand science, judgment, and skill, in their application. In many cases their power to cure, if rightly used, corresponds to their power to injure if misapplied. In hundreds and thousands of cases, by the admissions of the doctors themselves, patients have been killed outright by the poisons of allopathy. It is not strange that the mistakes of Water-Cure physicians should sometimes be fatal. I have an unaffected admiration for the genius of Preissnitz, but it is not to be denied that he has sometimes made fatal mistakes in his practice which a thorough education might have prevented.

Yet, curiously enough, a flying visit to Grafenberg has been thought an important qualification to a Water-Cure physician!

That I may not needlessly alarm the timid and deter the afflicted from seeking relief, I will specify some of the cases in which errors in Water-Cure may be attended with mischief. In all consumptive cases great care must be taken to adapt the degree of cold to the reactive power of the patient. In dysentery of a low type, very cold water applied to the surface, may increase the congestion of the inflamed organ. In diseases of the heart and in cases of tendency to apoplexy, the more powerful of the Water-Cure processes must be ventured upon with great caution. The treatment of pneumonia or lung fever, when violent, is a matter of some delicacy, Where uterine hemorrhage has produced excessive weakness, the Water-Cure may be the only hope, if properly applied; if applied recklessly, it may increase the danger. In aged and infirm persons, with a tendency to eruptive disease, there is danger from too violent treatment, the use of too cold water tending to produce uncontrollable crisis; and where cold foot baths are much used in such cases, they may produce obstinate ulcers. In congestion of the lungs, a cold sitz bath may produce fatal hemorrhage. In scrofulous disease of the viscera, congestions may be produced by ignorant and empirical treatment. In obstetric cases, the vanity of getting a patient up quickly may lead to unpleasant consequences; and the use of the cold sitz bath without the vagina syringe may be prejudicial, when there is congestion of the uterus and low reactive power. In short, the very power which water has to cure the disease may, by ignorance, be turned against the patient. The difference between Water-Cure and allopathy, in this respect, is, that while the former, in incompetent hands, may be injurious in some cases, the latter, in any hands, can hardly fail to do more or less injury in all. Competent physicians and intelligent patients will, I trust, appreciate my motives in making these remarks. To some they may seem impolitic; but the true interests of Water-Cure do not require concealment or misrepresentation, nor will they ever be safe in the hands of routine, ignorant, and empirical practitioners.*

* I do not wish it to be understood that I think no man can practice Water-Cure who has not received a regular medical education. I have seen too much of medical students and medical professors to have any very lofty idea of their inevitable wisdom. What I wish to assert is, that a man should have knowledge and judgment; I care not how or where he gets them.

THE PLEASURES OF WATER-CURE.

To persons of diseased nervous systems, the Water-Cure seems a chilly and disagreeable business; but they soon change their opinions. After the momentary shock of the cold bath, comes a delightful feeling of glowing invigoration. After the first chilling five minutes in the wet-sheet pack, there comes a calm, soothing, and delicious repose, and often sound and refreshing sleep. Coming from the douche, a patient feels like jumping over fences. With a Water-Cure appetite, the simplest fare is eaten with the greatest zest, while the air, exercise, a purified system, and the consciousness of returning health, give elasticity to the spirits, and continual enjoyment. I have never seen happier persons than those who were recovering from long, miserable diseases, under the Water-Cure. As melancholy, petulance, and despondency come from disease, they fly at its cure, and give place to buoyant hope and serene happiness. In Water-Cure, we escape nauseous drugs, tormenting blisters, and disgusting setons; we enjoy cleanly and refreshing baths; above all, we lay the foundation of all happiness, in a renovated constitution and vigorous health.

CONCLUSION.

THERE may arise a question as to the motives which have induced me to write and publish this work. I will frankly avow them. I have devoted my life, to such extent as it may please Providence, to the work of healing the sick, and hope that this pamphlet will aid me in that purpose, by calling attention to the system I have endeavored to explain, and whose merits are becoming every day more widely appreciated. It is my desire to do all in my power, not merely to cure the sick, but to prevent sickness by promoting the public health, and I know of no more efficient way of doing this, than by extending a knowledge of the principles of Water-Cure, which are those of health. This system is based upon the laws of life, and an observance of those laws will secure the health of the community.

Doubtless the publication of this work may be of some personal advantage. It can scarcely fail to increase my work, and correspondingly its emoluments; but there is a satisfaction in thinking that a thorough and competent Water-Cure physician earns his money, and that his patients get the worth of theirs, in what is above all price. The system is one of singular economy. The medicine costs nothing, and neither prolongs a disease nor prepares the way for a new one. Health, once thoroughly gained, is accompanied by the knowledge of the way to preserve it, and Water-Cure patients often become their own physicians. Mothers, especially, learn to treat their children. In a mercenary point of view it is a bad system for the medical profession, and will, doubtless, put an end to it as soon as the world gets some wiser; but we have the consolation of knowing that what, in a low sense, is bad for us, is, in the highest sense, good for the world.

My past and future labors must be the test of my sincerity and zeal in the health reform, which I hold to be at the basis of all reforms, and the first right step to be taken in our progress to that state of universal happiness and peace which may God hasten.

THE END.

EXPERIENCE

IN

WATER-CURE:

A FAMILIAR EXPOSITION OF THE

Principles and Results of Water Treatment,

IN THE CURE OF

ACUTE AND CHRONIC DISEASES,

ILLUSTRATED BY NUMEROUS CASES IN THE PRACTICE OF THE AUTHOR; WITH AN EXPLANATION OF WATER-CURE PROCESSES, ADVICE ON DIET AND REGIMEN, AND PARTICULAR DIRECTIONS TO WOMEN IN THE TREATMENT OF FEMALE DISEASES, WATER TREATMENT IN CHILDBIRTH, AND THE DISEASES OF INFANCY.

BY MARY S. GOVE NICHOLS,
WATER-CURE PHYSICIAN,
AUTHOR OF LECTURES TO LADIES ON ANATOMY AND PHYSIOLOGY, ETC. ETC.

STEREOTYPED.

NEW YORK:
FOWLERS AND WELLS, 131 NASSAU-STREET.
LONDON: JOHN CHAPMAN, 142 STRAND.
1850.

To my Husband,

WHO HAS A MIND TO UNDERSTAND

THE WORK OF HUMAN ELEVATION,

A HEART TO LOVE IT,

AND ENERGY TO LABOR FOR IT,

I Dedicate

THESE RECORDS OF MY EXPERIENCE

PREFACE.

I HAVE determined to add another book to the many already published on WATER-CURE. I think I owe a record of my experience to my friends; I trust it may be of service to the profession; and I am anxious to extend, as widely as possible, a knowledge of the principles and practice of the Water-Cure, and the blessings of restored health and prolonged usefulness.

My distant patients, who never see me, but who rely on my letters for instruction and direction in their cure, will, I trust, find the full and particular directions in this book of essential service. I have endeavored through the whole book to give general readers an understanding of the causes of disease, and the means of cure opened to them in the processes, diet, and regimen of Water-Cure. As far as possible, I have endeavored to make my instructions practical, to help those who are beyond the reach of personal advice. But no general rules, and no number of examples, will apply to the peculiarities of every case. Next to personal consultation, that by letter is to be desired; and by the publication of my "Experience," and by a daily increasing professional correspondence, I find my sphere of usefulness continually widening.

I by no means expect this little work to take the place of the valuable Water-Cure books now in the market; but it contains more particular directions to women, and treats more of their peculiar diseases, than any work I have seen. My mission has been to instruct and help woman. After spending several years in giving lectures to women on anatomy and physiology, I published the substance of these lectures in a book, as I now do the results of my subsequent labors in the cure of disease. I advise ladies who are interested in hygienic reform, to read all the Water-Cure books they can obtain. I have seen no book on the subject that was not valuable. Dr. Gully's I think the best, and yet there are errors in that which I would like to see corrected. The "Introduction to Water-Cure," written by Dr. Nichols, contains a brief and thorough exposition of the principles and results of the hydropathic treatment.

It is a great error to suppose that Water-Cure can only be used successfully in Water-Cure establishments. Such have their advantages, and, in many cases, I would greatly prefer to have a patient under my daily supervision and constant care. In some cases this personal supervision is indispensable to a cure. Aided by my husband, a medical graduate of the University of New York, but, notwithstanding, a thorough Water-Cure physician, I shall have, henceforth, increased facilities for each of the four branches of practice: the reception of patients in our city establishment for full board treatment; the care of those who reside here, and come for day treatment; the care of patients who are treated at their own residences; and answering letters of consultation from a distance.

Patients at a distance should give a full and clear account of their diseases, the time they have been affected, the health of their parents, if dead, of what diseases they died, and at what age, and all facts which may throw light upon the case; especially those relating to diseases, medicines, habits, and temperature, or reactive power against cold. The usual fee for consultation is five dollars. This should be inclosed in the first letter, and one dollar in subsequent letters, if any such are required.

I am aware that there are cases in this book which will hardly be credited by many who are unacquainted with the Water-Cure; but though, from motives of delicacy, the names of patients are not given, yet names and particular references are at the service of any who wish them for a useful purpose. Many of my patients in this city will be happy to give a verbal account of their experience in Water-Cure to those who are sufficiently interested to call on them.

The education of earnest and capable women for physicians is an object near my heart. I have had some worthy students, and hope for greater facilities. Some of our colleges have been opened to them, and we may in time have others for their exclusive benefit. At present we must compensate ourselves by energy of will and perseverance in action for those advantages which are granted to men, but denied to us. "God helps those who help themselves."

MARY S. GOVE NICHOLS.

WATER-CURE HOUSE,
No. 87 West Twenty-second Street, New York.

EXPERIENCE IN WATER CURE

CHAPTER I.

PRINCIPLES AND PROCESSES OF THE WATER TREATMENT.

BEFORE giving an account of my own experience and practice, as a Water Cure Physician, it may be well to give the reader some general idea of the character and claims of the system of medical treatment which has been termed Hydropathic, Hydrotherapeutic, and other terms perhaps, but which I prefer to designate, in plain English, as the Water Cure; and for this purpose I copy here the body of a little tract, which I have prepared and printed for gratuitous circulation, and which may be obtained free of cost, by any who believe that the promulgation of its truths will benefit the world.

THE WATER CURE.

HEALTH is the result of the natural performance of all the functions of life. It gives development, beauty, vigor, and happiness; and is characterized by strength of body, power and serenity of mind, and a keen enjoyment of all the blessings of life.

DISEASE is the result of any disorder of the natural functions. It hinders development, mars beauty, impairs vigor, and destroys happiness. It is characterized by indolence, weakness, pain, and misery; and brings a wretched life to a premature and painful death.

The NATURAL LIFE is one of health, with all its pleasures. There is no *natural death,* save the gradual and painless wearing out of the vital energy in old age. Health is the law of all organic life. Disease is the result of accidental, ignorant, or wilful violations of the laws of nature.

Health, as defined above, is maintained by a simple nourishing diet, pure air, exercise, cleanliness, and the regulation of the passions. Men cram themselves with the impure flesh and fat of diseased animals, heating condiments and spices, spirituous drinks, and the poisonous narcotics, as opium, tea, coffee, and tobacco—injuring their digestive powers, and filling their systems with poisonous matter; and to these are added a long list of vegetable and mineral poisons, given as medicines, not one grain of which can be taken without permanent injury to the human organism; we inhale poisons in filthy streets and unventilated buildings, and these poisons are kept in the system; and the skin—the great purifying organ of the body—is weakened, by a neglect of personal cleanliness, which cannot be maintained in perfection without daily bathing in cold water. The poisonous matter thus brought into, and kept in the system, weakens its powers, interrupts its functions, and produces a state of disease. Nature makes a violent effort to cast out these evils—and we have pain, inflammations, fevers, and the whole train of acute diseases. The poisons in the system, and the bleedings and poisonings of the doctors, weaken the powers of nature—and we have the less violent, but more protracted agonies of chronic disease. Such violations of the laws of God, have filled the world with disease and misery. Diseased parents bring forth sick and short-lived children, half of whom perish in infancy, and not one hundredth reach old age. Thus, 'sin came into the world, and death by sin.'

The struggle of the system to cast out its diseases, goes on as long as the vital power remains. Every effort of nature is for health; all pain is remedial; and all the symptoms of disease are caused by the reactive powers of the system. It is the work of the physician to assist and facilitate these efforts; but this cannot be done by drawing out the vital current, and thus weakening the reactive powers of nature; nor by giving additional poisons, to task still more the vital energies. Doctors with lancets and poisons, have joined Disease in a war upon Nature—instead of aiding Nature in its struggle with Disease.

The Water Cure is the scientific application of the principles of nature in the cure of disease. It is not the mere application of water, but it enters into all the causes of disease, and assists all the efforts of nature for its cure. It prescribes a pure and healthy diet, carefully adapted to the assimilating powers of the patient; it demands pure air and strengthening exercise, with other physical and moral hygienic conditions. The applications of water, according as they are made, are cleansing, exciting, tonic, or sedative. Water clears the stomach better than any other emetic; produces powerful and regular evacuations of the bowels; excites the skin—the great deterging organ of the system—to throw off masses of impurities; stimulates the whole absorbent and secretory systems; relieves pain more effectually than opium; dissolves acrid and poisonous matters; purifies the blood; reduces inflammations; calms irritations; and answers fully all the indications of cure—to fulfil which, physicians search their pharmacopias in vain. The proper application of the processes of the WATER CURE never fails of doing good. Its only abuses come from ignorance. The Water Cure physician requires a full knowledge of the system, and a careful discrimination in applying it to various constitutions, and the varied conditions of disease.

Medicines, too often, instead of aiding, check the curative processes of nature. They deaden and stifle diseases, instead of casting them out. Often they change acute affections, which, left to their own course, would result in health, to chronic and incurable diseases. The patient, after being rid of the particular action of the disease, still retains the cause that produced it, with the addition of the medicine he has taken. Often, in the Water Cure, patients throw off large quantities of mercury and other poisons, which have lain in their systems for years, producing rheumatic, neuralgic, and other nervous and chronic diseases.

As nature is making constant efforts to free the body from disease, and as the Water Cure strengthens and invigorates all the powers of nature, and assists in its great processes of dissolving and expelling morbid matter, it is applicable to every kind of disease, and will cure all that are curable. It cools raging fevers, and gives tone and energy to the most exhausted nervous system; it soothes the most violent pains, and calms the paroxysms of delirium; it brings out the poisonous matter of scrofula, and gives firmness to the shaking hand of palsy.

Unassisted Nature, where there is a large stock of vitality, may triumph over both disease and medicine. The success of the Homœopathic practice shows, that the less medicine taken, the oftener Nature asserts her rights. But the Water Cure equalizes the circulation, cleanses the system, invigorates the great organs of life, and, by exciting the functions of nutrition and excretion, builds up the body anew, and re-creates it in purity and health.

Health, once established by the Water Cure, is maintained by it ever after. It is rare indeed that a Water Cure family ever needs a physician the second time. The system threatens in this way to destroy all medical practice. Mothers learn to not only cure the diseases of their families, but, what is more important, to keep them in health. The only way a Water Cure physician can live, is by constantly getting new patients, as the old ones are too thoroughly cured, and too well informed, to require further advice. This is a striking advantage to Water Cure patients, if not to Water Cure physicians.

The efficacy of the water cure depends always upon the amount of vital energy or reactive force in the patient; and this in low and chronic diseases must be economized with the greatest care. Mistakes and failures in water cure, have come from not knowing how to adapt the treatment to the patient's reactive power. The same treatment that would cure one, might fail entirely with another. The practice of this system, therefore, requires profound science, the best judgment, and the finest discrimination. These are especially needed in chronic, nervous, and female diseases. In all these, the water cure is the only effectual remedy. Thousands of women are every year doctored into premature graves, who might be saved by a knowledge of the water cure. The world is scarcely prepared to believe that its processes relieve childbirth of nearly all its dangers and sufferings—yet this truth has many living witnesses.

The writer has had a large obstetric practice for several years, and has never had a patient who was not able to take an entire cold bath, and sit up and walk, the day after the birth of a child. I need not say, that life would often be the forfeit of even rising from the bed, at an early period after delivery, where patients are treated after the old methods. The water treatment strengthens the mother, so that she obtains a great immunity from suffering during the period of labor, and enables her to sit up and walk about during the first days after delivery. In all the writer's practice, and in the practice of other water cure physicians, she has never known an instance of the least evil resulting from this treatment.

Dyspepsia yields readily—slowly often, but very surely—to the water cure. There is no patching up, but a thorough renovation. Some of its greatest triumphs are in nervous and spinal diseases; and cases of epilepsy and insanity are cured in so many instances, as to encourage hope for all. In all diseases of the digestive organs, and the nerves of the organic system, medicines are worse than useless. The only hope is in some application of the water cure—the more scientific, the better.

The diseases of infancy, as croup, measles, scarlet fever, &c., lose all their terrors under the water cure system. Death, by any such disease, in this practice, is unheard of, and could only result from the grossest ignorance in the physician, or some terrible complication of hereditary disease in the patient. Colic, diarrhœa, and dysentery, in children and adults, are perfectly manageable in the water cure, and yield to its simplest applications, where the organism is not remedilessly depraved. Fevers and inflammations are controlled with so much ease, and are so shortened in duration, as not to excite the least uneasiness. The small-pox yields readily to the water cure, and is cured without leaving the slightest mutilation. In typhus and ship fever it is equally effectual; and in cholera, the writer has not seen a case that did not yield readily to its applications; though fatal cases must occur in a general practice, with bad patients. The water cure is a perfect preventive.

It may be proper to state, that all these acute diseases are shortened, because the system, in the water cure, is enabled to throw off as much bad matter in three or four days, as it could get rid of in as many weeks, if left to itself, or weakened by medication. Thus, fever-and-ague is cured in four or five days, without danger of relapse, as frequently happens after the poisoning of quinine. In all acute diseases, the water cure operates so promptly and effectually, and Nature, when not weakened and interfered with by bleeding and drugs, carries on her work so beneficently, that there is not the least fear of an unfavorable termination.

The writer has treated lung, typhus, scarlet, ship, and brain fever, and has never lost a patient; and in only two cases has the fever continued over six days. In measles, varioloid, and small-pox, she has found the treatment equally effective. In one instance, where the patient was fast sinking from suppressed measles—not having slept for seven days and nights—a single wet sheet pack induced sound sleep, and brought out the measles thickly all over the surface of the body; and in three days' treatment, the patient was comfortable and out of danger. In severe pain, in neuralgia, or tic doloreux, in delirium tremens, and in other severe nervous affections, the wet sheet pack has a more certain soothing effect, than any preparation of opium, or other anodyne, without after bad consequences.

Consumption is considered an incurable disease; but there have been many cases in the practice of the writer in which it has seemed to be permanently cured, and others in which existence has been greatly prolonged. Her own case is one of perfect recovery from consumptive tendencies of the most alarming character; and there is little doubt, that in most cases the disease might be arrested in the earlier stages of its progress, by the water cure, while drug medication never fails to aggravate the disease and hasten its progress.

The processes of the water cure, skilfully directed, are never painful, and seldom disagreeable. If irksome at first, they soon become pleasant, as the nerves acquire tone. They may be gone through at all seasons, and in many cases without materially interfering with the ordinary business and amusements of the patient. They can be applied in all situations where it is possible to get pure water, fresh air, and a proper diet. It is desirable, in many cases, to live at a water cure house; but many of the best cures are made by patients who apply the water at home, under competent advice. Summer is favorable for some cases, winter for others, and spring and autumn for all. A few days' treatment suffices for an acute case, but a chronic one may require weeks and months of persevering attention, according to the vitality of the system and the nature of the disease.

The great trouble with Americans, is, they are in too great a hurry. They are in a hurry to eat and drink and to get rich. They get sick as fast as they can, and they want a short cut to health. Chronic disease that has been inherited, or induced by wrong doing through half a lifetime, cannot be cured in a day by any process now known to the world. What we want for water cure, is a fair trial for a sufficient length of time.

The water cure is the most economical system of medicine. It supports no druggists, and requires few practitioners. Water is everywhere free, and the best diet is cheaper than the worst. The universal practice of water cure would lead to universal health. A single consultation and prescription is often all that is necessary; and, contrary to every other system of medicine, the means for gaining health are also the means of preserving it. For these reasons, water cure is destined to be the greatest blessing ever bestowed upon a diseased and suffering race.

This introduction will not be perfect, nor will the subsequent pages—especially the accounts of cases—be as well understood as I desire, without a brief description of the most common of the processes used in water cure.

WATER CURE PROCESSES.

QUALITIES OF WATER.

Soft, fresh, spring water is to be preferred for all the applications of the water treatment; and all water is good in proportion as it possesses the same qualities. Rain water, fresh from the clouds, is pure, soft, and full of vitality; but, after standing for some time in tanks or cisterns, it loses much of its living quality. Water that is hard, from the presence of lime, or brackish, from saline matter, is less beneficial than that which is pure and soft; but I have no hesitation in prefering it to that which is dead and stagnant. River water is good in proportion to its freshness and purity; but *any* water is better than *none;* and there is little room to doubt that the benefits derived from bathing in salt and mineral water are to be attributed far more to the virtues of the water, than to any operation of the minerals it holds in solution. There is something in the effects of "living water" beyond its cleansing qualities. There is little doubt that the skin absorbs oxygen from it, and perhaps some other vital quality, which, for want of a better word, we may call electricity. The strength and vigor often gained by a single bath, can scarcely be accounted for by its cleansing qualities or the tonic power of cold.

BATHING.

People excuse the filthiness of going without a full daily bath, on the ground that they have no conveniences; but this is an idle excuse. Wherever a pail or even a pitcher of water can be obtained, a cleanly person will have a bath, by means of a towel, a sponge, or by standing in a tub, and pouring it over the person. The pouring bath, by means of a large sponge or otherwise, is one of the finest that can be taken. The shower bath is never used in water cure processes. It is superseded by either the plunge, the pouring bath, the dripping sheet, or others to be described hereafter. It answers well enough for persons in full health and strong reactive power, but is found too chilling for invalids.

The duration of a full bath must be graduated by the reactive power of the patient. Where this is aided by exercise, as in swimming, it may continue for a considerable period, but a common plunge bath requires to be taken quickly, according to the temperature of the water and the season.

Water in its natural state varies in temperature from 48 to 70 degrees. Sixty degrees is a proper temperature. In winter, baths may be taken much lower, and a quick bath, near the freezing point, produces a brisk reaction. Tepid baths range from 70 degrees to blood heat; but cold and warmth are relative terms. Water which feels warm to a person in health, gives the sensation of cold to a man in a high fever. All baths should be of clean water, freshly drawn, and only one person should bathe in the same water, unless the quantity is very large, nor then, if there is the least risk of taking infectious diseases.

As a general rule, no bath should be taken until two hours after eating.

THE PLUNGE BATH.

This bath is used for general daily ablutions, and to follow the wet sheet and blanket packings. The best method of taking it, is by filling the common bathing tub sufficiently to immerse the entire person. In this, as in all other cases, the head should be wet before immersing the body.

THE POURING BATH.

After wetting the head and face, the patient stands or crouches in a tub or any convenient place, while the attendant pours over him one or two pailsful of cold water; or the patient may easily give himself this bath, without assistance.

A pleasant way of taking the pouring bath is, to have a sponge large enough to hold several pints of water. The bather can stand up, express the water with both hands upon the back of his neck, and get a refreshing bath over his whole body.

THE DRIPPING SHEET.

This convenient and powerful bath can be taken any where. Let the patient wet his head; then dip a common sheet in cold water, and envelope the patient as he stands up, rubbing him all over briskly outside and with the sheet. This bath is of great use in fevers.

THE DOUCHE.

A stream of water, from half an inch to three inches in diameter, and falling from five to twenty feet, constitutes a more or less powerful douche. The head may be wet first, or the stream allowed to break over the hands, held above the head for a moment, but the full force of the douche should never fall upon the head, but upon the back and limbs. This is a very exciting application, acting powerfully upon the whole system, and useful in many forms of chronic disease. It is used locally to discuss tumors, rheumatic swellings, and for spinal and nervous diseases.

THE SITZ BATH.

This is one of the most efficacious of the water cure processes, and also one of the most convenient for general use. A common washing tub may be filled, say a third full of water, in which the patient is to sit, having first removed his clothing as much as is necessary; the feet, of course, being left outside. It is common to begin with tepid water, and make it colder each bath, so that at the end of the week it is of the natural temperature.

The sitz bath is used in a great variety of cases. Where it is prescribed for its stimulating and tonic effect upon the nerves of the bowels or pelvic viscera, the usual time is from ten to fifteen minutes; but where it is used for its derivative effect in lessening inflammations of the head or chest, it is continued for half an hour, or even longer.

THE SHALLOW, OR HALF BATH.

This is a bath in which the patient can sit, with the water, tepid or cold, four or five inches deep, so as to be rubbed by attendants. Such a bath is of great service in cooling the heat of fevers, or relieving congestions. If more convenient, it may take the place of the plunge bath, following the wet sheet.

THE WET SHEET PACK.

This has been called the sheet anchor of water cure, as it is the most powerful and universally applicable of all its processes. It is used in almost every form and stage of disease. It cools febrile action, excites the action of the skin, equalizes the circulation, removes obstructions, brings out eruptive diseases, controls spasms, and relieves pain like a charm. Far from being disagreeable, it is a most delightful application. After the first shock of the cold sheet, there comes a pleasant glow, a calm, and usually a profound sleep.

Lay upon a bed, one or two comfortables and two or more woollen blankets. Take a sheet, large enough to envelop the whole person, or as much as is necessary; dip it in cold water, and wring it out until no more runs from it. Spread this upon the blankets. Let the patient extend himself on his back, upon the sheet, and wrap it quickly and tightly about him, arms and all, from head to feet, leaving the face free. Bring the blankets, one after another, tightly about him, one at a time, and pack him like a mummy or a baby for a winter's day out. Either a small feather bed, blankets, or comforters may be laid over all—enough to make a thick covering. If very weak and chilly, bottles of hot water may be put to the feet, and even under the armpits; but the use of artificial heat is seldom necessary, and always is as much as possible to be avoided. If the head ache, a towel wet in cold water must be applied.

The patient should remain in the pack until warmth is fully established, and the whole skin is in a glow, and just ready to burst into a perspiration. But if he is nervous and uneasy, he may be taken out at any time. Sometimes it is desirable to sweat the patient. This in most cases is readily accomplished.

On coming out of the pack, the patient must go as quickly as possible into a plunge, pouring, or other cold or tepid bath. This rule is invariable, except when, in cases of high inflammation, one wet sheet follows another in quick succession.

THE BLANKET PACK.

The patient is packed in dry blankets, instead of the wet sheet, and remains until a perspiration is excited, which is continued or not, according to the nature of the case. A cold bath follows.

On coming from any of these baths, the patient should be well rubbed with coarse towels, a brush, or the hand, or with all these; and sometimes much friction is necessary to excite the skin, quicken the circulation, and produce a healthy reaction.

Hand baths, foot baths, &c. are too easily understood to require any explanation.

Further remarks on baths, as well as directions for diet, exercise, clothing, &c. will be found in other portions of this work, particularly in the chapter on Consumption.

CHAPTER II.

FEMALE PHYSICIANS—MY EARLY EXPERIENCE AND STUDIES.

In giving to the world some few of the results of my work, I make no attempt to explore or define the sphere of woman. Each individual must do this for herself. But I assert, that woman in her nature is eminently qualified to heal the sick. If it were thought needful at this day to bleed and poison people into health, I would by no means recommend woman for the work. *This* is clearly not "woman's sphere."

Woman has great quickness in understanding principles. I do not say in discovering them. The first, and more rugged processes of intellection belong to man. Woman reasons well from principles, and acts wisely and kindly, particularly where affection induces her to act, and affection should be the prime moving power in constituting woman a physician,—a teacher—an artist, or indeed, to qualify her to act usefully or successfully in any sphere. She feels quickly and tenderly. She sees and comprehends with a rapidity that makes the conclusions of reason seem intuitions. By all this she is fitted to be a physician. Then there is a propriety, a delicacy, a *decency*, in a woman being the medical adviser of her own sex—which most people can see.

Many delicate ladies have said to me, that they would die before they would submit to examinations needful to their cure, by a male physician. We have reason to believe that many women, with that innate and shrinking modesty which is an ornament to the sex, do give up their lives a prey to hopeless disease, simply because women are not qualified to act as physicians. They cannot commit their cases to those who should care for them—they cannot persuade themselves to submit to exposure to men, and they linger a few years in untold and unconceived misery, and die when they should be in the full flush of life, and in the midst of usefulness.

Alas, for woman! her lot in this age, as in all previous ages, has been one of suffering, and the depth and bitterness of that suffering is known only to herself and to God.

The general prevalence of those diseases peculiar to woman, constitutes a fearful necessity for the education and training of women for physicians. The Healing Art opens a broad field of usefulness to our sex, but no woman can enter this field and be really useful, without deep devotion. We must desire above all to be of the greatest use, and then we shall seek to be prepared to accomplish the end we have in view.

At this day it would be a matter of much difficulty, if not of impossibility, for women to enrol themselves as members of the medical profession, by studying the Healing Art. We cannot receive a diploma from an Alma Mater, that has borne us through a course of study like an infant in arms. No long established institutions, no ancient and honorable societies offer us support and facilities on our untried way. Single-handed, we must grapple with iron prejudice and a time-honored custom, grown hoary in a dotage of error. We have work to do to strengthen our hands. We may be thankful that work will strengthen them. We have difficulties to overcome, that would sharpen meaner wits than ours.

The discipline of self-culture is wholesome. The labor of self-education goes far toward creating the mind it is meant to improve. At first thought, the obstacles interposed between woman and one of the learned professions, seem absolutely insurmountable. But it is not so. "There is not anything denied to persevering and well directed effort." Men cannot concede to us our position, but they can help us to secure it, when the purpose to attain it has come fully into our hearts. Men are willing to do this individually, though not yet corporately.

I am a witness of the truth of this assertion, for scientific men have acknowledged my earnestness of purpose, and assisted me in the attainment of knowledge, and rejoiced in my usefulness, though they could give me no diploma—albeit diplomas are *sold sometimes,* to men whose wit, worth, or scientific attainments do not move the especial reverence even of us women.

Fulton did not get a certificate to prove that he could build a steamboat. He built it. Priessnitz has no diploma—but he has won name and fame by his deeds without it. Men love justice, and when woman is truly qualified for the responsible work of curing disease, she may not only accept, but give diplomas.

The necessity for female physicians being sufficiently apparent to the most careless observer, the question very naturally presents itself for an answer, how are they to be educated for the work? The answer must be different in each individual case. It is a great mistake to suppose that men, and particularly scientific men, are opposed to the education of women. They are ready and willing to help all who can and will profit by their assistance. Let woman have the living germ of success in her heart, and she will succeed. "God helps those who help themselves"—and man does the same. It would be the poorest economy to waste effort on the mass of idlers.

Though I do not feel bound to apologize for being one of the first women to devote myself to the work of the physician, I may be excused for giving a few explanatory words respecting my choice of a profession, and my public lectures and labors.

I think it needful to do this, in order more fully to gain the confidence of the public. I want to be heard by the people, because I have most important truth to tell them—I want to labor for them, because I know I can do their work well, and I have plenty of witnesses to the truth of this assertion, though it may seem a little egotistical. I have not come hastily or lightly into my present work. My preparation has been going on providentially, as I believe, many years. I have lived to outlive the ignorance and consequent reproach of a great many people.

I took my place in the great field of labor which I now occupy, from a necessity of my being. I first received benefit from the practice of water cure in my own case, and then I sought to benefit others.

Years since I had a sister. I remember when the red deepened on her cheek, when she began to press her hand upon her side, and to cough—a hollow, boding cough; and then came physicians, and all the effort was made to save her, that could be made with the knowledge they had. But she faded away and died. I saw her in her coffin, so beautiful that she seemed not dead, but sleeping. The hectic red was still upon her cold, dead cheek, when they laid her in the grave. And then my brother, who had studied medicine, and was just beginning the world, sank with this disease. He was attacked with violent bleeding at the lungs, and a hard cough, but such was his strength of constitution, that it was four years before he could die, though he was subjected to all the poisonous medication of the allopathic profession in which he was educated. But he sank at last, and not long after his death I was attacked with cough and bleeding at the lungs. At the first attack I felt that I was doomed; that I must speedily go down to the grave as my brother and sister had gone. I remember well, though some ten years have since elapsed, laden with many joys and many sorrows—I remember my feelings when my lungs were first ruptured. The blood rushed rapidly into the trachea, and as I threw it off by violent coughing, the thought of my work, my great work for woman, rushed through my mind. The darkness that then shrouded the land on the subjects of health and disease was palpable, and I felt the importance of my mission to be in proportion to the evils I sought to remove. The thought of leaving my mission unfulfilled, of leaving woman to suffer and die under the black pall of ignorance that enveloped her then, was more than I could bear. I fainted and fell as if dead. It was at a lecture. The people gathered about me, and carried me into the air; and after a time I revived. With life came hope, or more properly speaking, trust. It was only for a moment that my faith had failed, or my trust been disturbed. God knows best, was then, as it has ever been, the watchword of my soul. After this bleeding, I had a severe cough, and all the symptoms of consumption. By constant bathing, exercise in the open air, and very simple and careful living, and ceasing entirely from my labors, I became rapidly better. My cough disappeared. I regained my strength, and my lungs seemed able to bear exertion. I again commenced speaking in public, and all the arduous duties connected with my profession. Various causes combined to make me labor far beyond my strength, and affliction came upon me with a crushing weight. Under the joint pressure of labor and sorrow my lungs again became ruptured, and this time the very fountains of my life seemed to be poured forth. In about four days I bled almost three quarts from my lungs. I was reduced to infantile weakness. In this state I sent for a German water-cure and homœopathic physician, who attended me with great care and kindness till the bleeding ceased. As soon as I was able, I commenced a regular course of water cure treatment, which I kept up with the most untiring zeal, until my lungs seemed fully restored. It is now five years since I have been able to sustain the full burden of the labors of my profession. Four years I have labored in this city, and I am willing to compare my work with that of the strongest man.

I have now good health, but I have a strong tendency to pulmonary difficulty. Great mental suffering will induce congestion of my lungs, and exposure to the bad air of an unventilated and crowded lecture or concert room, will inevitably make me cough next morning. But by proper care in my general habits, and the necessary applications of water cure, I maintain comfortable health all the time, and a power of endurance surprising to those who know me best.

It is not my wish to speak of my own course any further than is needful, in order that others may be benefited by my experience. It would be wrong for me to withhold facts that might be of use, from fear that I should incur the charge of egotism.

When a young girl, at school, an incident occurred, which, though slight in itself, and apparently worthy of no particular notice, probably determined my position in life. I was away from home. The gentleman where I boarded had some medical works in his library. I read them from curiosity, and was much interested; so much that I was constantly thinking how I could procure more books. I read what I found in my friend's library secretly, and after some months I returned home. I found my eldest brother engaged in the study of medicine. He had Bell's Anatomy at home with him occasionally, and sometimes left it for some days at a time. Without his knowledge, and unknown, indeed, to any of the family, I commenced studying these books. Time passed, and I became deeply interested in the subject. One day my brother was explaining the circulation of the blood, and fœtal circulation was incidentally mentioned. He was not master of his subject. He made some mistakes which I corrected, and finished his explanation for him. He stared at me with much astonishment, and asked me if I had been reading his books. I was obliged to confess the truth. My brother was much dissatisfied with my unwomanly conduct, and was determined that I should read no more. He ridiculed me, as the most effectual means of influencing a timid young girl. He told me mockingly, that he would bring me a book on obstetrics. I blushed scarlet and could not talk with him; but nothing broke my habit of reading his books till he hid them. Finding no opportunity to gratify my love for medical study, I turned my attention to the study of French and Latin, the best preliminary studies for me, though I was not aware of the fact.

Shortly after this period I married and went to live in New Hampshire. I now procured medical books from editors for whom I wrote; these I exchanged with a physician in the town where I resided. It happened that one of the books* that I had the good fortune to procure, was devoted largely to the illustration of the sanative effects of cold water: its use was particularly recommended for children. About this time I read Dr. John Mason Good's works, and my attention was arrested by his remarks on the use of water for the cure of fevers. I read these books in 1832, sixteen years before this present writing. About this time I had a child, and began the use of water by having her bathed in cold water daily from birth. Soon after, I commenced using water in hemorrhages and fevers. The physician who had loaned me the books, also used water in fevers, I think in all cases, giving little medicine. The patient was bathed during the accession of the fever in cold water—ice-cold, for it was drawn from very deep wells, and cloths wet in cold water were laid on the head. The patient drank plenty of cold water. This practice was wholly successful. At this period I only used water in fevers and hemorrhages, and with children, and with the last rather with the intention of preventing than curing disease. My warrant for this practice was obtained wholly from the before-mentioned books. It was not till years afterwards that I heard of Priessnitz and Water Cure as I now practice it.

From this time I was possessed with a passion for anatomical, physiological and pathological study. I could never explain the reason of this intense feeling to myself or others; all I know is, that it took possession of me, and mastered me wholly; it supported me through efforts that would otherwise have been to me inconceivable and insupportable. I am naturally timid and bashful; few would be likely to believe this who only see my doings without being acquainted with me. But timid as I was, I sought assistance from scientific and professional

* Book of Health, published at London, being a sort of Domestic Materia Medica.

men. I went through museums of morbid specimens that but for my passion for knowledge would have filled me with horror. I looked on dissections till I could see a woman or child dissected with far more firmness than I could now look upon the killing of an animal for food. My industry and earnestness were commensurate, notwithstanding my health was far from being firm. I had innumerable difficulties to contend against. When I am dead these may be told for the encouragement of others—not till then. When I retired to rest at night I took my books with me; the last minute I could keep awake was devoted to study, and the first light that was sufficient, was improved in learning the mysteries of our wonderful mechanism. My intense desire to learn seemed to make every one willing to help me who had knowledge to impart. Kindness from the medical profession, and the manifestation of a helpful disposition towards my undertakings, were everywhere the rule.

After my marriage, I had resided for several years in New Hampshire, and then moved to Lynn, Mass., near Boston. Here I engaged in teaching, and had many more facilities for pursuing my studies than ever before.

In 1837 I commenced lecturing in my school on anatomy and physiology. I had before this given one or two lectures before a Female Lyceum formed by my pupils and some of their friends. At first I gave these health lectures, as they were termed, to the young ladies of my school, and their particular friends whom they were allowed to invite, once in two weeks; subsequently once a week. In the autumn of 1838 I was invited by a society of ladies in Boston, to give a course of lectures before them, on anatomy and physiology. I gave this course of lectures to a large class of ladies, and repeated it afterward to a much larger number. I lectured pretty constantly for several years after this beginning in Boston. I lectured in Massachusetts, Maine, N. Hampshire, Rhode Island, New York, New Jersey, Pennsylvania, Maryland and Ohio, and also on the island of Nantucket. Physicians were uniformly obliging and friendly to me. I do not now recollect but one exception, and this was a "Doctor" who I believe honestly thought that knowledge was, or would be injurious to women, and therefore he opposed me in my efforts to teach. I have forgotten his name, and I presume the world will do the same. But I have not forgotten, and never can forget, the many who have held out the hand of help to me, and through me to others, for I have never learned selfishly; what I have gained for myself I have gained for others.

The passion that has possessed me from my first reading on pathology I consider providential. I believe fully, that I have been set apart from my birth for a peculiar work. I may be called enthusiast and superstitious for this conviction, but it is mine as much as my life. My ill health from earliest infancy, the poverty and struggles through which I have passed, and the indomitable desire which I have had to obtain knowledge, all seem to me so many providences. During the time that I studied alone my enthusiasm never for one moment failed. Day and night, in sickness and in health, the unquenchable desire for knowledge and use burned with undiminished flame. I studied day and night, though all the time I had to labor for bread, first with my needle and later with a school.

It may be said that I was an enthusiast, and that my enthusiasm sustained me. I grant this, but will those who make this assertion define the word enthusiasm? To me it means, as it meant through those many long years, an unfaltering trust in God, and an all-pervading desire to be useful to my fellow-beings. If these constitute religious enthusiasm, then I am an enthusiast.

CHAPTER III.

MEDICAL PRACTICE.

It is not my object to attack any school of medicine. I wish to give a very brief history of the principles and practice of the scientific schools of medicine, and also to give some results of my own labors in water cure.

I know that it is considered by some, presumption for a woman to come before the public as a physician. It is very unpleasant to some to see long established customs broken, and long cherished prejudices set at nought, even when a great good is to be achieved. But this is by no means the only class of persons in the community.

"Upward and onward," is the governing thought and the impelling motive of thousands. To these I speak—to these I bring the results of my investigations and my labors. The thought and the deed commend themselves to such as these, with no hindrance from respectable custom or grey-headed prejudice.

In looking over the history of medical science, we find that Allopathy has great claims on our respect. The Allopathic school has always insisted on its professors being educated.

Whatever has been known of anatomy, physiology, and pathology, in the past, has been taught by the Allopathic school; and there is no difference between the professors of Allopathy and Homœopathy in this respect. Both insist on thorough education. Both schools have been laborious in noting the characteristic symptoms of disease, and the effects of what they considered remedies. Perhaps the Homœopathic school has been most earnest and assiduous in this last work; but Homœopathy being of recent date, must rest its claims to our gratitude more on the zeal and minuteness of its observations and discoveries, than on the length of its days, or the voluminousness of its records. The members of the Allopathic profession have differed with regard to the primary cause of disease. Those of the homœopathic profession, I believe, have been united.

Amongst the Allopathists, one portion have advocated what was termed the Humoral Pathology, and another, the Nervous Pathology. Of all the nervous pathologists, Dr. Billings is clearest. He says, "all diseases have exhausted nervous influence for their cause." He says further,—

"During health, the capillary arteries go on with the work of nutrition and secretion, the muscles are fed, the mucous surfaces are lubricated just enough to prevent any sensation from the substances that pass along them—the serous surfaces are made sufficiently soft to slide upon each other without sensation, and the skin is kept soft by an insensible vapor. All this time, there is another process going on, which is the removal of superfluous matter by the absorbents."

After demonstrating that all these processes are carried on by the nervous energy, Dr. Billings shows by irrefragable argument, that the loss of this energy must produce disease.

Bœrhaave seems, in the latter part of his life, to have had a glimpse of this doctrine; indeed, he admitted the agency of the nervous power. In proof of this, we may mention that in the 755th of his aphorisms, where he lays down the proximate cause of intermitting fevers, he makes a change in the fourth edition. Hitherto it had stood—"Whence, after an accurate examination of the whole history, the proximate cause of intermittents is established to be viscosity of the arterial fluid." To this in the fourth edition is added, "Perhaps, also, the inertia of the nervous fluid as well of the cerebrum as of the cerebellum destined for the heart."

This theory of disease is shadowed in Cullen. According to Cullen, the system is superintended and regulated by a mobile and conservative energy seated in the brain, acting wisely but necessarily for the good of the whole. This energy, he considers to be distinct from the soul, and acting not only for the preservation, but the recovery of health.

Faint traces of this theory of disease may be found in the Brunonian system.

Darwin carries the idea farther, under the name of sensorial fluid. Broussais comes next to Brown with his theory of "organic contractility."

Humoral Pathology asserts, that morbid changes in the blood are the cause of disease.

Homœopathy asserts that psora is the cause of disease.

A little reflection shows that all these statements are true, and that it would be an error for either school to assert that the evil it sees is the only cause of disease.

It is clear, that if all the functions of the system are carried on, and the whole maintained in a state of health by the nervous energy, then if this nervous energy is wasted by any abuse, either by too much labor, too much thought, the domination of passion, or by taking poisonous stimulants, the nervous power, being thus wasted, cannot maintain the system in health. The consequence is disease, and the deposition of morbid matter in the system, which would have been thrown out if the nervous power had been left to do its work.

Thus we see that the observations of nervous and humoral pathologists and homœopathists, have all been valuable and truthful.

The practice of both these schools is understood. It is to give as remedies the most virulent poisons known to us.

The extreme minuteness of the doses used by homœopaths, has been a great recommendation to those who have seen the bad effects of allopathic doses, and yet have not lost their faith in medicine.

I have used homœopathic medicine with care and in entire good faith, upon myself and my patients. The result of my trials with it has been to convince me, that though it has been, and is, a great negative good to the world, it has no positive efficacy. But the hygienic rules insisted on by Homœopathists are worthy of all praise.

With regard to allopathy, I must say that I studied it honestly, and because it poisons and oppresses the human constitution with drugs, and debilitates it with bleeding, I consider it one of the greatest evils that now rests upon the civilized world. But I do not attach the blame of this evil to individual practitioners of the art. Monarchy and despotism are bad—gigantic in their badness, but kings and despots may be good men.

These evils have their origin with the people, and our only hope of removing them is in promoting the intelligence of the people.

I maintain that the cause of disease is one—the want of nervous energy. Numerous occasions spring from this cause. In the fact, that diseasing matter is left in the system, not only for years but for generations, is seen the foundation of the assertion of the homœopathic school, that *psora* is the cause of all disease.

The great questions for humanity are, What is the cause of disease? and what remedial treatment is best?

As a water cure physician, I maintain that nervous energy is restored, and morbid matter cast out of the system, by means of the proper application of water cure.

We see that in case of disease, morbid matter must be expelled from the system, and by means of the nervous energy. It becomes important, then, to know whether we shall add to the evil already in the system, and to the labor of the already enfeebled vital energy, the most virulent poisons known to us, and which are called medicines, and thus still farther waste the vital energy by compelling it to strive to expel the poison of the disease and the poison of the medicine at once.

I contend that we can add to the vital power continually, by the water cure.

With regard to the evils of blood-letting, I have only to say in the language of Scripture, "the blood is the life." The regular medical profession is rapidly purifying itself from the heresy of blood-letting, or taking the life of patients.

Majendie, Marshall Hall, Eberle, and many others, are doing this work, and there is no doubt that the good sense of the community is aiding in it more than physicians or people are aware.

It is impossible to do any justice to the subject of blood-letting, in a paragraph, and I shall not therefore attempt it.

In my "Lectures to Ladies on Anatomy and Physiology," page 226, some interesting facts and authorities are given. The regular profession of medicine has been and is, the depository of much knowledge. My hope is, that it will not lag behind the age.

It is known that the faculty bleed less, and give less medicine, and use more water than formerly. I see no good reason why this reform should not go on progressively with the intelligence and consequent demand of the public.

The greatest men in the profession have sanctioned the use of water. Hippocrates, the father of medicine, used water in his treatment of disease. His works bear testimony to the cure of cramp, convulsions, gout, and tetanus by water.

Galen, who lived in the second century, cured fever with water only.

Celsus recommends water for the cure of certain diseases.

Bœerhaave recommends water to make the body firm and strong.

Hoffman, a contemporary of Bœrhaave, wrote on water for the cure of disease. He said if there was a universal medicine, it was water. Hahn also wrote on water cure, and one of the best water cure works was written by Currie, a Fellow of the Royal Society, Liverpool, and published in 1799.

In 1749, Rev. John Wesley published a work on water cure. He gives a list of eighty diseases curable by water.

Dr. Billings and others have had a correct theory of disease. Their error has been in introducing medicines into the system, which they thought increased the nervous or contractile power. The medicines being poison, and recognised as such by the vital organism, have aroused all the energy left in the body to cast them out. The poison has not increased the power, but stimulated what remained, to action, and has thus resulted in still greater waste to the system. Increase of action has been mistaken for increase of power, and the stimulation of poison for the tonic or strengthening effects of medicine.

The frightful effects of various kinds of medicines can hardly be exaggerated. One of the most common is calomel.

Salivation and the destruction of the organs of speech, and of the nose; incurable rheumatisms and paralysis, with rottenness of the bones, have been caused by calomel, and minor ills produced by it are everywhere. But with regard to the effects of medicines, a volume would not do them justice.

Of homœopathic medicines, I must say, that if I believed in

their potency at all, I should believe it an evil potency, because they are the poisons of allopathy. Chalk, charcoal, and cuttle-fish, and several other substances used by the homœopathists, are exceptions. These, surely, cannot do injury. I should not fear to drink the water of Lake Superior, if a few grains of arsenic had been mixed with the whole of it. On the same principle I have never feared homœopathic medicines.

The darkness of this civilized era, with respect to the effects of medicines upon the human system, and the blind faith of even educated people in physicians, is to me one of the most astonishing phenomena in the world. But there is encouragement. Light—more light, is the anxious cry of many.

Some years since, I passed through the Albany Medical College. I saw there human bones that had rotted down under the poison of mercury. I saw uterine tumors, ranged in glass vases, weighing from one to more than twenty pounds. Doctors had doubtless done all they could to cure these diseases. With what they had done, or in spite of it, the victims of ignorance and abuse had died. Knowledge would have saved them from sufferings which cannot be described, and from premature death. When I saw these things, and many more that I cannot speak of, in that College, a devotion to woman—to the work of spreading light on the subject of health and disease, was kindled in my heart, that death only can quench.

I felt then that I would lay myself on the altar, and be burned with fire, if woman could be saved from the darkness of ignorance, and the untold horrors of her diseases.

CHAPTER IV.

GENERAL VIEW OF MY PRACTICE AND SUCCESS.

In 1843 I obtained books from England on the Water Cure, and much practical information from Henry Gardner Wright, an English gentleman, who spent some time in this country during that year. He brought several works on Water Cure, and being in bad health, he applied the water in his own case successfully at my father's house, where he remained some months. The books that he brought, the accounts that he gave me of Priessnitz' practice, and Water Cure practitioners in England, and his application of water in his own case, added to my practical knowledge and conviction on the subject, removed the last remnant of my faith in drugs, and induced me to practice water cure alone in every case that came under my care. I soon saw what qualifications were requisite to make a successful practitioner of water cure. There are no rules of practice applicable to all cases, but the water cure physician must have judgment to adapt the treatment to the vital or reactive power possessed by the patient. A practice that would be eminently successful in one case, would surely destroy life in another. Care and ability in the diagnosis of disease, and skill in adapting the treatment to the strength and peculiar idiosyncracy of the patient, are indispensable to success in water cure.

In 1844, at the opening of Dr. Wesselhoeft's water cure house in Brattleborough, Vermont, I went to that place. I boarded near the water cure house for three months, and observed the practice very carefully. I also gave lectures to classes, composed of ladies who were under water treatment, and others. From Brattleboro' I went to Lebanon Springs water cure house. They had no resident physician, and I concluded to remain for a time in that capacity. I took charge of the patients there for three months with the best success, and then came to New York, in the latter part of the autumn of 1844. I went to Dr. Shew's water cure house in Bond-street, and remained for some weeks and saw his practice. I then took rooms, and gave lectures to classes of young ladies, and advice to patients, and attended to out-door practice till May, 1845, when I went to reside at my late water cure house, 261 Tenth-street. There I have given lectures to classes of ladies, and have taken board and day patients, and have also attended to out-door practice as at my present residence.

The first two years I had a large number of board-patients, who came from a distance, from Connecticut, Northern New York, Rhode Island, Ohio, Kentucky, and several from the Southern States. During the past year, my practice has changed its character. Water cure houses have been established in different parts of the country, and patients can be treated nearer home ; consequently I have not had so many board-patients. I have now a much larger practice in the city, which is doubtless owing to the spread of intelligence respecting water cure amongst the people, and also to the fact of my having become known.

I have looked over the records of my practice in this city,

noting all failures and deaths, and their causes. Only two patients have died under my care—both children; one died in the summer of '47, the other in the summer of '49. The first died of disease of the brain and dysentery, the last of dysentery. Both were about nine months of age; both were born of unhealthy mothers, and were scrofulous. They seemed not to be organized to live any longer. The water greatly relieved them, and they suffered very little. The suffering was not to be compared, for a moment, with what is endured in these diseases under drug treatment. I had a little patient about five years of age, who had hip disease. It was the worst case I ever saw. He was treated under my direction, and I saw him occasionally for about a year, with the most remarkably beneficial results. At the end of this time, his mother fell very sick, and the child went into the care of a very ignorant black woman. I had not seen him for some weeks, and knew nothing of the hands he was in. One day I was called in haste, and found the child very low from the effects of retained pus, several outlets in his hip being closed entirely, whence had flowed pints of scrofulous matter within a few months. I probed and syringed the cavities of these abscesses, and the child revived from a comatose state, but he was too far gone for hope. I told the parents this, and they called an allopathic physician. The child died under his care not long afterward. I have thus carefully chronicled the failures of my practice, with what I consider their causes.

It may seem strange, that with a large practice, I have had so few deaths. I do not attribute this to my skill altogether, though I believe that I understand my profession; but it has so happened.

Several persons who had consumption have been treated by me for the alleviation of their symptoms, when their cases were hopeless. Four of these have died, but at the time of their death they were not under my care, and in each case I told them there was no hope of cure, but that they could be relieved, and they were much relieved in each instance.

I have treated with entire success, the following diseases: Brain Fever, Typhus Fever, Lung Fever, Ship Fever, Delirium Tremens, Small Pox, Scarlatina, Measles, Chicken Pox, Varioloid, Inflammatory Rheumatism, Spinal Disease, and the whole train of Female Weaknesses, and Uterine Diseases.

I have treated Hernia, injuries of the lungs, and other injuries; and I have a large and most interesting obstetric practice.

I have treated Fever and Ague, Croup, Influenza, Diseases of the Eyes, Jaundice, Dysentery, and Cholera, and have been equally successful with all.

I find that the confidence of the people of New York, and the public generally, is daily gaining strength in water cure. I direct the treatment of patients by letter in different parts of the United States, and I believe the day is not far distant, when intelligent persons everywhere will be their own physicians to a great extent. I have already educated a great many mothers in this city, so that they are physicians in their own families, and successful ones too. Occasionally they call for advice, but in the main they do not need me.

I am now looking toward the education of women as physicians, and particularly to attend to obstetric practice. If our medical colleges are not soon opened to woman, others will be founded where she will be educated. The spirit of the age will not any longer submit to bonds.

CHAPTER V.

WATER CURE IN ACUTE DISEASES.

Many persons who have become sensible of the excellence of water cure in chronic diseases, know nothing of its wonderful uses in acute diseases, and frequently ladies who are under water treatment for chronic ailments, have sent for a physician, and submitted their children to a course of drug practice, when they have been attacked by fever, or some other acute malady.

They have thus laid the foundation with their children, in the most tender and susceptible period of life, for chronic disease, perhaps of a very obstinate character. Mothers who are so ignorant as to injure their children in this manner, only need to be enlightened. A few cases of fever, measles, or small pox, or any acute disease successfully treated with water, either seen by these persons, or accurately recorded for their perusal, will save children and others from the evils of drug treatment.

The effects of water cure in acute disease, have only to be seen to inspire the fullest confidence; for so rapidly are fevers and all acute maladies subdued by judicious water treatment, that the remedial effects thus obtained seem absolutely miraculous.

If people only knew the remarkable and almost marvellous way in which all violent and febrile diseases yield to a judicious application of this cure, drugs would be at a discount, and blisters and the lancet among the thousand horrors of the past. In my water cure experience, I have had abundant evidence that depletion by bleeding or purgatives is never required, that counter-irritants are unnecessary tortures, and that all the indications of a rapid cure, without unnecessary weakness or poisoning can be attained by this mode of treatment. If a patient has vitality enough to have a fever, he has life enough to be cured, and always can be, except in fatal lesions of vital organs.

In illustration of the foregoing, I will give cases that have occurred in my practice during the three years last past.

CASE OF CROUP.

This affection of the mucous membrane of the larynx, so often fatal to children, is the terror of parents, and the dread of the faculty, from the suddenness of its attacks, and the rapidity of its progress to a fatal termination. A boy, ten years old, the son of a distinguished allopathic physician, had a tendency to the disease, which had apparently been strengthened by the usual treatment in his previous attacks. When called to him, his croupy, rattling breathing, and dry, barking cough, could be heard over the whole house, and he had not apparently an hour to live, unless immediate relief could be afforded.

The boy, as is usual in such cases, was of a full habit, and possessed of strong reactive powers, and the treatment was made proportionally active. Placing him in a tub, I first poured over his throat and chest two pails full of cold water, and then rubbed the parts until the skin was quite red. He was then packed in the wet sheet, and well covered with blankets. With the glow and perspiration came the relief to his breathing, and freedom from the choking distress. As soon as the perspiration was fully established, he was taken out of the sheet, and drenched with cold water, followed by rubbing with coarse towels, after which he was put into bed, quite free from the croupy symptoms.

The inflammatory action, however, was not entirely subdued, and on the afternoon of the same day the symptoms began to return, when he was again packed in the wet sheet. This was followed by a pouring bath as before, and the cure was complete.

There is no doubt that a similar treatment, varied to suit the constitutions of different patients, would cure every case of this disease, except in the last stages of its most violent forms, which may be beyond the powers of any remedial agents.

SMALL-POX.

Mrs. D., a very beautiful woman, who had been in feeble and delicate health from her childhood, was taken on the 6th of April, 1848, with small-pox. She is a catholic, and had kept the fasts of the church faithfully. She had been for a short time previous under water treatment, and it being Lent, was living on a very spare and temperate diet. This was exceedingly fortunate for her, as her system was filled with scrofula, and she had a strong tendency to inflammatory action.

Mrs. D. was seized very violently. The chills were excessive, the fever was burning. It seemed that the flame of Vesuvius was kindled in the system, at the same time that the frosts of a thousand Laplands were freezing her. The pain in the bones was most excruciating, and her head she declared was "splitting" all the time. Her face became frightfully swollen.

The first day she was enveloped in a wet sheet, the disease as usual not having declared itself, and the other treatment was adapted to what seemed a "crisis" in the technical language of water cure. The second day, the fever, the chills, pain in the head and bones, and swelling of the face, made me very certain that it was a case of small-pox. Still, as ship-fever was at the time very rife in the city, I would not give the disease a name until the third day. The family knew very little of water cure. What they knew was from reading and report. They had not seen any cases treated by water.

Under these discouraging circumstances it is not at all wonderful that they should be exceedingly anxious. The morning of the third day came; the eruption had not appeared. The disease had received no name, and the patient was in the hands of a woman who had no diploma, and was treated according to a new system, of which they really knew nothing.

The husband, with the tenderest love for his wife, was in an agony of anxiety. He wished to call in a physician; and the man who was their family physician, before this experiment in water cure, was an allopathist. Of course I was greatly distressed at the thought that this delicate, weak and beautiful creature, should fall under allopathic treatment at such a frightful moment as the present. I doubted not that she had smallpox, and I had just as little doubt that with the poison of medicine, added to the terrible disease raging in her system, she would either lose her life or be badly mutilated. I felt almost certain of the first, quite certain of the last. In the short time that the lady had been under my care I had become tenderly attached to her.

I spoke earnestly to the anxious husband. I told him what madness it would be to subject his wife to the poison of medicine, and the terror of her disease at the same time. I told him of the uniform success of proper water treatment in these cases. I begged for time. He left all to his wife. She decided to try the water a little farther. He consented very cheerfully, on condition that I would be willing to have another physician called in. I begged to be allowed to consult with a water cure physician. They consented. I called in Dr. Shew, who was very attentive, and behaved in the most gentlemanly manner. We, of course, agreed as to the treatment. Dr. Shew called several times, and reassured the family very much.

The fever became so intense the third day, that instead of enveloping the patient in a single wet sheet, she was covered with four folds of wet linen at the period of the greatest heat, and two and three folds, and then one fold, as the heat abated.

These folds of linen were covered by thick blankets, and removed at proper intervals, and the patient sponged with cold water, and then fresh linen was again wet and applied. The efflorescence began to appear the third day, but was very full on the fourth. The pustules were most abundant, the disease assuming the confluent form on the face.

The bowels were kept open and free with water injections, and the patient took the juices of fruit for nourishment. The fever was subdued by the constant application of the water; the itching, so frightful usually during the recovery, was not even uncomfortable in this case. The face was kept covered with wet linen. The room was much darkened, though the windows were kept open, and a current of fresh air was all the time admitted.

The patient, lovely character of Mrs. D. doubtless assisted

materially in the favorable issue of the disease. It was enough for her to know that any process was necessary, however disagreeable; she submitted so sweetly and cheerfully, that all felt that the beauty of her countenance must be preserved as a correspondent to her beautiful spirit, and with pleasure I record that it was preserved. *She was not marked.*

Very terrible boils on the head and limbs attended Mrs. D.'s recovery. These were lanced in several instances, and large quantities of scrofulous matter evacuated. These were treated with water only.

CASE OF MALIGNANT TYPHUS.

In December last, Mrs. B., a young married lady, in Hudson-street, who had been weakened by uterine and spinal disease, was attacked with typhus fever in its most malignant form. When called to see her, I found her suffering from a violent pain in the head, and lying in a very low state, with the characteristic effluvia, and other symptoms of typhus. It was a case such as, under allopathic treatment, no one would expect to recover in less than from twenty to forty days. Some idea of the malignancy of the disease may be formed from the circumstance, that the mother-in-law of the patient, a strong, healthy woman, from merely assisting in the first rubbing bath prescribed, was attacked with headache and vomiting, and was very ill for many hours.

The rubbing baths and wet sheet packings, administered at short intervals, cooled down the parching fever, brought out the morbid matter in the system, and in six days the fever was conquered. During the time that the fever was at the worst, she was immersed in the sitz bath, or in the wet sheet pack, or enveloped in wet bandages all the time. It was the most severe weather of the winter, and yet she was kept in a room without fire, and the window was open all the time.

She was able to go about the house in two weeks, and her health became much better than before her illness.

CASE OF SHIP FEVER.

A young Irishman, aged seventeen, was seized with ship fever directly after landing at New York. He was fat and full of blood, and the fever seemed as violent as was possible. He was first put in a tepid bath, and rubbed until the skin was perfectly cleansed—a ceremony that had not probably been performed before since his birth. After this, he was sponged in cold water, and then packed in a very wet sheet. When he came out of this, he was put under a dripping sheet, and rubbed for some time. At the third pack the peculiar eruption appeared. His tongue was very foul, and his mouth very sore. During the day he had, in the morning, a dripping-sheet bath, then a wet-sheet pack, and then again a dripping-sheet bath. He then lay enveloped in a wet sheet and very slight covering besides, and drank water till afternoon. He was then packed again, and again put under the dripping sheet. During the night, he lay in a wet sheet, slightly covered. This sheet was several times wrung out of fresh water during the night. For five days he took nothing but water. The sixth day he ate a bowl of gruel during the day, and went out of his room. The seventh day he went out doors, and after that was free from fever. He was very weak, and greatly emaciated, but immediately regained his health and strength, taking only one bath a day after the fever was subdued. The treatment was graduated to the degree of fever.

This case is a fair sample of ship fever in the average, when submitted to water cure. It is never dangerous when taken by contagion and properly treated with water. If those physicians who have fallen victims to it had known of the efficacy of water treatment, and been allowed to try it, they would without a doubt have all been saved.

VARIOLOID.

Mrs. ——— had varioloid. She was attacked with great pain in the bones and intense chill, with considerable fever. She was put first under a pouring bath and rubbed into a glow. A cold wet bandage was put about the abdomen, and another about the head; then she was wrapped in blankets till profuse perspiration was induced. She was then well rubbed with the cold dripping sheet. This treatment was substantially repeated until the third day. The fourth she was about the house as if she had not been ill.

SCARLET FEVER.

Miss ——— was taken with a very malignant form of scarlet fever, which was then rife in the neighborhood. She was delirious, and the fever was of the worst type, and ran very high. She was first put under a pouring bath, then packed in the wet sheet. The wet sheet packs, and dripping sheet baths succeeded each other rapidly, for several days and nights, before the fever was subdued. The throat sloughed horridly, and large quantities of matter were thrown off. She took nothing but water for ten days, and four wet sheets in the twenty-four hours. She lay enveloped in wet linen when not in the wet sheet. The fever was then subdued, the appetite returned, the throat got well, and the patient fully recovered, with no drug poison in the system, and with health greatly better than she had ever before enjoyed.

SCROFULA.

Miss L. S—— was a child of diseased parents; the father a drunkard, the mother died young of consumption. This child was attacked with purulent ophthalmia at two years. The glands of the throat were also affected. Health conditions at her home were almost all wanting. The food of the child was very bad, pork and lard making a considerable portion of it. At the age of ten years she went to reside with a relative, who fed her on plain substantial food, giving her no flesh but the lean muscle, and this but once a day. She was bathed daily in cold water. The first year after being thus treated, she had a fever. In the course of the next year, she was affected with scrofulous sores in the head. A large quantity of matter was thrown off. Shower bathing, and constant bathing of the head and syringing the ears, were resorted to. The first attack was in autumn. The next autumn she passed through a similar affection of the head, with the same treatment. The third year, after sea bathing, she was attacked with scarlet fever. The writer was called early one morning, with the information that L. S—— was ill and delirious. Found her in a raging fever, the scarlet rash appearing like a flame over the whole surface of the body. She was immediately undressed and put in a common shower bath, and a large quantity of water poured over her. The steam arose as if the water had been poured on hot iron. After this bath she was thoroughly rubbed, and wrapped in a wet sheet, and put in bed. The heat continued intense, the throat was terribly swollen, but the delirium was gone. The wet sheet was wrung out of a tub of cold water once in fifteen minutes, and the tub of water changed once an hour.

(It would have been better to have had clean water for each application.) This process was continued unremittingly the first twenty-four hours, and in all cases should be continued till the heat abates. The next morning after her first attack, she was washed in Castile soap-suds. After this, clean water was poured over her as she stood in the tub, and then she was thoroughly rubbed. After the first twenty-four hours, the fever had so far abated, that frequent changes of the wet sheet did not seem needful; but for several days almost constant bathing of the head, arms, and feet were resorted to, and the sheet was renewed once an hour. After the fever abated so that the patient could be put in dry clothes, she was wholly bathed several times in the day, and she bathed constantly her arms, chest, and head. The quantity of scrofulous matter discharged from the throat was almost incredible. The throat was gargled at first with Castile soap-suds, and afterward with clear cold water very frequently. This fever might well be termed a *crisis*, in which the system relieved itself of psoric matter. In three weeks the patient was convalescent. During the whole illness, the only substance used which could be called medicinal was the soap. The food was gruel made of wheaten meal, and bread of the same.

After she became convalescent, a physician called and advised a cathartic. I objected strongly, and none was taken, or needed. The triumph of cold water was complete in this case, and the cure created much remark where the scrofulous habits of the patient were known. After this fever, she had no more affections of the head, nor, indeed, any indications of scrofula.

Before this fever, this child was very dull and stupid, particularly at the period when the head was affected; at those times she seemed almost idiotic. After this last crisis, she became active and bright, so much so as to be remarked as a very bright girl.

This case was treated several years since. I should not now use soap as I then used it.

INFLAMMATION OF THE LUNGS FROM INJURY.

Miss H., of Waterbury, Conn. This was a case of inflammation of the lungs, from repeated blows received in the region of the lungs and stomach, from the handle of a machine used in the manufacture of buttons. When she came under my care, the inflammation was so exceedingly violent, that only just sufficient air to sustain life was admitted into the lungs. The portion of the chest involving the lower part of the lungs was swollen, so as to resemble a large breast. The breath was drawn with the utmost difficulty, and the swelled portion of the chest was so tender to the touch, that it seemed at first impossible for her to bear the pressure of the wet sheet, and pack. But she breathed easier on the first application of the wet sheet. Each succeeding application was equally useful with the first. In a few weeks the swelling over the chest disappeared, the inflammation was subdued, the breathing became easy, and the strength greatly increased; and the young lady returned home, with directions to continue her cure, with entire confidence that health would be attained at no very distant period. She had continued to improve, as we anticipated, when I last heard from her.

FEVER AND AGUE.

A child of four years of age, living on Long Island, in a portion of the island pretty well adapted to the production of this disease, was attacked and suffered regularly, and greatly, for three weeks. She was brought to me at the end of that time. When the chills came on, I placed her in a bath, and poured two pails of cold water over her. I then rubbed the whole surface of her body for several minutes, and put a wet bandage around the body. She lay down, was covered, not at all heavily, fell asleep, and began to perspire. This bath and bandage broke the regularity of the fits. When the fever came on, she was bathed and enveloped in wet linen. During the cold stage she was treated as above. Her food was measured to her according to my judgment of the quantity proper, for her appetite was inordinate. The bowels were kept open by injections, till they became regular. In ten days she was cured.

TYPHUS FEVER.

I was called in the winter of '47–8 to a case of typhus fever. The patient, a young woman, was given up to die. I had so little hope, that I asked the mother if she was prepared to see her daughter die, whilst we should be putting her in the wet sheet. She said that she was prepared to see her die if she was not put in, and was also prepared for the worst if she was;

and added, that no blame should be thrown on water cure in case of her death. I immediately prepared to put her in the sheet. The mother assisted. We stopped once after the process was begun, thinking that she was dying—but as she continued to breathe, we finished the envelopement. She began to revive in ten or fifteen minutes after she was enveloped. She continued to revive under the treatment, and ultimately recovered.

BRAIN FEVER.

Miss ———, aged 24 years. I first saw this young lady on the 24th of June, 1848. She was then entirely delirious from brain fever; her whole system seemed on fire, particularly the brain. Her employment was that of musical and mathematical teacher, and she had made great and long continued exertion in both departments, and had acquired a high reputation. Her system was infected with scrofula, though she was very energetic and persevering. These two excellent qualities had well nigh wrought her death.

When I first saw her, she was entirely insensible to the fact of her illness, and thought her fever and difficulty of breathing owing to the heat and closeness of the room, though every window and door was open. I first put her into a shallow bath, and rubbed her for some minutes. This slightly abated the heat. I then took a large heavy linen sheet and dipped it in cold water, wringing it only so as to keep it from dripping. She was enveloped in this for an hour, then put in a cold pouring bath and rubbed for two minutes, and then put in a deep hip bath for half an hour. The fever was abated, but the delirium continued the same. During four nights I watched by her, giving her the following treatment. When the fever fit came on, I put her in the wet sheet as above. She was generally peaceful and silent for an hour in this. I then took her out of the sheet and put her in a cold pouring and rubbing bath; out of that she went in a deep hip bath for thirty minutes, out of that into a wet sheet as before for an hour, and sometimes an hour and twenty minutes. Then out of the sheet into the pouring bath, then into the deep hip bath for half an hour, and then under a dripping sheet. All these processes consumed the night, and as morning came, she would fall asleep cool and quiet. During the day she usually had one wet sheet pack, and two or three hip baths. The fever was much more violent in the night. After these four nights of watching and unintermitting treatment, the fever was broken and sanity began to return. In eight days she was sane, but not free from fever. On the tenth night from the commencement of the treatment, she had a violent accession of fever, but no delirium. The eleventh day she was slightly feverish, but perfectly sane. The twelfth day she had no remains of the fever; she was perfectly sane and had no return of insanity, or aberration of mind in the slightest degree.

INFLAMMATORY RHEUMATISM.

Mr. ——— was suffering from an attack of inflammatory rheumatism and the poison of tobacco leaves, which he had applied by the advice of some quack. Thorough bathing and bandaging the swollen limbs with wet linen, the fomentations being often renewed, soon cured this attack.

DELIRIUM TREMENS.

I have treated several cases of delirium tremens, substantially the same as brain fever, and with the same results. The worst cases of delirium were calmed and soothed in ten minutes after being enveloped in the wet sheet. The length of time required to complete the cure, varied, of course, according to the intensity of the disease. The cases that I have treated have been those of literary men, and passed mostly under the name of brain fever.

CASE OF DYSENTERY.

Mrs. ——— was attacked with dysentery. She was a woman of full habit with much reactive power. Much blood had been evacuated from the bowels when I saw her first. She took first a tepid bath, followed by the douche upon the bowels, then the abdomen was enveloped in four folds of wet linen, which was wet in cold water, and renewed once an hour. After each passage, an injection of cold water was given. A wine-glass of water was drunk each hour. The diet was very sparing, consisting of gruel, or dry toast. In three days the dysentery was entirely cured.

DYSENTERY.—A CASE ILLUSTRATIVE OF THE DANGERS OF INJUDICIOUS TREATMENT.

The great danger of unskilful water treatment is from congestion, and here you will mark well what I tell you. Take for instance, a case of congestion of the lungs. A patient who knew little of water cure, had congestion of the lungs. She took a cold sitz bath for half an hour. There was no reaction, she was so feeble. She was greatly chilled; the blood was driven forcibly to her lungs, and she bled profusely, and narrowly escaped with her life. Another case.—Last summer, the dysentery was very prevalent and fatal. A gentleman had lost one child, of dysentery, under allopathic treatment, and when his only remaining child was attacked, he sent for a water cure doctor. This physician, though a man of skill, and success in the main, has the German mania for "forcible treatment." He saw the child but a few minutes, and wrote his prescription hastily. This prescription involved treatment with very cold water. The consequence was, congestion. There was not reaction. The surface was chilled, and the blood driven inward upon the bowels. The congested vessels burst, and the hemorrhage from the bowels was frightful. The water cure used in this case was pretty nearly the water kill. I found the patient bleeding profusely. I immediately put her into a bath of 92 degrees, and put bandages about the bowels of the same temperature. I used cold injections to stop the bleeding from the bowels, after each evacuation; I also poured water from a pitcher upon the bowels once an hour, and twice a day she was immersed in the tub of water at 92 degrees. The bleeding from the bowels ceased as by a charm. The whole surface, and particularly, the abdomen, was rubbed much with the bare hand. The child recovered as by a miracle.

Now the same care and discrimination should be used in cholera as in dysentery. The first symptoms of cholera are analogous to dysentery. Those water cure doctors who use as much cold water for the weak as for the strong, who take no account of the reactive power of a patient, will succeed with one class of patients and fail with another. They lack discrimination, and though they will inevitably do much good, they cannot fail of doing some harm. Those who have judgment to adapt their treatment to the vital power of their patients, will cure all curable cases.

CHAPTER VI.

WATER CURE IN CHRONIC DISEASES.

The treatment of chronic disease, requires for the best success, that the physician should understand the degree of recuperative power possessed by the patient, and what organs are most oppressed by disease. Congestion is particularly to be guarded against. Water cure processes, which would be most beneficial in one case, will produce death from congestion in another. In no disease is water treatment more beneficial than in consumption, both in curing the disease, and alleviating it, where it cannot be cured; but the treatment may be so unskilfully applied, as to aggravate every bad symptom. So of chronic diarrhœa, dysentery, &c. These may be aggravated, and rendered fatal, by unskilful treatment.

The chief conditions of cure in chronic disease are, first, that the physician should know how to adapt his treatment to the state of the patient; secondly, that there be pure water, pure air, proper diet, and exercise, and all those means that are really as much a part of water cure as water itself. Having all these, the patient must have a *good disposition*. By this I do not mean a quiet temper, though this is desirable; but that the patient should be disposed to profit by the cure, and to second the efforts of the physician in every possible way. The great foe of water cure in America, is the restless hurry of the people. Many of them are enemies to all fixity constitutionally. If they have been ten, twenty, or fifty years getting sick, they want to be cured in a month, and often think it very hard if the water cure physician will not promise them a cure, of perhaps a life-long disease, in that time. A few patients have a sufficiently clear understanding, and firm purpose to go on for years in the cure. I have had patients who have been one, two, and three years in regaining their health. They have persevered like sensible people, and they have their reward. It is true, that some benefit always is experienced, where water cure is properly applied, in chronic diseases, in a few weeks; but sometimes it is so small, that the patient's faith is severely tried, if he has not a clear understanding.

I think the most common errors in the treatment of chronic

disease, are too forcible treatment, and too abundant use of proper or improper food.

A great many diseases can be cured by simple abstinence from bad forms of food, or by taking small quantities of good food. Dyspepsia, chronic diarrhœa, gout, and other diseases, may be brought as instances. In all things we first want to know our duty, and then we must have the will to perform it, or the knowledge is of no use. Patient perseverance in a right way, brings reward sooner or later. The writer took daily cold baths for seven years, before full reaction took place after the bath. But reaction came at last—a warm, delicious glow, that was a full reward for years of chills.

It is a great mistake to suppose that one cannot cure chronic disease, unless they go to a water cure house, or are under the immediate care of a physician. If a patient thoroughly understands his or her disease, and has the requisite energy to accomplish a cure, it may be done almost anywhere, and with very meagre advantages. I have known delicate and feeble women, who have done wonders for themselves, at home, with no physician but their own clear understanding, and no help but their own indomitable energy.

It is very necessary, that water for the cure of disease, should be pure and living, and in most cases cold. All water used for water cure processes should be fresh drawn from the fountain. Water soon loses its life by standing. Hence, rain, or cistern water is not as useful, as even hard water that is living from the fountain. If tepid water is used, it should be water fresh drawn with warm water poured in to make it the desired temperature. There are many cases when only tepid water can be used for a time.

No person should go into a bath that another person has used, unless it is as large as a pond or river. The practice in some water cure houses, of having ten, twenty, or thirty patients go into the same bath, cannot be too severely reprobated. They take the life from the water if the bath is small, and they leave their own impurities if the bath is large. We have only to suppose a case of contagious disease, such as syphilis, or small pox, or a patient with cancer, going into the same plunge with us, to make us feel the horror of the impurity.

The conditions of cure, then, in chronic diseases may be briefly enumerated,—skill, patience, perseverance, pure living, cold water, proper exercise, pure air, and good food, in proper quantities.

CASE OF DYSPEPSIA AND GREAT COLDNESS.

Mrs, ——— had been long afflicted with dyspepsia, accompanied by such intense coldness, that it seemed next to impossible to bear any treatment in which cold was an ingredient. A single wet towel over the chest, and a dry blanket pack made ever so close and warm, caused the most entire chill for a long time. But this sort of packing was persevered in, accompanied by the dripping sheet when she came out of pack, and long-continued rubbing with the hand. This pack, gradually increasing the towel till we used a half, and then a whole sheet, and the friction, together with strict attention to diet, the use of the vagina syringe and sitz bath, and after a time the abdominal bandage, so far restored vital heat, that after three months treatment, she was able to take the douche, and then she rapidly recovered her natural strength and heat. The dyspepsia got leave of absence, and good health came in its stead.

SPINAL DISEASE AND DISTORTION.

Miss ———, aged 18 years, of very delicate and frail organization, came to me in the summer of 1847. She had spinal disease, and distortion of the chest, from tight lacing—the false ribs lapping over each other. She had been suffering from cough, and seemed strongly tending to confirmed scrofulous consumption. She was very weak, and obliged to refrain from exertion, and lie in bed much of the time. Her appetite was poor, and very capricious. She was put through a careful course of treatment, which was gradually increased in force, as her strength increased. She took gymnastic and calisthenic exercises daily, under careful supervision. In nine months, her chest had enlarged five inches, her ribs had resumed their true position, her health was firm and good, and her strength would allow her to walk several miles without stopping, and without fatigue.

SCROFULA.—CASE OF AN INFANT.

A babe of six months, who had been nursed by a scrofulous nurse, came under my care. I had seen the child of the nurse, and accidentally remarked, from its appearance, that the infant was scrofulous, and that unless the matter was thrown off by boils, it would lose the use of its limbs. This seemed remarkable to those who heard the observation, as the babe, though quite old enough, had never been able to stand, and had then boils. This made them think that the other infant, who was nursing the same mother, might owe an illness with which it was afflicted, to the milk of the scrofulous nurse. The other babe was brought to me. According to my advice, a healthy nurse was procured for it at once. The child was suffering from indigestion, emaciation, and general irritability. She had a very large brain, and active nervous temperament. I advised a quiet nurse, with good temper, and little intellect.

I put the child daily in a wet sheet pack, and dripping sheet bath when it came out. In less than two weeks, a large portion of the surface was covered with a scrofulous eruption. Continuing the treatment the eruption disappeared, and the child recovered good health, under the care of its quiet nurse.

DYSPEPSIA.

Mrs. ——— had dyspepsia and chronic inflammation of the stomach, of the most alarming character. She had been the mother of a large family of children, and was also afflicted with falling of the womb and flooding.

At the time I was called to her, she was reduced, by large loss of blood in repeated floodings. She was apparently dying when I first saw her. There seemed no heat, or vitality in the exhausted system, except at the pit of the stomach, where there was burning inflammation. She had been treated by water, but very injudiciously, ice and ice water having been constantly applied over the region of the stomach. The blood was thus drawn from the surface to the centre, there being scarcely any reactive power, and the congestion was very frightful when I was called. The limbs were cold as death, the pulse low and fluttering, and the prospect of life seemed very doubtful. I applied hot fomentations to the stomach, and active friction to the limbs, for a long time before much apparent effect was produced. At the end of six hours almost unremitting exertion, with two efficient assistants, the circulation was established—the whole body was comfortably warm, and the patient could look about and speak with considerable ease. The treatment in this case was by much friction, the application of the wet sheet, ice water thrown upon the uterus with the vagina syringe, and the most careful attention to the nourishment of the patient. For days she took food by the tea-spoonful, and sipped water to cool the burning inflammation of the stomach. The improvement was immediate and steady. The inflammation was subdued; then she regained her strength, and then her emaciated frame began to be covered with flesh. In a few weeks she had gained twenty pounds. She went into the country as soon as she was able. Some eight weeks passed, and she returned so renovated in health and appearance, that when I called to see her, I did not recognise my emaciated patient, in the full, rounded form of the lady before me. Had I not heard her voice, I might have left without being at all aware that I had seen my patient. I had never seen her until I was called to her in her illness.

This case shows that water cure, like all other modes of practice, may be so injudiciously administered as to become a means of great evil, instead of good.

CASE OF NEURALGIA.

Miss ——— had been ill from birth—had taken a great deal of calomel and other medicine during her early years. The consequence of the errors in the training of this young lady, and the constant medication to which she was subjected, was general derangement of the health, very bad eyes, and finally prolapsus uteri and spinal disease, accompanied by the most distressing neuralgia, which seized upon different portions of the body at different times. At one period the nerves of the face and neck would be the seat of pain, at others, the lumbar region of the back, or the sacrum, or the uterus. Her sufferings during these accessions of pain, were absolutely frightful. She had also constant dyspepsia, fluor albus, and vomiting of bile in the morning. Her spirits were greatly depressed, and although one of the most benevolent and self-sacrificing persons in the world, and one of the most deeply pious, there was an irritability that showed itself almost beyond control, with those nearest and dearest to her. Such a complication of miseries I have seldom seen.

At the time she came under my care, she was suffering from an attack of acute inflammation of the uterus. She could not stand upright, or walk across the room. Her physician said to me, that there was nothing for her but to die.

She was treated for this attack, and relieved, and shortly after came under regular treatment at my house. She remained three months with great advantage to her health. Indeed, the worst symptoms were overcome during this time, but it remained for her to follow out my directions, to complete her cure at home, at a great distance from me, and amongst those who had little knowledge and less faith respecting water cure. In less than a year from the time she commenced, her health was very firm and good—so much so that she could walk miles, or for hours, without a pain of any kind being induced by the exertion.

TIC DOLOREUX, OR FACIAL NEURALGIA.

Mrs. ——— came to me with violent tic doloreux in the face. She had suffered for months with it, and was given up to great discouragement and depression.

She passed through a course of tonic treatment by water, consisting mostly of wet sheet packing during the paroxysms, dripping sheet, and sitz bath. She was packed once a day, remaining for an hour in the wet sheet, after the pain was relieved. In one month she returned home free from the disease.

A number of cases of chronic disease, with complications of a sexual character, will be found under the head of female diseases.

CHAPTER VII.

CAUSES, PREVENTION, AND TREATMENT OF THE DISEASES OF INFANCY.

This is a subject of the first and last importance; and whoever has the instinct of paternity or philanthropy in his heart will feel that he has duties connected with it. Last year, during the four hot weeks of July, 1,702 corpses were buried in the city of New York, and 802 of this number were infants, under five years of age. In 1847, out of 15,788 deaths, 7,373 were of children under five years old, and of 3,519 deaths in July and August, the number of 1,848, or more than one-half, were under the same age.

Here is this frightful infantile mortality staring us in the face, and who raises the voice of explanation or reprehension with regard to its causes? And few are awake to the subject, and know that "the curse causeless cannot come," but the majority know nothing of causes or remedies. They only know that they suffer, and they go on beseiging the doctors for poisonous drugs, and Heaven with prayers that their children may be saved. As the fatal season to infants approaches, many an anxious mother is casting about for the best preventive of disease. One gets some soothing syrup, or some lozenges, another some tincture of rhubarb or blackberry cordial, or some of the many patent nostrums which enable quacks to build themselves palaces with the money of the ignorant. Some of the orthodox in the medical faith give their children mercury in the form of the blue mass, or send for a doctor at the slightest appearance of illness. What we wish to understand and explain to the public is, the origin and nature of the fatal diseases of infancy; their causes, appearances, progress, and results; the treatment usually pursued in these cases, and the reasons why it is unsuccessful; and lastly, the means of avoiding or preventing such diseases, and the proper mode of treating them to produce a successful result. If the different schools of medicine would investigate the subject, and give the people the information they so much need, they would show cause why the public should honor the medical profession.

A large proportion of the causes of infant mortality begins with the constitution of the mothers. The ignorance and constant violation of the laws of life by mothers, insures the death of half the children in the civilized world, before they have reached the age of five years. Ignorance of our duties to ourselves and our children is steadily, day after day, month after month, and year after year, doing its work of death in the world.

No mother can give health to her child unless she is herself healthy. Women enter the married state weak from the confinement of a boarding-school, and often squeezed into the vice of corsets till their poisoned blood has been unable to circulate sufficiently to nourish the body, much less to keep it in health. They have half-breathed and half-lived, and been crammed with useless knowledge, and regular or quack medicines, till life is as much a burthen, as death is a terror. With no dependence for health, but upon a doctor, who cannot create it in the midst of their wrong habits, they marry and enter upon life. They are old in their youth—they are sick and languid—they want to lounge upon a sofa because they have no strength for the duties of life. Many have spinal disease and falling of the womb to begin the world with. Women who have to bear the responsibilities of maternity are afflicted in almost nine cases out of ten, with headache, or languor, and a sort of lazy debility, with pain and weakness of the back, especially at the monthly period. Very likely the sight is impaired; then, there is the faint, hollow stomach, especially in the morning, which is accompanied with a debility of the abdominal muscles, and a dragging down of the internal viscera, which causes the sufferer to bend forward, and thus cramps the lungs and prevents their being properly inflated. Instead of four pints of air, perhaps three are inhaled, and thus one-quarter of life is sacrificed at every breath—years are thus taken from life, but what is the loss of years to the loss of health, which is the crowning joy of human existence? When these sick ones, who call themselves well fifty times a day, if they are asked as many times "how do you do?" are afflicted with dyspepsia, and costiveness, and piles, and a general weakness and inability to depend on themselves, which are most painful to bear, and then when they begin to become conscious that another being is growing within them, instead of feeling a thrill of joy that a new love is nestling under their heart, they feel a more deathly sickness than I can describe. Most truly it may be said, that children are born at fearful cost. The mother wrestles with pain, and nausea, and weakness, through the period of gestation—and often with death at the time of birth—and she knows no way of escape. She complains to her friends, perhaps, and they smile and say that "women must have a thousand and one pains if they have children; these things are to be expected; they are a matter of course; who ever heard of having babies without suffering?"

The doctor recommends patience; takes a little blood, that is, takes a little of his patient's life when she so much needs all she has, and cheers her as much as he can; and the hapless mother suffers on the allotted time, and then, perhaps, has milk leg, or puerperal fever, or an abscess in the breast, or a permanent falling of the womb. And women think that all these horrors are the legitimate consequence of the fulfilment of the command to increase and multiply. And they are not aware that they cannot give a healthy life to their children, whilst thus prostrated in their own best energies by disease. How many times must the plain truth be uttered in the world's ear—ye cannot give away what ye do not possess?

It is not one class, or two classes of mothers who are thus

afflicted, and who bear babes to swell the frightful mortality. Those who live in luxury and idleness, and those who live in want and hard labor, are the most diseased and the most wretched; but everywhere, those who violate the laws of life, suffer the inevitable consequence of wrong. The feeble mother, of necessity, gives birth to a child more or less diseased, or with tendency to disease. It is true, that the vital powers of the sick mother are exerted in the best possible manner for the child, so that often comparatively healthy children are born of sickly mothers. But after all, the children are only comparatively healthy, and great care is needed in the first years of their life to preserve them from the often fatal diseases of infancy. The child is born, and consigned to some ignorant nurse, who swathes its body tightly with a band, so that it cannot breathe with any healthy freedom. Its stomach is nauseated with an unmentionable potion, and its head is smothered in bed clothing, so that the close air of the sick room is rendered closer and more unhealthy still, by being breathed again and again, under smothering clothes. Its dress seems purposely contrived with pins, and straps, and belts, and many garments, to make it uncomfortable; and its feet are rolled close in a pinning blanket, so that it cannot get the benefit of the little exercise of kicking its little feet. But, perhaps, the worst wrongs that baby has to encounter, are the poison of drugs, paregoric and the like, and its sick mother's milk. It is not a month since I was called to lance an abscess on a poor woman's breast, and her babe was nursing from the same breast. She had what the doctors call a milk leg, which ultimately ulcerated and broke, and discharged some pints of corruption. Can we expect a babe born of such a mother and nursed on such food to live many months? Will not the filth of the city, sending up its plague steams in the hot summer weeks, poison the last wretched remnant of its little life? We may be sure of it.

Those children who are thus born and reared, cannot live. The dysentery with them is death. The ill-made vital organism is worn out. The disease is the sure prognosis of death in many cases. No earthly means can save. I have been called on in hot weather in several instances to such cases among the ignorant poor. The mother, a pale, consumptive creature, or a bent bilious-looking being, who seemed hardly to have strength to hold her miserable infant in her arms; the child, with the stamp of death on every feature, as the mother thought, perhaps, only slightly sick of summer complaint. They had heard of water cure, and though not in a state to fulfil one of the conditions of the cure, they had sent for me, with a vague sort of notion that I would work some miracle for their child, and keep off death from it. I always deal frankly in such cases. I say, your child *must* die in the city, and probably will die in the country; but your only chance is to take it into the pure air of the country, and to take it from the breast, and feed it on good milk, and care for it properly. They would listen to me, and presently ask me if I would not take charge of the case, though I had just assured them that the child must die in the city. Perhaps they would go into the country for a day or two, well supplied with paregoric, and when the child grew worse, they would return, and send for two or three doctors.

Intelligence is as necessary to the proper treatment of children and the adoption of the water cure, as the water itself; and though a great number of intelligent people may resort to drugs and doctors, yet no really ignorant person will be devoted to water cure.

The *first* cause, then, of infant mortality, is the ill health of mothers—the fact that children are born with half lives, and less than that. Then they are fed on the sick milk of the mother, or the milk of unhealthy cows, or on other bad food. I have known mothers who were well informed on most common subjects, who still did not know any better than to give their young children flesh as food, and even pork; and when fever comes to the child, or the ulcerated sore throat of scarlatina, or when they have scrofula in its many loathsome forms, destroying the beauty of the skin by foul blotches, taking away sight and hearing, and producing death by consumption, king's evil, or some other disease—they never once think that they have brought these ills upon their children, by depriving them of their natural and proper food, and giving them the fat and flesh of sick animals. For let it be known everywhere, that a large portion of the flesh of animals brought to market is diseased; and we have good reason to believe that all pork, fattened as it is ordinarily, is full of scrofula.

The air that many children breathe is close and unhealthy. The open air of confined localities would be bad, even if they were suffered to go out and breathe it; but they are shut up often in what is worse, without the benefit of exercise. Sometimes they live through the first months with no apparent disease—they are only what is termed "very cross children;"

but when the period of dentition comes, then the time of trial begins. Then comes the dreaded diarrhœa, which is met with quack medicines, the base of all of which is opium; or with doctors' drugs, which, whatever they may be, can hardly be worse. The poor child, with its half life, is doomed to do battle with fearful odds—all the evils of city life, and medication besides. If it lives through the dysentery or summer complaint, there are measles, whooping-cough, scarlatina, and other maladies, and death often comes as attendant, or consequence to these diseases.

The first duty of mothers is to render their own health firm. By practising water-cure through the period of gestation, the nerves are strengthened so that the suffering from nausea and weakness and other evils of pregnancy is escaped, and the pains of parturition are greatly abridged; and sometimes an almost entire immunity from suffering is obtained, and the health of the infant is secured as much as that of the mother. The confinement and dosing of the sick room are also escaped at the time of birth. In all my obstetric practice for several years in New York, I have never had a single case where the mother was not able to walk from the bed to the cold bath the day after the birth of her babe, and in no case has any after ill consequence come to the mother or infant from this course; and the children of such mothers have passed through teething without difficulty, have escaped dysentery altogether, or have had it lightly; have had whooping-cough, measles, and scarlatina with no danger at all, and but slight inconvenience.

In the management of children, the first rule is, avoid drugs of every kind and quantity. The nursing infant takes medicine whenever its mother takes it. Get pure air, and plain, simple, healthful food for your child. In his first years the child should eat no animal food. Bread, fruit, milk, and vegetables should constitute the infant's nourishment. Flesh, gravies, grease, sweets, pastry, and condiments should be especially avoided. Grown people should be sparing in their use, but they should give none of them to their children. The clothing of children should be loose, easy, not too much nor too little, and flannel should not be worn next the skin. All clothing worn during the day by infants or adults, should be removed on going to bed, and one long cotton garment should be worn in the night. Day clothing should be thoroughly aired at night, and night clothing during the day. When flannel is worn by infants or adults, it should not be worn next the skin. It irritates and harms the skin. Exercise in the open air is as healthful for infants as for grown people. Thorough cold bathing should be used daily for children from infancy, and if they have any illness, the water cure will assist nature to throw it off rapidly, and in a manner to secure the future health of the child, whilst drugs remain to poison and oppress the system for we know not how long.

One of the pleasantest fruits of knowledge is that we become self-dependent. The mother who has had her health restored by water cure, and who has learned to prevent and cure disease in her family, is relieved from a thousand nameless fears. She is not frightened out of her common sense at the illness of her infant, but she manages it wisely, and its sickness is soon past. And the saving of expense for doctors is no trifling consideration.

From long experience and wide-spread observation of disease, I have become fully convinced that, to children born of healthy parents, and fed on simple, proper food, and bathed daily in cold water, all the diseases of childhood are divested of terror. Such children have them very lightly, and without danger. But the mother asks what *is* proper food for her infant. If the mother is healthy, if she retires to bed as early as ten o'clock, if she rises at six and takes a cold bath, and breakfasts with no drink but water, and with no rich or indigestible food, such as flesh meat, hot bread, &c., if she have exercise and a proper industry, if her mind is free from dominant passions or corroding cares; if she eats a dinner for health, and not for a morbid gratification, and a supper like her breakfast, to be digested, then the mother's milk is the best food for the infant, not at all hours of the day, but at regular periods, separated by an interval of three hours, when the child is young. As soon as a child will sleep through the night without food, it is well for it to do so; no fear need be entertained of a hunger that does not disturb sleep. If the mother's milk be insufficient, cow's milk, diluted with water, with the crust of bread boiled in it, or rice water, or thin gruel, is good food for the child. It is too common for children to be fed on what is on the table, and a great many things are put on the table that had better be buried than eaten by any one, and especially, by children. A potato, ripe and mealy, may be very good food for a child, but covered with butter, salt and grease, it is very bad food. If people will eat condiments, such as mustard, pepper, oil, grease, pickles, spices, old cheese, and smoked food, and salads, and drink tea and coffee, let them prize the health of their children enough to spare them the evils of such feeding.

Babies are almost always fed too much, and with too rich food. A cow's milk is much richer than the milk of the mother. An infant of a day old, when its mother's milk is wanting, is often condemned to have its delicate stomach filled with rich pap, wholly unfit for its digestive powers. A few tea-spoonsful of sweetened water would be far better nourishment, whilst the little one is waiting for the milk of the mother.

Last year I was one Sunday at Fordham, waiting for the cars, when an accident had detained them. We had to wait till deep into the night. A great crowd was assembled at the station-house, and in it was a nurse, who had brought a babe three weeks old to the chapel at Fordham, to be christened. The babe had had no nourishment since the morning, and its cries were piteous. I obtained some water and white sugar in a tumbler, and a tea-spoon. I warmed each spoonful of this sweetened water a little in my mouth, and then gave it to the baby. After being thus fed, the child's hunger was perfectly satisfied, and it fell into a sound sleep. We should have found it difficult to have obtained milk, and if we could, the sugared water was the best for the babe.

A friend of mine was separated by ill health for more than a year from a young infant, being ordered to travel by medical men. The child was fed so badly as to be an idiot when restored to its mother. Its frightful illness continued for years, and was only removed by the most wise and resolute care on the part of the mother, who substituted plain food, and the cold bath and exercise in the open air, for flesh, milk punch, paregoric, a close room, and a total neglect of bathing. The reason and health came in time to bless and reward the mother's efforts. Another child was fed on pork till scrofulous ulcers were made to cover the throat, and the doctor was called to cure what was termed "king's evil." I was at one time called to prescribe for a child who was fed much on pork and fat food, whose eyes were nearly destroyed by scrofula. The child was cured, and the eyes restored, by simple food, bathing, and general attention to the habits. I have seen the worst forms of scrofula overcome in children by these means. Children are more readily cured of disease than grown people. Their bodies more rapidly change by growth, and the growth is in their favor. Children born of very unhealthy parents may, by wise treatment, have their health constantly increased, so that their lives may be insured for a much greater length of years than those who are born strong and well, and brought up in an unwise and unhealthy manner. I have seen a child, who, at the age of two years, was almost devoured with scrofulous sores in the head and eyes, and other parts of the body, and yet, by careful training, living on vegetable food, and constant application of the commonest processes of water cure, she was at the age of fifteen perfectly cured of the disease. She is now over eighteen years of age, and for the last three years I have not known her to be sick a day. Though it is so short a time since water cure has been generally known in this country, yet I have practised it in a considerable degree for nineteen years, and I know a physician in New England, who used branches of water cure practice as many years since; for we consulted together over a case of typhus fever some sixteen years ago.

Any course which tends to render the general health of a child firm, diminishes its danger in the diseases of childhood, or exempts it from their attacks altogether. And any course that weakens and deteriorates, exposes the child to disease and death in early years. Scarlatina is particularly fatal to children who are fed on a rich and animal diet, and who are seldom bathed. Though I have never had a case of scarlet fever that I have not cured, I have still seen great suffering from the ulcerated sore throat, in my patients who have been fed on rich food, and not bathed, whilst those who had been bathed, and fed on simple, plain food, have been scarcely affected at all in the throat. The average duration of scarlet fever in my practice, is from three to six days. I once had an extreme case of scarlatina that lasted two weeks, and it was only on the twenty-first day that the patient was able to walk about out of doors. But in this instance the whole organism was deeply infected with scrofula from birth, and the child had been fed on pork, and in its early years the parents would as soon have thought of drowning the child as bathing her. Ordinarily, the duration of the scarlet fever under my treatment has been from three to six days, but in children who have been badly fed, even if they have had daily bathing, the sore throat continues after the fever is entirely removed.

To give the treatment in one case of scarlatina—we have not given the treatment in all, because water cure must always be adapted to the vital or reactive power of the patient, and the violence of the fever determines the amount of virulence.

A. B. was a case of malignant scarlatina. The disease commenced with delirium. The patient was bled, had an emetic, and Dover's powders, and was laid on a soft feather bed. After this, calomel was given; on the third day the patient died. Three other fatal cases that came under my observation were treated with like allopathic wisdom. Dropsy of the chest succeeded the fever, consequent on bleeding and purging. The patients lingered longer but died. The fourth case was of the most malignant character, accompanied by delirium. The patient did not sleep for an incredibly long time. A physician was called, who put a broad wet bandage around the stomach and abdomen, and another around the head, and directed the patient to be sponged. He gave some medicine, but I did not have an opportunity to see what it was. I was told, however, that little medicine was taken. The patient fell into a quiet sleep, directly the wet bandage was applied, and awoke without delirium. The cure was rapid. The child who took the fever from this patient, and who had been fed on vegetable food, and daily bathed, was under my care, and was only confined a week to the house, and was able to play a portion of each day.

My treatment in scarlet fever has consisted of packing in the wet sheet, and pouring baths, sponge baths, and sleeping in a wet night dress, wet bandages, and if the extremities are cold, much friction with the bare hand. Drinking water constantly and gargling the throat with cold water, and often cleansing the mouth and throat, a very slight nourishment, with frequent changes of clothing, and fresh air, constitute the treatment in scarlatina; also, injections, to open the bowels. Last winter I was called to a very violent case of scarlatina, which the father of the child was himself treating, having a good knowledge of water cure. The fever was so violent that it was not readily subdued, and the mother becoming alarmed, I was called in. I asked the father how much he had done. He said he had packed the child once a day. The patient was fat and ruddy, and full of blood and life. "You should pack him once in three hours," said I, "if you cannot overcome this fever without. Please get ready a pack instantly." He went to the pump out doors, and wrung out a very heavy linen sheet. It was folded so as to present four thicknesses to the child, and was frozen when he brought it in. I smiled, as he proceeded to envelope the child, because the severity of the fever fully warranted the application, and because this heroic treatment was worthy of Priessnitz, and not one water cure doctor in a dozen would have dared apply it. "This treatment," said I, "in a different form of scarlatina, where the vitality was low, and the extremities were cold, would kill the patient." "I know it," said the father, quietly; "I applied the water according to his fever."

"If you know so much," said I, "you have no need of me." And the event proved that it was not necessary for me call again.

Water cure doctors would have small practice if all parents were as well informed as this gentleman.

There is not one of the diseases of childhood that yields more readily to water cure than measles. Parents who have a moderate knowledge of water treatment need no physician.

A few weeks since I was called to a case of suppressed measles. The child was not weaned, and another child of the same family had died a short time previous of the measles. It was only from the fact that the disorder was in the house, that they knew that this child had measles, the efflorescence upon the skin not having appeared. The fever was intense. The child seemed to be in great pain, especially in the head. For seven weary days and nights this babe had not slept. Worn with watching and anxiety, and grief for the loss of the other child, the parents wished to try water cure. The doctor, a very estimable and inquiring man, sent for me, wishing himself to see water cure tried.

I took the child, which was moaning in pain and fever upon the mother's lap, and prepared to envelope him in a wet sheet as large as his little body. The grandmother exclaimed, "You will not put the child in a sheet wet in *cold* water?" I asked the parents if they were afraid. They said, No, and the doctor very kindly assisted in the envelopment. Within five minutes from the time that the wet sheet and blankets were wrapped about the babe, he slept a tranquil, sweet sleep. This continued an hour. In less than an hour and a half he was taken out and put in a tub, and pitchers of cold water poured over him. When I took him from this bath the measles were out upon him as thick as snow-flakes in a storm.

For several days he had two packs a day, and two in the night also. Then he was put to bed in a wet night-dress, which was wet once or twice during the night, and he was often sponged. A wet bandage was kept around his chest, day and night, as he had the peculiar cough that accompanies measles badly.

In five days he was convalescent, and his recovery was rapid.

In ordinary cases of measles, I have found two or three visits enough to put the patient on the sure road to health.

In whooping-cough I have found water cure equally beneficial. I have reduced the most violent case of whooping-cough by one week of constant treatment, so that the cough was not even an inconvenience. But to do this we must have thorough treatment and no child's play. The pouring bath twice a day, two wet-sheet packings, and constant bandaging, will produce rapid results in this disease, and make it break through all scientific rules of duration. Some cases, however, hold the patient much longer than others, with the same amount of treatment.

I have treated varioloid and chicken-pox with as entire success as whooping-cough, scarlatina, and measles. The treatment is substantially the same.

CHAPTER VIII.

FEMALE DISEASES.

To all who are interested or uninterested in water cure, I have something to say; for all are interested in health. We fall little short of the truth when we say, that the whole world is sick. I have hesitated somewhat as to what portion of my experience I should give to the public in the present volume. I have decided to speak to women, and mothers particularly, being satisfied that I cannot achieve a higher good than to enlighten these as widely as possible with regard to the conditions of health and disease. I have endeavored to give plain, practical, *home* directions. Many women are ill and wretched, and feel life to be a burden instead of a blessing, who cannot go to a water cure house to recover their health. But they have wells and springs of pure water at home. What they want is instruction. Many of them display a heroism in the endurance of suffering equal to that of Washington or Bonaparte; and give them knowledge, and that same heroism will save them—will restore them to health and usefulness.

And for every individual thus relieved, an added joy will spring in my life, whether I know the fact of such relief or not. "We are members one of another," and the universal life-spirit circulates in every heart more freely and joyously, for every new influx of wisdom, and goodness, and consequent health, that is received by the world.

The following directions and cases are written for my sisters in all plainness of speech. I love truth too well to conceal it, and thus obstruct its blessings.

PARTICULAR DIRECTIONS TO WOMEN.

Women have too long contemplated their diseases as the atheist contemplates the world—as coming without a cause. There is much hereditary disease, and tendency to disease; aside from this, we are responsible for our illness; and this responsibility, which I am now contemplating, is not removed from us because we are ignorant of the laws and conditions of health. If we take poison we are responsible, whether we do it ignorantly or advisedly; that is, the body is responsible, and we cannot escape. Our ignorance of physical laws never lessens our suffering when we violate them.

Women have many troubles, of which they know neither the cause nor the cure. They think these things come upon them because they are women.

The most common diseases of women are painful and obstructed menstruation, fluor albus, and prolapsus uteri. Properly speaking, these are all symptoms attendant on a weakened or prostrated nervous system.

The causes of these affections are various. Hereditary disease comes first, then the ignorance and errors of mothers, as to the training of children; tight dressing, impeding the circulation of the blood and nervous energy; excessive amativeness and its indulgence, either social or solitary. All these causes, and many more, waste the vital or nervous power, and the result is, what are called female diseases, such as fluor albus, or whites, obstructed or painful menstruation, piles, prolapsus uteri, or falling of the womb, and general neuralgic affections, such as tooth-ache, and other facial pains, pains in the spine, and a great many other miserable aches.

The question first to be answered by each woman who finds herself suffering from either of the above maladies is—What is the cause of my disease? Is it tight dressing, improper food or drinks, late hours, the round of fashionable dissipation; or is it excessive labor, or mental anxiety, or excessive indulgence of amativeness?

We must not hide from ourselves the fact, that solitary vice in young persons, and the too great indulgence of amativeness by married partners, are powerful producing causes of all nervous diseases. We must look life in the face, and meet its evils. In all cases of female weakness, the cause or causes must be first ascertained and removed; then the different applications of water are rapid in curing the disease. In whites, and falling of the womb, the sitz bath, vagina syringe, and wet compress about the abdomen, will often cure without other applications of water, when the cause is removed.

Interrupted menstruation is often a cause of great alarm, but it is only a symptom of weakness, or disturbance in the vital economy, and as soon as the strength is restored, or the disease overcome, the vital energy is again at liberty to cause this secretion. In water cure, menstruation is often suspended for some months, with much advantage to the patient, as the nervous power required to produce this fluid is employed in building up and restoring the body to health, when the menses will again become regular.

The different processes of water cure, with the exception of the douche, are passed through at the period of the menses, not only with safety to the patient, but with great advantage. Ladies have often made inquiry of me relative to the use of baths during the menstrual period, and I take this method of replying to all at once. Baths, with the exception of the douche, should be used more at this time, if there is any difference, than at any other.

CASE OF UTERINE DISEASE.

Mrs. ——— had been several years afflicted with falling of the womb and nervous debility. She was a woman of great natural energy, had borne several children, and felt the strongest wish to take proper care of her family. But her unfortunate disease baffled all her wishes, and the skill of the physicians to whom she resorted. She had constant leucorrhœa, piles, and pain across the back, with the dragging-down sensation in the abdomen and back, which so generally attends prolapsus. She had also painful and irritating dyspepsia, whatever she might eat. So capricious and unhealthy was her appetite, that she took whatever she fancied, and suffered accordingly.

When she came to me for advice, she said she could not go from home to a water cure house to be treated. Whatever she did, must be done with such slender means as she could have at home. I saw at once that I might trust to her energy, when once she had the requisite knowledge.

I gave her advice. The following is a copy of the directions in her case.

Thorough sponge bath on rising, with much friction with a soft flesh brush.

Put a wet bandage about the abdomen; pin it quite low, so as to support the uterus. Wet this bandage three or four times a day. Mid forenoon take a sitz bath, beginning with tepid water; take it fifteen minutes and gradually cool the water. In a week use the water cold. Mid afternoon repeat this bath. Move the bowels with a syringe every morning; use the vagina syringe four times a day, injecting a pint of water each time, cold.

Eat no pork, fat meat, or gravies; no pastries, and no condiments, except a little salt.

Drink only cold water. Eat fruit and brown bread. Sleep on a mattress. Wear no clothing in the night that you have worn during the day. Ventilate your rooms thoroughly. Make all your clothing loose.

These directions the lady followed to the letter. In a few weeks an eruption appeared upon the abdomen, which was succeeded by a plentiful crop of boils, which extended over the surface covered by the wet bandage. The bowels recovered their tone and regularity. The piles ceased. The distressing leucorrhœa was cured. The digestion became good. The uterus recovered its contractile power. The pain in the back, the languor and weariness were gone. In a word, the patient was *well*, and that by a course of domestic treatment, and in less than five months.

CASE OF UTERINE AND NERVOUS DISEASE.

Mrs. ———, a lady of large brain and very active temperament. She was piously educated, and with large benevolence and conscientiousness, had the most intense desire to be useful. But all her wishes were rendered abortive by the state of her health. In early childhood she became addicted to the solitary habit, so prevalent amongst children and young people, and so very hurtful. The result was, that at the period of maturity there was entire prostration of the tone of the nervous system. The uterus was so weakened, that there was flooding about three-fourths of the time. The commencement of the menstrual illness was marked by severe pain, and the dulness, languor, weakness, and despondency which were present the remainder of the time, kept the patient much of the time confined to her bed. I first saw the patient in the summer of 1840. She was then florid from determination of blood to the head, and a good deal bloated from a dropsical affection, owing to the loss of blood. A superficial observer would have called the lady very healthy. The pupils of the eyes were much dilated, owing to the weakness of the nerves of vision. This gave the eyes a very brilliant appearance, and added to the general impression that the lady was in good health.

She had attended one of my lectures, in which I spoke of the effects of solitary vice upon the nervous system. This was the first light she had had on the subject. She was interested and appalled. She seemed to herself to have taken the very first lesson in self-knowledge. She immediately came to me for advice. With the frankness and earnestness of a true woman and a Christian, she told me everything in her case that seemed needful to be known. I gave her general directions, such as she could follow at home. The principal of these were, to lie on a hard bed, to resolve firmly not to be seduced into a single repetition of the fatal practice, to live on simple diet, to drink only water, and bathe daily. In the winter of 1846, she again called on me. She had married meanwhile, but had not waited till her strength was restored. The consequence was, she had suffered a miscarriage in an advanced stage of pregnancy, and was reduced to great weakness. Her state was about the same as when I first saw her. This condition of weakness and uselessness, to one who has the nature of an apostle, who would do and suffer all things to make the world better, was very terrible. If she only had been obliged to submit to suffering and privation in consequence of her illness, she would have borne it very patiently, but the sting of her disease was that it hindered her from doing the good that her heart continually impelled her to do.

I was greatly affected by the earnestness and loveliness of spirit, and at the same time, the utter powerlessness of this dear lady. I recommended her to come at once under full water treatment at my house. She came, and began immediately to gain strength. She went on progressing very rapidly for some time, when she became pregnant. She then returned home and kept up mild treatment, suited to her state, till the seventh month of pregnancy, when she was seized with whooping-cough. Thinking it only a cold, she neglected to call on me till she became very bad ; she then came to me. At this period I never saw whooping-cough so violent. The accessions of the cough were such, that I feared miscarriage momentarily. I put her under treatment, which consisted principally of a succession of wet sheets and pouring baths. In one week the cough was so far cured, that it was not even an inconvenience. But the concussion of the cough had been too violent for the weakened and delicate uterus. She was taken with labor in another week, when seven and a half months advanced, and bore one dead and one living child. The labor was four and a half hours, and *very* severe. The birth of the children was greatly complicated by the rupture of the membranes, which occurred at the very commencement of the labor, and the fact that there was unnatural presentation with both. A quarter of an hour after the birth, she was washed in cold water, and slept. The next day she arose and walked to the sitz bath, and after the bath she sat up some time.

The lingering illness of the infant was a very great injury to her health, as she exerted herself greatly in its care. Its death occurred after some weeks, and then she immediately recovered her strength by the proper application of water.

The year after she bore another child, with comparatively light suffering. She was able to walk to the cold bath the next day after the birth of this child, and to go out of her room in one week. She now enjoys excellent health.

CASE OF RUPTURE AND PREMATURE DELIVERY.

The following case is illustrative of the terrible sufferings to which women are liable from their diseases, and the malpractice of physicians ; and though in some of its features it is of an extraordinary character, it is but one of hundreds, in which women unnecessarily suffer, first from their own ignorance of the laws of their being, and next from the deplorable and inexcusable quackery of pretenders to medical science.

Mrs. D., a lady of New York, was afflicted with inguinal hernia (rupture in the groin), during the seventh month of her pregnancy. The family physician was consulted, and instead of using the proper means for reducing the hernia, he decided that it could not be done without first bringing on labor, which he proceeded to attempt by the administration of ergot! The operation of this poison upon a diseased nervous system, was terrible and disastrous. The unnaturally excited efforts of the uterus to expel the fœtus, did not produce the desired effect, but brought on the most frightful convulsions, and after three days of indescribable sufferings, the whole system sunk, and the action of the uterus entirely ceased, nor could the deadly ergot excite it to another effort. At this stage the fœtus was extracted with instruments.

After this scene of wrong and outrage, in which this delicate, diseased, and nervous lady had been a victim, and in which she had suffered a thousand deaths, besides the wholly needless murder of her offspring, I was called to attend her in a second pregnancy. Her recent sufferings had weakened an already diseased constitution, and the retchings and vomitings were so severe as to threaten abortion. She was treated with the half pack in the wet sheet, constant fomentations of wet linen to the stomach, sitz baths, and injections. In a week the sickness of the stomach was gone. In the seventh month of pregnancy the intestine again descended, and symptoms of miscarriage appeared. Pressure immediately reduced the rupture, a wet bandage and wet compress were applied, and secured so as to fit properly. The half pack was again resorted to. The nervous system was thus soothed, and strength restored. The patient, from being in much suffering and unable to sit up at all, became very comfortable in health, and able to sit up, and walk about without any inconvenience.

Those who had recommended doctors, and trusses, and medicines, were greatly disappointed and troubled, when they saw her supported by a simple compress and bandage, fashioned of cloth, (properly, of course,) and saw her pain relieved, and her strength restored, and only by the aid of water in its various applications.

The delight of my patient at this happy change may be easily imagined, for the remembrance of her former sufferings was awfully vivid, and no persuasions could induce her again to trust herself in the hands of a physician, though but few, holding the same rank in the regular profession, it is to be hoped, would treat a case of hernia with ergot and a miscarriage. For the honor of humanity, it is to be hoped that more would vote for the indictment of such a practitioner, than would defend his practice.

I attended the case to its termination. A constant and persevering application of the proper processes of water cure increased the health and strength of the patient. Her labor was attended with but little suffering, and no inconvenience from the rupture; and she was able to leave her room on the third day after delivery, and mother and child have got on as well as could be desired.

Those who accuse water cure physicians of speaking harshly of the poisonings and malpractices of allopathic doctors, need but to be acquainted with such facts as the above, to sympathize with us in our impatient feelings, and with their abused patients in their needless sufferings.

INFLAMMATION AND ULCERATION OF THE UTERUS AND RENAL ORGANS.

Mrs. C. had been injured in delivery, the os-uteri being torn on each side. She was very scrofulous, and inflammation of the uterus, including the whole renal system, was the consequence of this injury. She was well-nigh doctored to death according to different systems, after the negative good of homœopathy had been tried for some time. The urethra was ulcerated through to the vagina, and one of her physicians thought proper to inject into the vagina a strong decoction of capsicum, (red pepper,) in the ulcerated state of the parts. The burning agony of the sufferer during this worse than savage infliction, may be conceived, but cannot be described. When we think of this most delicate and sensitive portion of woman's organism, subjected to actual cautery and lavements of nitrate of silver, (lunar caustic,) and capsicum, (red pepper,) we see the need that some one speak so that the voice be heard. This lady, a sweet, darling woman, the idol of her husband and parents, was given up to die; and her suffering was so great that she could almost look to death with joy, as her only relief. For ten months she did not set her foot upon the ground. She lay in hopeless torture a great part of the time, given up by her friends, and experimented upon by doctors. At last some one recommended water cure. The homœopathic physician who had attended her, thought it might be well for her to try it. But most of her friends thought it would be useless, and her mother said to me, "If you cure my daughter, it will be a miracle." I examined the case carefully when first called, and gave it as my opinion that the lady could be cured. I can never forget the mingled look of suffering and of joy that struggled in the face of this young creature, when she thought that there was a possibility that she might be restored to health, to be a blessing to her kind and manly husband, instead of a burden; and that she might once again be a mother to her little ones. That look haunted me till the young mother was fairly in my house and under my care.

She was treated by wet-sheet packing, sitz baths, injections of water, fomentations with wet linen, and a very plain, bland diet. Her recovery seemed little short of miraculous. In one month she walked two miles with ease, and went home to have the supervision of her family and continue her cure. I saw her a short time since in excellent health.

UTERINE DISEASE.

Mrs. ——— had been fifteen years laboring under disease of the womb, and general nervous prostration. The period of the appearance of the menses, was always marked with great pain and violent symptoms of hysteria. The menses generally appeared once in three weeks. The hysterical symptoms were of such a violent and convulsive character, that the patient was often entirely exhausted by them.

"She suffered many things of divers physicians, and was nothing bettered." Homœopathy was at last resorted to. For a time she seemed much relieved by the prescriptions, and then she relapsed again into her former greatly suffering state. The symptoms of hysteria seemed entirely at variance with her general character and temperament—she being not at all "nervous," or imaginative, in the usual sense of those terms, but possessed of much energy of character, and calm common sense. She saw her own case clearly, and exercised great self-control, and knew perfectly when she was about to be overcome by the convulsive spasms, which were wearing away her strength, at once a cause and consequence of her illness. On a careful examination, I found the uterus much diseased—much prostration in the tone of the nervous system, and strong tendency to bilious derangement.

Latterly the hysterical symptoms had been somewhat relieved by magnetism.

She was brought to me by the advice of her physician, in a very weak state, during the accession of the spasms. She was carried to her room by her husband and the physician, being unable to walk, and dreading a recurrence of spasms every minute. I found, by laying my hand upon her, that I had magnetic control over her, quite equal to that exercised by the magnetizer who had relieved her. I could calm her when her mind began to reel. I could induce a sound magnetic sleep in five minutes, when she was lying in convulsions, throwing over bath tubs, or tearing her clothes. When the sleep was established, she would obey my will by going to bed, and remaining perfectly still, and apparently sound asleep, for two hours.

The treatment of this case was complicated and long continued. It consisted of the following processes administered at different times, as the symptoms demanded :—

Tonic wet sheet—wet bandages about the abdomen—the use of the rectum and vagina syringe—sitz baths—the douche and sweating blankets. The first month of the treatment was greatly beneficial. All the bad symptoms were relieved. The uterine evils, such as a distressing prolapsus, leucorrhœa, and sinking faintness at the pit of the stomach, with occasional vomiting, were all abated. These symptoms had been so severe as to be almost intolerable. But in one month's treatment they were all abated so as be quite endurable.

The suffering at each succeeding menstrual illness decreased, until she was able to pursue her ordinary avocations at that period with slight suffering.

In a year her health was so far established, that she might much more properly have called herself well, than nine out of ten who do so. Still she continues portions of the treatment. Her case is a constant surprise to those who have known her sufferings these many years; and the incredulous in water cure amuse themselves by prophecying that it cannot last, and that she will sink back after a time into the miserable way in which she formerly lived. Those who know what water cure can effect, have no such fears.

SPINAL DISEASE AND PROLAPSUS UTERI.

The following notes were given me to prepare a notice of the case from them. I think it better that the patient should speak for herself.

"Report of Myself by Myself.

"I was twenty-seven years of age when I placed myself under Mrs. Gove's care. I had been ill nearly six years with disease of the spine. My medical treatment was cupping, blistering, wearing plasters, liniments, &c., with the use of Saratoga Water for two months. I became better, but after some months the disease appeared again, and extended the whole length of the spine. At first it had been confined to the region of the shoulder. I had also prolapsus uteri. I suffered great pain, could take no exercise without palpitation of the heart. I had a severe cough, pain in the chest and side, with entire loss of appetite. I resided for three months under Dr. Brewster's care in New York. While there my disease was checked. On its reappearance, I tried homœopathy without effect. In the fall of 1846, I went to Mrs. Gove's water cure house, with all my former symptoms in an aggravated state. The faithful use of the wet sheet, douche, sitz bath, and plunge bath, with vegetable diet, and gymnastic exercises, for four months, so far restored my health, that I was able to return home. Since my return I have continued to use the plunge, douche, and sitz baths. My health has steadily improved, and now (Aug. '47,) I am entirely free from pain, and call myself well, though still obliged to be more careful of my health than before my illness. I attribute my recovery to the water cure alone. No other course of treatment is, in my opinion, so worthy of confidence, so certain of success.

"I am not sure, dear Mrs. Gove, that I have written all you wish—I have made a plain statement of facts and trust to you to put it "ship shape." Thanks to you, dear friend, I am quite well. What a glorious mission is yours to relieve so much suffering. You will have the satisfaction of a well spent life, and the grateful love of many a sufferer relieved by your care.

"To all invalids I recommend the Water Cure, and my father, made a convert by my case, brings in people to talk with me, and the family laugh at my eloquence. I am rejoiced to hear that you are doing so much good—I wish I could walk in, and breakfast with you. The oatmeal would have a relish. I am a pretty good girl about my diet. Whenever I transgress, I pay the penalty, and under the infliction make many resolves for the future."

ULCERATION OF THE WOMB, &C.

Mrs. —— had been a very free liver—with every want ministered to. Her health being delicate, and her life monotonous, having a large fortune, and no occasion for exertion, she became depressed in spirits. This form of illness was met by her husband with excessive indulgence. She was petted until she became like a sick and spoiled child. Under these conditions her husband died suddenly. The blow fell on the weak and sickly wife with stunning power. She was completely miserable.

Her physician unfortunately saw fit to meet her difficulties with brandy and laudanum. She took them until she felt unable to live but under their influence. Meanwhile her health sank frightfully. (Confirmed Leucorrhea, and ultimately ulceration of the womb, with the most offensive discharges, was her portion.) She continually assuaged, and increased her miserable disease by taking brandy and opium, and finally morphine. She was reduced to the weakness of an infant, and her suffering could hardly find a parallel in the regions below, or in any state, or place that we can imagine. At this juncture she heard of Water Cure. It is very strange that one in such a condition should have courage to rise from such a bed of torment, and at the same time stupefaction, and go to a Water Cure House. But this patient's natural energy and understanding are seldom equalled. At a time when she was a little better, she resolutely made her preparations, and without taking even a servant, she came to me. She told me her whole life, and all her sorrows, and temptations. She renounced every hurtful thing at once, and went into forcible water treatment. In a week the abdomen was covered with a purple efflorescence. In a month she had forty biles on the back and abdomen. Her strength increased continually and there seemed not even a wish for brandy or opium in any form. Her recovery was gradual, but sure. Nearly two years elapsed before her health could be called really good, though in a few months she was quite as well as most people, who tell us that they enjoy good health.

The recovery of the tone and elasticity of her spirits, and her moral freedom from habits that she abhorred, though she had seemed to herself to be hopelessly enslaved by them, was to her the most important portion of her cure. Life became a boon for which she could thank heaven, instead of being a bitter curse.

INFLAMMATION OF THE UTERUS.

The inflammation in this case was very violent, and accompanied with spinal irritation. There was much general weakness and indigestion—pain in the back and abdominal region, a sense of sinking at the stomach, with inability to hold the body upright. Patient could walk very little. The treatment consisted of wet sheet packing on alternate days, and douche intermediate days—sitz bath and abdominal bandage, wet often—and strict diet. In three months she considered herself well. No perceptible crisis.

UTERINE DISEASE.

Mrs. ——— had disease of the womb. Dr. Cheeseman had pronounced it ulceration of the womb. There was general derangement of the nervous system, and the head was affected with a painful congestion and confusion. The eyes were almost useless. She was not able to read or pay continuous attention to anything. The only kind of work she could do was knitting. She was so afflicted with general nervousness as to be unable to see company, and sometimes felt compelled to lock herself into her room and see no one, such was her extreme nervous susceptibility. She commenced treatment in the winter of 1847. In less than a year she was *entirely well.*

SYPHILIS.

The following case must serve as a representative of a class. I cannot be willing to give such cases. It is very painful to make such records, and only my wish to spread light, and ameliorate suffering, could induce me to do it.

Mrs. ——— had been for a considerable time separated from her husband, for what seemed good and sufficient reasons. In an evil hour she was persuaded again to live with him. Not long after she came to me for advice, having as she supposed the worst form of leucorrhœa. She watched my countenance as she told me her symptoms, and seeing me look very grave, as I could hardly avoid, she begged to know if she had the "bad disorder." I evaded her question, telling her that whatever her disease was, I could cure it. She said it was not possible for her to remain with me—her home was at a distance, and she must be there. I then wrote for her careful directions. Her sufferings from the inflammation of the uterus and vagina, the constant and excoriating discharge, were intense. I was not able to treat the case as I wished, but I gave the best advice I could under the circumstances.

In the first place I put her upon a diet of bread and fruit, with a little milk, and only cold water for a drink.

She slept on a hard bed, enveloped around the abdomen in four folds of wet linen, with a dry covering over these. She took a wet sheet pack an hour in the forenoon, and had pails of water poured over her during the day. She used the sitz bath twice a day, for half an hour, and the vagina syringe many times in the day. She wore also wet bandages during the day about the abdomen. In six weeks the disease was conquered and cast out. The application of the four folds of wet linen about the abdomen and the inflamed portion during the night, was probably as efficient for the cure as any portion of the means used, if not more so.

She had been told that she could not possibly recover without the application of caustic, but the event proved that this was not true.

DIABETES AND PRURIGO.

I have treated both these diseases most successfully by water, but the limits of this work will not allow of any lengthy notice of cases.

The last case of diabetes was relieved in two weeks; the patient's strength restored, and the quantity of water was natural in three months.

Prurigo being a symptom of general depravation of the blood, and the presence of much morbid matter in the system, is a disease that requires time, and generally a large amount of treatment. I have found the time required for a cure to vary from one month to a year, or more.

CHAPTER IX.

WATER CURE IN GESTATION AND PARTURITION.

One of the most important and wonderful uses of water is to promote health during gestation, and to diminish the pains of parturition. Many will not believe that an immunity may be obtained from a large portion of the suffering of childbirth. But why not? Gestation and parturition are as natural functions as those of digestion, and unless the nerves be diseased, we know we can digest our food without pain, and we know also that we have intense suffering when they are diseased. A luxurious civilization increases all diseases, and particularly those of gestation and parturition. The common Irish, the middle classes of the Scotch, the Indians, the slaves at the south, and others who might be mentioned, have little suffering in child-bearing.

The Indian woman bears her babe, washes herself and her infant in the next running stream, and the travelling party to which she belongs seldom waits more than half a day for her. Why this exemption from suffering? God has made of one blood all the people who dwell on the face of the earth. Then why should one class be afflicted with suffering a thousand times bitterer than death, whilst another class is entirely exempt from such misery? The Indian woman is subject to many hardships, but tight lacing and breathing impure air are not among them; and the exhausting influence of the undue indulgence of amativeness, social and solitary, which a luxurious and voluptuous civilization causes and perpetuates, is unknown amongst the Indians, and all people who are exempt from the sufferings of birth. The great truth must be uttered in the ear of the nations, that exhaustion of the nervous system, either from being born of weak and diseased parents, from undue labor, or licentiousness, is the great one cause of suffering in gestation and parturition. And let it be known that marriage does not change the laws of the human constitution. Licentiousness is the same with or without the marriage sanction Women attempt to give life to children when they have not half enough for themselves. The consequences to the children I have detailed in my chapter on Infant Mortality. The consequence to the mother is a suffering to which the rack or the fire could add little poignancy.

The course to be pursued to obtain immunity from suffering in child-bearing, is, to restore the integrity of the nervous system. Give tone or strength to the nerves, and you take away suffering just in proportion as you do this.

The treatment I have adopted, most generally, in pregnancy, has been daily wet sheet packing, which is a powerful tonic to the nerves. The patient has remained in this pack till a warm glow was established over the whole body. This is usually accomplished in an hour and a half, and sometimes in half that time. They have sometimes used the plunge bath, and sometimes the dripping sheet after the pack. The sitz bath once or twice a day, cold water enemas to keep the bowels open, if inclined to costiveness, and vaginal injections of cold water, particular attention to diet, pure air, and exercise, have also been carefully enjoined. Peculiar cases have needed peculiar treatment, but the above treatment has been used in a majority of cases.

The consequence has been, that the duration of labors under my care has been from 20 minutes to 4½ hours. With one exception I have had no labor over 4½ hours. Ladies who have had long and severe labors before they came under water treatment, have had their time of suffering reduced from 48 hours to one hour, and in several instances the time of labor has been reduced to a few minutes. These are facts that the world is interested in knowing.

A few days since I was called to a lady who had been treating herself according to the principles she had learned at my Lectures. Her labor was very light, and was from 20 to 30 minutes in duration, for the disagreeable feeling she had occasionally had for an hour previous, could not be called labor. She went immediately into a cold bath, and then was laid in bed. She was told to take a daily morning bath, and two sitz baths a day; to wear the cold abdominal compress, and to go about the house on the third day. In a large obstetric practice for years I have known no ill effect from this treatment. All my patients without one exception have been able to go into the cold bath, and walk the day after the birth, to be about the house the first week, and all with one exception have been able to ride out in a week or two. I have had a patient who when her babe was one week old spent an hour in a park at some distance from her home, walking about with her other children. I was recently called to a lady who had been many years married without children, and whose health till she came under water cure some two years since, was wretched in the extreme. She was advanced in years so as to justify us in supposing that she would suffer a good deal. She was faithful in treatment and became very strong. Her labor was light. She was bathed after the birth, wore the wet bandage, and was about the house in a week as if nothing had occurred.

My practice at the period of birth is as follows: when the delivery is perfectly accomplished, which includes of course the placenta, I allow the woman to rest for ten minutes. I then with a vagina syringe throw a quart of cold water upon the uterus. This greatly facilitates its contraction, and gives immunity from after pains, which are caused by the efforts of the uterus to contract; and it is a law that diseased nerves give pain in contracting. This ready contraction of the uterus secures the woman against flooding and prolapsus. As soon as I have thus used the syringe I put a broad bandage wrung from cold water around the abdomen, and pin it closely, compressing the abdomen. I then wash the woman thoroughly in cold water with a sponge or wet towel and change her clothes, and put her in bed. She generally sleeps six hours. When she wakes she rises and goes into a sitz bath and is bathed over the whole surface, and has a fresh bandage. She is able to walk and sit up, for a time after this bath, in ninety-nine cases out of a hundred.

Several cases have been given in the last chapter, in which pregnancy was attended by female diseases; and a few more are here added. Where the results are constantly the same, there is little need of accumulating cases.

WATER CURE DURING GESTATION.—CASE FIRST.

Mrs. ——— had been for a long time in delicate health, and had borne one infant, which died soon after its birth. She had passed through great suffering in this confinement, and when she again found herself pregnant, she concluded to try the water cure.

She came under treatment and remained two months, daily improving. At the end of this time, she felt so strong and well, that she concluded to go into the country. There she was obliged entirely to suspend her treatment. When her pregnancy was five months advanced, she unfortunately suffered an injury which was sufficiently violent to separate a portion of the placenta from the uterus. The consequence was the death of the child, and violent hemorrhage. I was called, and by sitz baths, bandages, and injections, I succeeded in arresting the flooding for the time. But it soon returned and labor commenced, but the contractions of the uterus were without pain. The child was born, with a very slight degree of suffering; flooding was entirely prevented by the use of the vagina syringe, with ice water, and a close wet bandage. The patient immediately recovered, and in a few weeks was able to go again into the country.

CASE SECOND.

Mrs. ——— came under treatment during pregnancy. The confinement was attended with very little suffering. Some of the family, including herself, had suffered from chills and fever. She seemed after the birth of her child to be almost as well as if nothing had occurred, but the third day she was seized with fever and ague. The fact that she had been in cold baths daily since the birth of her child, and had also been sitting up, and walking about, alarmed some of the family. However, she remained firm, and the unwelcome and intrusive company of chills and fever, met a very cold reception. She was treated with a succession of wet sheet sweatings and baths, and in four days the enemy was expelled, and the family convinced that the disease came as it had come to the rest of the family, and to Mrs. ——— previously, and that it was not *caused* but *cured* by the water treatment.

CASE THIRD.

Mrs. ——— had been the mother of one child, and had had a miscarriage. She was of a scrofulous family, and had suffered a good deal from scrofula. She had also nervous prostration and a falling of the womb, and was altogether in a very poor state of health, when she became convinced of the virtues of water cure. She was pregnant when she commenced treatment. She had been a great sufferer in her previous confinements, and of course, felt very anxious to escape, if possible, a portion at least of the suffering which she had hitherto supposed inevitable. She began treatment earnestly. She was daily enveloped in the wet sheet, till a thorough glow of heat was established over the system. She had a pouring bath, or dripping sheet when she came out of the pack. She wore a wet bandage constantly about the abdomen, and took sitz baths, and used the vagina syringe. She drank only water, and lived simply.

The consequence of this course of treatment, continued up to the time she was confined, was very marked. Her child was born in the night, and the day previous she had been in the wet sheet, and taken her other baths as usual. She was ill about twenty minutes, and the child, a fine boy, was born with three pains. She rested for a time after delivery, and then was thoroughly bathed and dressed, and went to bed. She slept well. The next morning she arose and walked to the bath with ease, took a sitz and sponge bath, and went across the room to look at her babe, then sat down in her arm-chair for some fifteen minutes. She had no ill turn, but went rapidly up to full health, and has since enjoyed very much better health than at any former period.

CASE FOURTH.

The last birth that I attended was really a very pleasant occurrence. The mother of the babe had been under her own care during the period of gestation. She had attended many of my lectures, and was well informed. Though by no means a strong woman, she manages so well, that she enjoys a good deal of health. She has been for years a vegetable eater, and a hydropathist. I did not know of her pregnancy till I was called to deliver her. When I reached her, she had been conscious that her labor had commenced for about two hours. But she could only be said to suffer about twenty minutes, and then very little.

The babe was a fine boy, and the mother was bathed in cold water about ten minutes after the birth, and a wet bandage was put about the abdomen. She was directed to take a cold bath in the morning, and two sitz baths a day, and to go about the house as soon as she felt disposed to do so. Her knowledge, and simple and natural habits, made this allowance perfectly safe for her. Where the uterus is made to contract by throwing cold water upon it, with the syringe directly after birth, and this contraction is secured by a close wet bandage; where, moreover, the tone of the whole nervous system is high, from good habits and tonic water treatment, a patient may safely, and even with advantage, take an amount of exercise, that would be surely fatal to a patient suffering from an exhausted nervous system, the consequence of the uses and abuses of the life usually lived by women.

In most cases of birth, the uterus is so weakened that very little contractile power is left in it. The relaxed organ cannot restore itself to its natural and true position, owing to the weakness of the nerves. And its feeble efforts at contraction are attended by intolerable pains, called "after pains," and which are very common. The organ sinks down, and if the patient stands upon her feet, the open blood vessels pour out the fountain of her life, and if she does not flood to death, she is greatly weakened by the loss of blood, and permanent falling of the womb is the consequence.

I would have no one attempt to do the works of the water cure patient, without having first strengthened and qualified the body for the undertaking. A fatal failure will be very likely the result if they make the attempt. But I would earnestly ask all women to look at these facts, and to ponder them till they influence their lives.

Any person who wishes information respecting this interesting subject, can know the names and residences of the patients whose cases I have given, and can see and converse with them.

CHAPTER X.

WATER CURE IN CONSUMPTION.

To me life seems valuable only when we use it for good—when we make the world better and happier by living. The calm of domestic life is the lovely and desirable sphere of woman—and not less desirable to me than to others. But its calm, its peace, its happiness is invaded by a fell destroyer; a most insidious enemy is lurking in its midst, and the loveliest flowers fade and wither, and drop into dust daily, before our eyes—and those to whom they are fairest and dearest, can do nothing to save them. Shall I live for myself at such a time? Shall I ask for quiet, and the cool shade of domestic life, when I have truth that can save many, if I will but bring it to the people? Many will accept it—a few may criticise and grieve me, and make me wish at times that I had no name, so that these could not speak it; but the blessing of one life saved for years of happiness and usefulness, will repay me for any misunderstanding or criticism.

I confess that I would willingly have done and suffered much, rather than appear in this manner before the public. But the belief that a great good is to be accomplished by bringing this subject before fathers, and mothers, and sisters, has reconciled me. I do not wish to die with one duty unfulfilled. The sweetest flowers of Paradise would be less sweet to me, and their beautiful hues would be darkened and stained in my sight, if I could look back to earth and see one pang endured that

I might have removed, and replaced with a joy. The balmiest bliss of Heaven would fall freezing on my heart, if I had made the earth more dark, or even less bright, by a life of selfishness.

God help me to live for others, that I may truly live for myself.

Let me commence this subject by the statement of one appalling fact. Every week, from thirty to fifty persons die of Consumption in the city of New York. In some sections of the country, the disease is still more fatal, and the number of deaths in New York may be considered as a fair indication of its average mortality.

The characteristic symptoms of Pulmonary Consumption vary very considerably. In some cases the cough is slight, and the quantity of matter expectorated is very small. In other cases the cough is violent, and the expectoration of purulent matter is large. Some cases are attended by profuse bleeding from the lungs; some have slight bleeding, and some none at all. In some cases there is much pain and difficulty of breathing, and much fever. All these symptoms are milder in many cases.

The organ of Hope seems strangely stimulated in most cases of Consumption; and the decay is so gradual, and the fever so simulates the hue of health, that often, very often, both patients and friends are deceived almost to the last hour.

Oh, it is dreadful to see decline and death so beautiful—to see a beloved child, or partner, or brother, or sister, surely sinking into the grave, with the mind as clear and brilliant as in firmest health, and to know that no human power can save, or even bring alleviation of the suffering; and it is often the case, that one after another in a family falls a victim until all are gone, and the stricken parents are left alone and desolate. It would seem cruel indeed to say to these parents, You have destroyed your loved ones, if no good were to be gained by the enlightenment.

I sympathise with those who are bereaved, and yet I must speak of the causes of sickness and death. The people have too long been left in ignorance on this subject. "Mysterious Providence," and "Inscrutable Dispensation," have too long headed obituaries, when their causes were as palpable to those who could read them, as hanging, or drowning. These causes must clearly, plainly, and fearlessly be set before the people. They must know what they do when they rear their children in the midst of wrong and enervating habits. They must not be allowed ignorantly to plunge themselves and their children into evil, whilst they pray to be delivered from it. There is such a thing as unpardonable sin. It is the sin against the Divine Truth—the law that God has given to govern our complex nature. If we hate, God cannot forgive us. Whilst we remain in the state, we must suffer its penalty; and so of the law that governs our material nature; if we take poison, we must suffer the penalty—whether it be the poison of bad air, or the poison of arsenic.

CAUSES OF CONSUMPTION.

It is the business of this age, more perhaps, than any that has preceded it, to unfold the causes of things. The causes of consumption often commence with the ancestors of a patient. We say such a one was born of consumptive parents, or he belongs to a consumptive family. Parents are little aware how many wrongs they inflict on their children by wronging themselves. We cannot give away what we do not possess. We can no more give health to our children if we have it not, than we can give them a fortune out of poverty.

As I remarked in a former chapter, there are causes that determine the specific character of diseases, that seem to lie beyond our ken. The causes that determine pulmonary consumption seem more obvious than the causes that determine some other diseases. We know that the lungs constitute a very large deterging or cleansing organ. You all can perceive that the lungs act largely in cleansing the system, by observing the breath. If a person is ill, and especially if the skin is in a bad state, there is a bad odor in the breath, and many kinds of poisons are plainly thrown off through the lungs. The drunkard's breath is proverbial. The lungs labor to throw off the poison of alcohol, and we are made sensible of the fact by the pungent odor. Other poisons are doubtless exhaled from the lungs, but being inodorous, we do not readily detect the process. The lungs then, being a great deterging or cleansing organ, large quantities of morbid matter are conveyed out of the system by means of the lungs. After they have thus labored for a time, often doing their own work and a large amount of labor for the skin, they fail, and become diseased. The millions of pores in the skin are the orifices of exhalent vessels, whose business it is to convey away effete, or hurtful matter from the system. If these pores become closed by diminution of the vital power, caused by excesses and by an unpardonable neglect of bathing, and thus cleansing and vivifying the skin, the morbid matter that should be thrown off from the skin is thrown upon the lungs, and especially is this the case, where there is tendency to disease of the lungs. As I before remarked, the lungs go on laboring for themselves and the sick skin, till they can no longer carry off all the morbid matter. The consequence is, that it begins to be deposited in the parenchyma of the lungs, at first, in very minute quantities. The first deposition of matter in the lungs, is called tubercles. They are of different sizes, some of them being of considerable size, and others no larger than a pea, or even the point of a pin. They go on enlarging for a time, and almost as if endowed with intelligence, they suppurate, become pus or matter, as it is termed, and then this matter can be coughed up through the trachea. This process goes on till the lungs are partially destroyed, and then the blood is of course improperly formed, as the lungs are not in a state to perform their function in vitalizing the blood, and then the decay of the patient is rapid, for the system has to sustain the diseased action in the lungs and the diseasing consequence of half formed blood.

The first cause of consumption is deficiency of vital energy from birth, or the waste of this energy from excesses and abuses. Whatever excess or abuse weakens or lessens the amount of vital power, lessens consequently, the ability of the human economy to maintain itself in a state of health. There are a thousand bad habits and deteriorating influences in our common and daily life, aside from the great and acknowledged causes of disease and death, intemperance and licentiousness.

Often one of the first causes of consumption has been lacing the female form—compressing the lungs till the blood could not circulate, and could not therefore come in contact with the air, and consequently, could not be vitalized by its union with oxygen, and could not throw off those impurities with which the blood always becomes loaded in its passage over the system. By this compression the blood becomes a poison instead of a healthful and nourishing fluid. The vessels of the lungs by this pressure, are collapsed and inflamed, and often the process of ulceration is thus begun.

When the muscles that support the chest and enable us to hold ourselves in an upright position, are weakened, either by compression, or excesses and abuses, the consequence is a weakness of the spine and all the support of the body. When the abdominal and dorsal support gives way from weakness, there is a sinking and consequent cramping in the position of the lungs. When this occurs, we do not fully inflate the lungs when we breathe. Many persons do not inhale more than two-thirds as much air as their lungs would contain in an erect or uncompressed state. If they inhale only three-quarters or two-thirds the quantity of air their lungs are capable of receiving, it is plain they thus defraud themselves of one-quarter or one-third their vital breath, their very life; and this fraud of air will produce disease that often destroys life in a comparatively short space of time.

Then when this weakness in the support of the lungs and chest is induced, the effort to speak is made wrong. There is no sinking of the voice—there is no strength in it—and speaking, which should be a healthful and invigorating exercise, becomes painful, fatiguing, and diseasing to the lungs, and often congestion and bleeding of the lungs is caused by the cramped position of the chest, and the wrong effort made in speaking. There is no ease to ourselves or others when the effort to speak is made in the chest and throat. A low abdominal effort in speaking is healthful and invigorating.

The silvery voice so much praised in women, has often its origin in tight dressing and consequent weakness, though at times, it comes from habit and imitation, and affectation becomes a disease.

Of the causes that induce consumption, there is first, weakness from birth; second, all the diseasing influences of civic life. Though their name is legion, we must still attempt to particularize some of them.

The ignorance of the public on the subject of health and disease, is nowhere more clearly seen or more mischievously felt, than in the bad treatment of babies. People do not know how to treat them, they do not deserve them, and in multitudes of instances, they are taken away from their ignorant care-takers who have killed them with kindness, and the parents wonder at the mysterious Providence. During three months of last year, 2,586 children in this city, died under five years of age, and doubtless many of their parents wondered why Providence saw fit to afflict them by taking their children. The true wonder is not why so many children die, but why so many live.

The first food of an infant is the milk of a sick mother, more suited to the production of disease than the sustentation of life. The first air it breathes is the pent up and impure air of the sick room; the first clothes it wears are much more remarkable for prettiness than comfort, and perhaps it is bound as tightly as the mother has been before it, and many people are as much afraid of putting a baby in a bath, as if it were made of sugar and were sure to melt under the operation. With all these evil and diseasing influences, if the baby complains or gets sick, it is silenced with a dose of paregoric or laudanum, or other poison. If the child is not carried off by disease or medication at an early age, the foundation of future disease is laid in the constitution. Then come the diseases of childhood,—measles, chicken pox, scarlatina, whooping cough, all of which are perfectly shorn of their terrors, to children reared with the diet and regimen of water cure. With these disorders there comes a course of drugging, domestic or otherwise, and the child comes forth from the sick chamber, if alive, often like a withered or blasted flower. I exempt homœopathy from all censure of this kind. The homœopathist poisons no child,—he allows his patients to get well, if they can, with rational diet and kindly care. As to his medicine, it seems to me about like the little end of nothing whittled to a point, and then split and sharpened. But for one, I say a blessing on homœopathy.

With allopathic medication I have so often heard mothers say of their pale, sickly children, "My child had the measles, or the scarlet fever, or something else, and the disorder did not leave him well, and he has never been well since." Neither disease nor drugs have left the child, but both remain, perhaps to lay the foundation of consumption in mature life, or perhaps to swell the overwhelming mortality among children.

If children escape the nursery and its medication, they must be vaccinated and sent to school. Vaccination is considered a great blessing, and so it may be with the present habits of society, if pure vaccine virus can be procured; but I hesitate not to say, that the virus of the most deadly diseases is introduced into the veins of children by impure vaccine matter. This is a terrible subject. It would take more than one chapter to do it justice. I do not know how the matter of vaccination is managed here, but I do know that in Boston a physician is paid for vaccinating all the children. They are brought to him, and he vaccinates them, and says to all, whatever taint of scrofula or other horror may be in the blood, "Come again when the pustule is full;" and he takes the matter and inoculates fresh victims with it, and this work of diseasing the public goes on at the public expense, from month to month, and from year to year.

It may be asked whether I vaccinate. I do, but I do not use vaccine matter from persons with scrofulous or still worse diseases.

With the school comes often crowding and bad air, although I believe the school-houses in New-York are better ventilated than almost any others. Great improvements are being made in this respect, but a vast deal remains to be done. I went some years since into a school-house in Baltimore, built on an improved plan, with a great number of ventilators in the ceiling over head. It was winter, and every one of the ventilators was carefully closed, by fastening sheets of pasteboard over them. With true Yankee economy they were saving the heat. But what are we to expect of people who do not know the constituents of air, or the relation it bears to the lungs? Many do not know that the air we breathe is deprived of its oxygen for the support of the blood by every breath we inhale, and that no air is fit for respiration a second time. We render several gallons of air unfit for respiration every minute; and ventilation must be in proportion to this depravation, and no one is safe unless it is. But bad air is found everywhere. It is in our homes, in our schools, it is constant at church; thus churches, no less than steamboats, railroad cars, all public conveyances, theatres, concerts, &c. &c. are almost all manufactories of disease and death, by their want of proper ventilation.

At school, children very generally sit in a cramped position. This impedes free inhalation of air, and becomes a source of disease and often consumption.

There are abuses and excesses in youth and maturer years of which I cannot now speak, but which it has been a portion of the mission which God has given me to fulfil, to bring before mothers. The numbers of ignorantly and wilfully licentious have glutted the ranks of lunacy, idiocy, consumption, and death. But day has dawned upon the nations, and those who dare to speak truth are neither stoned, sawn asunder, or slain with the edge of the sword. The good and the true form an impenetrable phalanx about them, and if any wish to speak evil of them for their labor of love, they are awed into silence by a public sentiment as honorable as it is pure and truthful.

There are a thousand errors that I might particularize if I

had time. I might speak of the health-destroying trades and occupations of men and women who labor for their bread, at once preserving and destroying life; and I might speak of the hurried, anxious life of our men of business—men who live by steam, every moment dreading the boiler's collapse, but time fails to number evils in civilization; they are countless as the sands of the sea shore.

I must speak, however, of the evil of a neglect of bathing—of proper attention to the skin. The skin is an immense deterging or cleansing organ; its myriads of pores are the mouths of exhalent vessels which should convey morbid and worn-out matter continually from the system. If the skin does not perform its functions, some other organ or organs has to do its work—just as many a hard-working man works himself to death to support an idle family, or a lot of loafers who have got control of his labor.

It is often true of patients who come under my care, that when once their pores are opened by bathing, the exhalations in this first action of the skin are so very offensive, that it is almost impossible for me to remain near them during the applications of the treatment; and when the skin is excited by the treatment to throw off the diseasing matter that has been afflicting the lungs or other viscera, the patient has at times very bad boils and even abscesses; though with careful treatment we avoid this sort of crisis much more than in the first days of water cure, when the patient ate everything, and was treated sometimes at randon, the only condition being that the treatment should be severe enough. Still there are cases where we cannot avoid producing these boils and abscesses. It must be seen from this, that the regular and due performance of the functions of the skin is all important in the preservation of health and in recovery from disease.

The constant and daily practice of bathing ourselves and our children, should be considered a religious duty. A bath is not only a comfort and decency, but it is indispensable to health. We would not appear in company with unwashed face and hands; we ought to feel quite as much ashamed of neglecting a thorough bath as of neglecting to wash the face. I know that there are now a great many more decent people in this particular than there were twenty years ago. We are daily gaining converts from the ranks of "the great unwashed," but we want them all. The world must be baptized daily, before it can be saved. People say, "O, it is too difficult; we have not time—

we have not conveniences." Begging your pardon, this is a miserable untruth. Anybody with life above a snail can get a pail or bowl of water and two towels, or one towel and a sponge, and ten minutes are all sufficient for a thorough bathing. Will you say that you cannot afford such a domestic bathing establishment as this, and that you cannot rise ten minutes earlier, and thus earn health enough to perform twice the work that you would get through without the bath, besides having the comfortable consciousness that you are a clean Christian?

Persons who sleep on a feather bed are not as willing to get up in season and take a bath, as those who sleep on a mattress, but they need the bath much more. Feathers are exceedingly unhealthy from various causes. Feather beds constantly absorb the exhalations from the body, and unless frequently aired and cleansed, they become poisonous from this cause; and when well cleansed, they still induce a feverish state of the body. Besides, they are kept for a long time, and very nice ones are handed down in families; and from their facility of absorbing exhalations from the body, they become "heirlooms" of filth and disease. It was once said of a certain paper in this city, that it was "a paltry concentration of nastiness." This would have been very just if it had been said of feather beds.

A good mattress made of hair, husks, straw, palm-leaf, moss, hard wood shavings, or even wool, and a thorough cold bath every morning, are among the best preventives of consumption.

Every house should be built with a bath—but if we have no bath, we can bathe. We have seen that it is not indispensable to a thorough ablution, to have a bath-tub, or a pond to bathe in. A pail or a bowl, and a sponge or towel, with a hearty "good will" to be washed, are excellent substitutes.

Purity is the great law of life. Internal and external purity—a pure love and pure thoughts—lead us to purify all the details of life. To bathe our bodies in pure water is a correspondence of truth received in the soul. One of the surest signs to me of mental illumination, is the fact, that baths and bathing-houses are multiplying everywhere. People ask for air and water as for daily bread.

It is a good rule to distrust dogmas in religion or philosophy that are promulgated from year to year in an impure and stifling atmosphere. It is reasonable to suppose, that if people know just what is good for the soul, they will at least know something of what is good for the body.

With regard to diet, one great rule to be observed in order to the preservation and recovery of health is this: avoid repletion. America is a land of plenty. Our street beggars often throw away food because it is not good enough to suit them. Every body eats too much—too much animal food, and too much of all kinds of food. Some people seem to think that if they avoid eating flesh, they may eat anything else and any quantity. This is a great mistake. With regard to the question, Whether man is anatomically constituted to eat flesh? anatomists have decided that he is not. Still every one will settle the question for himself. I have no doubt that, other things being equal, human life is lengthened by a vegetarian diet. It is now nearly eleven years since I have tasted flesh. I attribute the ready removal of my consumptive symptoms, in a measure, to my bland and unstimulating diet. My great power of endurance now, I attribute partly to the same cause, and my mental powers, I am sure, have been improved by this diet, and as farther improvement is very desirable, I intend to persevere in this mode of living. A diet of fruit, vegetables, and farinacea, is especially suited to the consumptive. Persons with consumptive tendency should be sparing in the use of animal food, and it would be better if they would resign its use altogether.

But people seem to think there is nothing left in the world to eat, if they give up animal food. But upon careful examination they will find that the world is filled with good things.

The great errors in diet, however, are not alone in the use of animal food. Made dishes, high seasoned, with admixture of oils, are particularly unhealthy. Oily food should be especially avoided by children and consumptives. Pork is one of the worst forms of food in the world, and the lard is even more unhealthy than the flesh. Hogs are almost always afflicted with scrofula, the very word, scrofula, being derived from a Greek word that means "swine evil," or morbid tumor, to which swine are subject. Scrofula is often the basis of consumption. Scrofulous swine's flesh and lard are very dangerous food.

If we would preserve our health and that of our children, we should first avoid eating too much; second, eating oily food and condiments. Plain, simple food, in which vegetables, fruit, and farinacea predominate, is most conducive to health. As I before remarked, tea and coffee are poisonous, and should be avoided altogether. Few people give their children tea and coffee, even though they still indulge themselves in their use. They are wise for their children, if not for themselves.

Thorough mastication of food is important to good digestion and good health. Americans bargain for dyspepsia and disease at every meal, by half chewing their food. And they get what they bargain for. About half of the people in this country are literally hurried to death.

With regard to the treatment of consumption by water, I can only say, it *must* be adapted to the vital, or reactive power of the patient. A water cure physician must know his business, or he is liable to do serious mischief. The treatment of my own case was by constant stimulation of the skin, by the application of the different processes of water cure.

Many persons knowing the consumptive symptoms in my case, and knowing also that I have been successful thus far in preserving my life, a large number have been induced to come to me. Thus I have had the opportunity of seeing all kinds of cases, from the incipient to the worst stage of consumption.

It is idle to pretend that consumption is curable by any kind of medication, after a certain point of decay is reached. There is a period when no earthly means can save. But this is not the period that many suppose. The amount of local disease, ulceration of the lungs, does not always determine the fatality of the case. The amount of nervous energy, and the tendency of the lungs to decay, does in reality determine the fatality of the case.

A large amount of ulceration may be present in the lungs, and yet the patient may be cured. The ulcerated lungs may be healed even when large portions of the air-cells are obliterated, and their places may be supplied with cartilage.

I have spoken of my own case in a former chapter; but it may be well to describe it more particularly, in this connection.

I was born under circumstances peculiarly unfavorable to producing a firm constitution. Soon after my birth, my mother had "spotted fever" of a very malignant character, which was sufficient evidence that her system was full of morbid matter. She could not nurse me, and I was delivered over to the wise ignorance of an old nurse, who fed me in a very unhealthy manner. I was also dreadfully poisoned with opium in the first months of my life.

During all my early years I was feeble, and often ill, having scarlatina, and all the disorders incident to childhood, in a very severe form. At thirteen, in obedience to fashion, I dressed very improperly, lacing my form in the closest way, till my lungs gave signs of being diseased. In 1839, I began to bleed at the lungs. Prior to this time I had thrown off my tight dress, but I was feeble and much bent. I had been lecturing, and had been subjected to very laborious exertion and much mental suffering. Both these causes continued actively operating during the several succeeding years. I, however, lived very simply, and bathed much in cold water, and drank only water. But labor and anxiety obtained the mastery over my feeble frame and injured lungs, and in the autumn of 1843, I was attacked, while giving a course of lectures, with severe bleeding. I attempted to go on, but was prostrated, and bled from my lungs, in one week, nearly three quarts. I was reduced to infantile weakness.

As soon as possible, I commenced exercise in the open air, and very active treatment with water. I used sponge and pouring baths, and wore constantly my whole chest and abdomen enveloped in wet bandages. I had my lungs examined with a stethescope. The physician decided that there was considerable disease of the upper portion of the left lung. During the winter, I used the water very freely as above. In the meantime, I exercised much in the open air, and lived very simply, taking no animal food, except a very little butter and a little milk. In the spring, I again had my lungs examined. All traces of disease had disappeared.

I have continued the use of the water since. I have had some slight attacks of hemorrhage since, on occasions of much mental suffering and much labor. I find myself perfectly able to control the bleeding, by the use of water. The cough, which I had at first, disappeared entirely under the water treatment. It returns now if I go into crowded assemblies, or in the impure air of a steamboat, or if I am unable to get proper daily baths. I can now live in a state of comfortable health, with one bath a day, and a wet bandage about the abdomen. I am able to walk ten miles without fatigue. My lungs give me no pain or uneasiness. If I can maintain tolerable health conditions, I have no fear of further hemorrhage from the lungs.

I have had three patients under my care who had pulmonary consumption, whose cases were hopeless when they commenced treatment. They however had confidence that they might be relieved, and I took charge of the cases with the understanding that they were not to expect cure, but only relief.

In all these cases the symptoms were much alleviated. In one case the effect of the treatment was so marked, that I thought then, and still think, if the patient had remained under water treatment, she would have added years to her life.

When she came to my water cure house, she had a violent cough, and raised large quantities of matter. The cough was almost incessant during the night, and she consequently had very little rest. This had reduced her strength very considerably. I commenced treating her with careful reference to the reactive power of her system. She was enveloped in so much of the wet sheet as would allow of reaction and consequent heat readily.

She had also wet bandages over the lungs and abdomen. She took, in short, just as much of the treatment as she could take, without inducing hurtful chills. I would here remark that, the first end to be attained in the treatment of consumption is, to restore the action of the skin. If water cure treatment is not adapted to the reactive power, it may be made to diminish still farther the already enfeebled action of the skin. This would be most disastrous to the patient, as it would hasten the catastrophe of the disease. Those who suppose that water cure consists of throwing cold water hap-hazard over a patient are much mistaken in their supposition, and if they undertake the business, they will be likely to be as successful as ignorance deserves to be.

(A man came to me sometime since, to know how long he would need to study to set up a water cure house. I told him three years. He was indignant. He considered three weeks long enough. I might have told him that his life would not be long enough to qualify him.)

The first effect of the water in this case was exhilaration of spirits. The patient became very hopeful. The next effect was a violent diarrhœa. If the skin and system had not been carefully guarded from chill, I should have set the diarrhœa to the account of the chill, and should not have considered it critical. As it was, I considered it a salutary crisis, and such it proved.

The diarrhœa was treated with warm fomentations to the bowels, injections, fasting, and water-drinking. She was greatly relieved by it. The next appearance was an eruption over the entire portion of the chest and abdomen, which was covered by the wet bandages. This eruption resembled a half drawn blister, and large quantities of thick, yellow matter constantly exuded from the abraded surface. This matter seemed identical with that raised from the lungs, and the cough now became much less. As the exudations went on, the cough continued to decrease, and in four weeks from the time that she commenced treatment, she coughed not at all in the night, but rested quietly. The cough came on in the morning *only;* at this time she raised a moderate quantity of the yellow matter. During the day and night she hardly coughed enough to consider it an inconvenience. Her strength was much improved. She now decided to go South to a warmer climate. I remonstrated, for thus far the beneficial effect of the water treatment had exceeded my expectation. But she felt greatly better, and very hopeful. She had relatives in the South on whom she was dependent. She left—subsequently went South, came under drug treatment, and died within a year.

Two other cases have been fatal that have resorted to water cure under my direction, though in both these cases, the patients died under drug treatment, and some months after they left my care, and in both instances I gave them no hope of ultimate recovery. I only promised relief, and this they obtained. But the persuasions of friends, and the promises of doctors, who either believed they could cure them, or wished to make them believe it, perhaps to try the good effects of hope on the disease of the patient, or the purse of the practitioner, induced the sufferers to give up the soothing and relieving processes of the water treatment, and submit to great suffering from the use of drugs.

Cases of prolongation of life for an indefinite period, and of ultimate cure of consumption, by water treatment, have come under my own observation, and are well authenticated in many instances that I have not seen. I have seen a case where vomica (encysted tumor) was formed in the substance of the lungs, and burst, and threw off half a pint of ulcerous matter at a time; and this process was repeated, and the substance of the lungs so broken as to cause hemorrhage, and yet the patient, under careful water treatment, has recovered. He was a teacher in a public school in this city, and is now enjoying rugged health in California.

I have now a case of consumption in my mind, where there was violent cough and raising of matter for some years, and the general symptoms were very discouraging, and yet the patient was cured by gentle and long-continued water treatment.

There is now residing in this city, in good health, a gentleman who commenced water treatment under my care last autumn. He had then well-developed symptoms of consumption—a hard cough, which had been upon him for months, languor, general weakness and weakness of the spine, and that stimulation of the organ of Hope which is the almost unfailing attendant of consumption. Owing to this hopefulness it was difficult to persuade him to enter upon the treatment. He was however persuaded before it was too late. He began treatment in autumn, and now calls himself well with more truth than two-thirds the people I meet. He has still the tendency to consumption, and through the winter will have to continue as much treatment as is consistent with a constant attention to a laborious business.

The economy of getting well under a treatment that allows the patient in very many cases to attend to business, should be taken into account. This gentleman was treated at home, and it cost him just five dollars to cure himself of consumption.

The facts that I give you in this chapter have occurred here in our midst, and I can give you reliable references to confirm their truth.

A case of neglected dyspepsia and spinal disease, which finally induced chills and fever, and then a severe attack of fever, with an amount of lung disease which promised pulmonary consumption, and that of a rapid kind, recently came under my care. This complication of diseases has been cured by water; and the diseased lungs, from which a considerable quantity of matter was constantly raised by a severe cough, have been cured by a determination to the surface. I counted ninety-five boils upon this patient when the lungs were entirely relieved—some of them very large, and all filled with yellow pus.

A lady at Albany, who has been a patient of mine, furnishes one of the most remarkable instances of the prolongation of life in consumption by water treatment that I have ever seen. She has been several years under water treatment. About two years since I examined her lungs, and found cavities—in one of them, a cavity larger than a dollar. The air rushed through these cavities in the most frightful manner. By a persevering tonic treatment by water, she has thus far preserved her life and improved her general health. The last letter I received from her, she was comfortable, and able to go out and walk some distance. Those who know her, know how valuable her life is, and rejoice in every day added to it by her perseverance in water treatment.

I could go on enumerating cases, but there is no use in accumulating evidence of a similar character.

CHAPTER XI.

CHOLERA.

Cholera has been considered the rock on which all medical professions were destined to split. There is no doubt that in many cases of cholera no effort can save the patient. The disease is simply death. It is the final convulsion of the wronged and outraged vital economy. Majendie has well said, "Cholera begins where all other diseases end—*in death.*" This is true in many cases.

I have seen nothing of the disease except this season and in this city. My theory of the cause of cholera is this:—Miasmata and deathly exhalations are constantly arising from the badly cultivated earth, cursed with war and famine and disease over much of its surface. This miasma moves in veins and parcels around the globe, and when it passes over a city or country which is enveloped with its kindred evil, it is attracted toward it. Like seeks like. Those who come within this evil influence must be strong enough to resist it, or they fall before it. The joint effect of death-causes within man, and this deadly miasm without him, is the disease known as cholera.

Persons suffering from nervous exhaustion, delicate and badly organized children, old people, and the ignorant and vicious poor, are known to be the classes which furnish most of the victims of cholera.

Camphor, opium, and calomel have been principally relied on by the allopathic profession for the cure of cholera. When we reflect on the large number that have recovered, in spite of twenty grain doses of calomel, and opium and camphor in proportion, we may easily believe that few, comparatively, would have died with proper water cure treatment. For myself, I am convinced that cholera is much easier to cure than dysentery. I have not had half the difficulty in curing cholera, as with bilious diarrhœa and dysentery.

Before I had seen and become acquainted with the disease,

I was much terrified at the thought of it. My first case alarmed me much. I feared that the water might not control it. The patient was a young lady, very nervous and delicate. She had been for some years ill of uterine disease.

She was violently seized at two o'clock in the morning, having had no premonitory symptoms. She vomited the rice-water fluid copiously, and purged violently a substance resembling coffee-grounds. She cramped terribly, and had a burning at the pit of the stomach like fire. There was pain in the head, and cold extremities.

She was first put into a tub of cold water, and rubbed until the vomiting ceased, and the cramps also. She had water to drink, and injections of cold water. As soon as she came out of the tub, four folds of wet linen wrung from cold water were put over the abdomen—two on the back. She was rubbed with the hands wet in cold water till the warmth of the body was restored.

At nine o'clock, A. M. all the symptoms remitted, but at eleven, A. M. vomiting again came on; but this time the ejected fluid was tinged with bile.

After this vomiting she was seized with shivering. She was wrapped in the cold, wet bandages, and enveloped in blankets, and soon became warm.

After the subsidence of the urgent symptoms, she was packed in the wet sheet. The third day she went to the door, and about the house.

My first thought when I saw her was, "She is so sick that she must recover;" that is, I saw the system making such violent efforts to relieve itself, that I felt sure, that with proper assistance, relief would be obtained; and the event proved that I was right.

My second case was of a lady who was afflicted with the premonitory symptoms for a week. She took laudanum, and kept about till about the seventh day, when she sunk at once, fainting nearly. A cold, deathly state came on, with no vomiting. She was put into a tub of tepid water, and rubbed for nearly half an hour; then taken out; the abdomen bound in bandages wrung from cold water, and she wrapped in blankets, when she became warm and revived. Purging came on again, and she had injections.

This treatment was repeated as often as she sunk, and became cold. In three days she was out of danger, and suffered only from the opium she had taken.

These were my first two cases. In one of these I used the wet sheet after the vomiting and purging were subdued. In the other I did not use it; but in my later cases I used it earlier, and with great advantage.

I had many cases where the premonitory symptoms were severe; but the cold or tepid half bath, and a half-hour's smart friction in this bath, with constant use of cold water enemas, and cold, wet bandages to the abdomen, with fasting, cured all these cases in twelve hours. When diarrhœa was not premonitory of cholera, but was bilious in its character, or tending to dysentery, the cure was nearly as rapid.

I did not realize the deadly nature of the disease, so rapid was the relief afforded by water treatment, till it was my fortune to see a patient treated with mustard plasters, and the congestive or heating treatment. At early morning I was called to a young lady who was violently attacked with cholera. The case was most alarming to me, because the lady was suffering from severe spinal disease. The rice-water discharges were so profuse, that I ventured upon no preliminary treatment, fearing greatly the consequence of congestion in her case. I had her enveloped at once in a full wet sheet, and many blankets. I left her to see some other patients, and found at a place where I was attending an infant with diarrhœa, that an older child had been attacked with cholera. The child, a boy of five years, was born of a mother who has been for years in ill health, and his organization must have been very frail and delicate. He had always seemed to belong more to the spiritual world than to this, such was the strange wisdom and beauty of his character. The evacuations had ceased when I saw him. A physician had been called, and had left him some time previous. He had given homœopathic doses of camphor, with some other medicines, and he had been enveloped in a multitude of blankets, with bottles of hot water, and a mustard-plaster to the stomach. He had been forcibly held in this apparatus for producing congestion, till he was exceedingly heated and sweating.

The father said that they had sent for me, but I had not seen the messenger, and was told at home that no one had been for me. He said that the doctor did not wish the heating treatment continued after reaction had taken place. The child begged most piteously to be relieved, and I removed the bottles and the clothing, and the mustard plaster was also taken off. I put a wet bandage about the stomach, and covered the child comfortably. I did not think he could die, he seemed so bright, and the heat of the skin and the pulse so natural, but the nurse of the babe told me that the doctor said he would die. I staid as long as possible, doing nothing more than to advise the family to give the medicine faithfully. I did this because the medicine was homœopathic, and I was sure could do no harm, and because they spoke of a willingness to combine water treatment with the medicine, and I hoped the doctor would extend the same courtesy to me.

I left at nine, A. M., and returned to my cholera patient. There had been but partial reaction in the sheet, but the most alarming symptoms had subsided. She was put under a pouring bath, and had enemas of cold water and cold bandages, and then was put again into the wet sheet; and I returned to the other, hoping that if any danger appeared, I should get liberty to do something. The doctor came shortly, and the parents did not introduce me to him, or ask my opinion, but told me that the doctor feared collapse, and had again ordered the congestive treatment. This seemed very bad to me, but I did not think the child would die even now. I turned to my husband with great sadness, but I said, "They can't kill him," and I fully believed that he would live through the treatment. If I had not thus thought, I should have spoken my mind of this dreadful mode of treatment, which I do not consider homœopathic or human. I do not object to homœopathic medicine; I believe the genuine article is harmless; but I felt that I could not stay to see that frail body heated and held by force in the hell the doctor had ordered. I had a solemn and tender love for the child that I could never explain, and I felt wounded professionally that my opinion had not been asked, nor any mention made to the doctor that I was then ready to administer water cure, although the parents had said in the morning that they were willing to combine the two modes of treatment. I left the house in great sadness, but comforted with the feeling that the child had been so carefully reared, that he would have strength to outlive the disease and the treatment. It was the greatest professional mistake that I ever made. He doubtless began to die from the moment that he was again enveloped in mustard, hot bottles, and piles of blankets. His last little life was extinguished in the struggle against these appliances, and the outward force that held him in them. His pure, heavenly instinct cried for water and a bath, and rebelled, as long as he was capable of effort, against the treatment. I am very thankful that I did not see this treatment administered, or the death of the child, which took place before five, P. M. He was seized at two, A. M. I again saw my patient about two, P. M. The second wet sheet pack, of little more than an hour's duration, had established full reaction; and just after the news of the child's death had reached me, I found her sitting up. Now I do not say that these cases were identical, but they seemed to me to be so at the time. I have since learned facts that make me think that no treatment could have saved the child for any length of time. His organization was most frail and delicate. He had an unearthly beauty and wisdom, that pointed unmistakeably to early death. And there doubtless was a deadly miasm surrounding the place where the family lived, at the time of his death. I have reason to think that the discharges were more copious than in the case I have given, and that even the most judicious water treatment could not have given back the life he had lost; although I think if he had been packed in a wet sheet when I first saw him, he might have lived longer, and died in a different manner. I wish to be understood with regard to the use of water and the wet sheet in exhaustion, from whatever cause. I believe the effect is a positive augmentation of life. Water is the material correspondence of the Divine Truth. Heat is the material correspondence of the Divine Love. Truth and Love constitute Life in the higher degrees, and the living element of the water unites with the heat of the system, aud gives life in the lower degrees to the patient. If the patient has no heat in the body, the water is of no use. If he have no love in the soul, truth is of no use. This I believe is the true philosophy of water cure. Those who believe in a New Heaven and a New Earth, will understand this philosophy, and will know by whom its first principles were revealed. No bereavement of my life has ever so strongly affected me as the death of this child, and yet I believe it was a Providence by which good must be effected. It teaches first, the lesson, that when life and health are not given from birth, they can be but partially attained even with the greatest care. Probably no child was ever more carefully reared than this. Again, it teaches the lesson, that deadly miasma arising from the boiling of dead animals, putrid and diseased, cannot be resisted by all those who live in their vicinity, even though their personal habits be as good as possible. Then again it teaches the lesson, that wars and famines, oppression and misery, ignorance and vice, on one side the globe, send their baneful miasma everywhere; that the human race is but one Man; and that congestion, or famine, or cancer of any one part of this great Human Body, affects the whole; that not one man on the earth can be healthy, holy, and happy, until all are.

In the treatment of cholera, I have relied upon cold and tepid rubbing baths at first; the wet sheet pack, after vomiting has subsided. Injections of cold water, drinking of cold water in small quantities, or large quantities when I wished to promote vomiting, and wet bandages and abundant friction, with fasting at first, and small quantities of the simplest food when the danger was past.

I have known several instances where judicious water cure treatment was administered by the friends of the patient, with eminent success. In one instance, the lady who was attacked was cramped so that the intestines were drawn up under the ribs. She was put into a warm bath and rubbed till the cramps gave way. She said, the sensation of relief was like that of the birth of a child. Hot flannel fomentations were put upon the abdomen, and she was in this manner entirely relieved, and in a few days was well again.

Another instance was the case of a child. This child was eight years of age, and had been some three years under water cure treatment whenever he was ill. He was taken very ill with cholera, and his mother feared the delay of sending six miles for me, and her distress and alarm were met by her boy. The little sufferer said, "Mother, I will tell you what to do—what Mrs. Gove did once for me when I was sick: she put me in a bath that was not cold nor warm, and rubbed me, and then wrapped me in a blanket without drying me." His mother immediately had a tepid bath got ready, and he was rubbed in it for some time, and then wrapped, dripping, in blankets. He soon sweat, and then had a cold bath, cold wet bandages, injections of cold water, and water to drink. This treatment cured the disease. The boy very likely saved his own life.

I might multiply instances of the domestic treatment of cholera by water, but will only mention one other. A poor Irish woman was taken with cholera in the street. She fell, and broke out several of her teeth, but after a time succeeded in reaching the house of a lady whose benevolence is only equalled by her skill in water cure. She took the woman in, applied proper water treatment, and cured her.

The latest cases of cholera which I have treated, were complicated with bilious symptoms. One of these cases presented some symptoms which I have seen in no other case. The purging was almost entirely without pain, and there were extensive painless cramps. From this state of things the patient thought herself in very little danger, whilst I apprehended much. The wet sheet packing, rubbing baths, and injections of cold water, soon overcame the disease.

I have had many cases of an attack of diarrhœa, and of vomiting and purging, which if the cholera had not been in the city, would have suggested no thought of danger to my mind, and which were just as readily cured as if there had been no epidemic. From the progress of exactly this class of symptoms, under ordinary medication, to collapse and death, I was always alarmed, and careful to do everything in my power.

My experience has convinced me, that with people of ordinary good health, with good habits, and with a resolute refusal to take medicine of any kind, preventive or remedial, cholera is by no means a disease difficult of cure. In its premonitory symptoms it is perfectly controllable, and with rubbing baths, cold water enemas, cold bandages, and fasting, I have seen no premonitory symptoms that could not be cured in twelve hours. Cases complicated with dysentery or bilious symptoms, are much more difficult, and take a much longer time.

With persons of low vitality, or who have been poisoned by living in unhealthy localities and on bad food, by drinking ardent spirits, with the general bad habits of the ignorant, and with persons who have lived in luxury and who have been long under the dominion of drugs and doctors, cholera becomes the most terrible disease that I have ever looked upon. Death is sure to many of these, under whatever treatment they may be placed. I have no words to describe my horror and detestation of the system of drugging resorted to by the people, almost universally, for the prevention and cure of cholera. It has done its work, and those who have escaped death, have laid the foundation of much sickness and suffering, and have prepared themselves to be more ready victims to the cholera when it shall come again to scourge us, and force us to learn wisdom by the things we suffer.

My small experience in cholera has been inexpressibly painful, and yet I cannot regret it. It is one of the many lessons of my life, and I trust it will not be in vain to myself or others. I now feel that I know the disease, and that I have the means in my power to cure all curable cases. I thank God more than ever for water cure, and I shall pursue my profession more reverently and earnestly than before I looked on this pestilence.

CHAPTER XII.

BILIOUS DIARRHŒA — COLIC — COMMON COLDS — PNEUMONIA — INFLAMMATORY RHEUMATISM AND GOUT — NEURALGIC AFFECTIONS — CUTANEOUS ERUPTIONS — APOPLEXY AND LIGHTNING — CRISIS.

HAVING a few words to say upon each of the above-mentioned subjects, I have reserved them all for this concluding chapter.

BILIOUS DIARRHŒA.

Numerous cases of bilious diarrhœa have come under my care. I have observed, that in most cases the patients who suffered from this form of diarrhœa, had taken a great deal of medicine.

I recently treated a case, which I give as an example of many cases, and which was cured after a large quantity of slimy membrane had passed off. This membrane had doubtless lined the stomach and intestinal canal, and was probably first formed to protect the delicate mucous lining of those organs from the acrid and poisonous medicines which the patient had taken for years. For some time previous to this illness, no medicine had been taken; and so much water treatment had been used, that I had no doubt that the diarrhœa was a crisis intended to throw off this membrane; and I predicted, that when the membrane had passed off, the diarrhœa would cease, and that the patient would recover at once. The result was exactly what I had expected—and had known in previous cases.

The reader will find much very valuable matter on the formation of false membrane, in order to protect the mucous membrane of the stomach and intestines, in Francke's, *alias* Rause's, works on Water Cure.

The "sliming up" of medicines, as the German calls it, is no doubt often resorted to in the stomach, when there is not sufficient vital power to carry the poison out of the system.

As this kind of protection from poisonous medicines betokens low vitality, so those patients whose stomachs are thus lined, are amongst the most difficult to cure. Diarrhœa is a hopeful symptom in the progress of their cure. But patients who have enough vitality to carry poisonous matters to the surface, in boils, or even to the mucous membrane, in salivation, recover much more rapidly than those who have no particular trouble, but a general weakness and want of tone. These last have not strength enough to be sick, and consequently to get well—for nature's mode of curing us, is to cast bad matters out of the system by a painful effort, which we call sickness.

In bilious diarrhœa, as in all relaxed conditions of the bowels, the skin should be stimulated by constant packing. If the patient cannot react against a full wet sheet, partial wet sheet packing should be resorted to, or a dry blanket pack should be given with as much wet linen over the chest and abdomen as can be borne, without a chill so excessive that it cannot be overcome.

The treatment of dysentery, diarrhœa, and cholera, are substantially the same, with variations to suit different conditions, for which no directions can be given, for they must depend on the tact and judgment of the physican or person administering the cure. To be successful in water cure, people must know *why* they do things. The physician can no longer say to intelligent believers in water cure, "It is for you to do what I tell you." He must give a reason—and if he cannot, they will find one for themselves, and dispense with his service.

In all cases of disease, and particularly in disorders of the stomach and digestive organs, very little food should be taken. This cannot be too forcibly impressed on the mind. Diarrhœa and dysentery and cholera, I am never weary of assuring you, may be prevented in a very great proportion of cases simply by fasting and bathing. It is astonishing how difficult it is to make people believe this. I recollect asking a lady of much intelligence if she had given her brother any food when he was suffering in a terrible congestive fever, under which I feared he might sink in a few hours. She named several articles that she had given him to eat during the day, and amongst the rest an ear of boiled, green corn. "You know," said she, "that he must have something to eat." This is the general idea, and it is very hard to dispossess people of it. It is difficult to convince even the intelligent of the fact, that fasting is one of the most potent remedies for disease.

COLIC.

When the pain is about the diaphragm, an emetic of warm water should be given. The throat should be tickled with the finger, or with a little skewer around which a piece of linen has been wrapped, to make the vomiting easy and effectual. The stomach should be thoroughly cleansed. If the pain is below the diaphragm, enemas of cold, or tepid water should be given until the bowels are perfectly cleansed. If any pain remains after these processes, put the patient in a wet sheet pack, partial or entire, according to the heat of the system.

COMMON COLDS.

It is often the case in a cold that the patient is very chilly, and unable to react against a wet sheet pack, and hardly any practice could be more injurious than to put such a patient in the wet sheet. A blanket pack, warm and close, with a wet towel about the head and lungs is the proper treatment, and the patient should be made to perspire. If the patient is full of life and heat, and can react quickly, a wet sheet pack is the proper remedy for a cold. After the pack a thorough cold bath should be had, and wet bandages put about the lungs.

PNEUMONIA.

The treatment of pneumonia is substantially the same as that of a common cold, only it must be longer continued to be effectual. Fasting entirely for a time, and then very little food until the complaint is removed, is an important part of the treatment.

INFLAMMATORY RHEUMATISM AND GOUT.

Inflammatory rheumatism is thought by many to depend on cold. There is no doubt that cold is a proximate cause, but the primary cause is the exhaustion of nervous energy by hard labor, undue license of the passions, luxury, care, anxiety, &c. I have cured several very severe cases of inflammatory rheumatism. I have had cases where the patients were not able to rise, or to step, and in a few weeks' treatment they were able to walk about and attend to the duties of life, and complete their cure at home and under their own care. In some cases relief and a cure may be obtained in a week; other cases require weeks or months to complete the cure.

The reliance for cure in this disease, and also in that of its first cousin, gout, is on constant wet bandages to the afflicted portions, made thicker as the inflammation is more violent, and wet sheet packings. In some cases the douche is very useful, in others it cannot be borne. In gout and rheumatism, fasting, packing, and wet bandaging are the most rapid and reliable means of cure, and the patient must have the same will as his physician, or he may undo a week's work, or make it of no avail by one "good" dinner or other excess, such as has caused his disease.

NEURALGIA.

Neuralgia, ear-ache and tooth-ache, are often comprehended under the head of colds, cold being a proximate cause of these affections. To ease all neuralgic affections, let the pain be ever so severe, I have found the wet sheet effectual. The pain is not always cured (except for the time) by one application of the sheet, but repeated applications not only ease, but cure the tooth-ache, the horrible pain of tic doloreux, ear-ache, and all pains comprehended under the general term, Neuralgia.

CUTANEOUS ERUPTIONS.

There is no class of diseases in which water cure is more efficacious than in skin diseases.

I had some time since a case of salt rheum which had invaded the whole system, but which principally made its appearance on the head and face. The ears ulcerated externally and internally, the lungs were badly affected. The patient, naturally a very pretty and pleasant woman, was reduced to a deplorable state of stupor mentally, and was much disfigured by the eruption. When she began treatment, one could hardly have seen a more discouraging case. The head was bald and smooth as the face, from the eruption, except where there were large scabs. The face was partially, and the ears wholly covered with the foul eruption, and the hearing was entirely lost in one ear. The body had no sores, but the skin was rough and grating to the touch. In three weeks after she began treatment, her whole body was covered with a raw efflorescence that looked like flame, and constantly exuded matter, and the head and face began to get better. You could not put down a pin's head on the body that was not covered with the eruption. After a time it disappeared, and then reappeared partially. There was several times crisis in the head. After months of treatment the evil was expelled from the system, the patient became healthy, pretty and cheerful, and her hearing was restored.

The skin was fair and smooth, and plenty of soft hair like a baby's, came out on her bald head. This was an extreme case. Many less severe cases have come under my care, reports of which I would give, if the limits of this work would permit.

I have treated salt rheum, St. Anthony's fire, prurigo, attended with diabetes, tetter, leprosy, and many other psoric eruptions with entire success.

Sore and inflamed eyes, blindness and deafness often depend on scrofula in the system. Where this is the cause of such affections, relief always, and often an entire cure is obtained from water treatment.

APOPLEXY AND LIGHTNING.

The treatment for a patient who is attacked by apoplexy and one who is struck by lightning, is identical. In both cases water should be poured on the head, and then over the whole body; and the patient should be rubbed with the bare hands of as many persons as can properly assist. Life has been restored in this way, after many hours of unconsciousness. The after treatment should be tonic, with particular care to equalize the circulation as fast as possible, and prevent the catastrophe of congestion, which is almost always more dangerous at each succeeding attack.

CRISIS.

Crisis is mostly of three kinds—fever, eruption, or boils, and diarrhœa. In the earlier days of water cure, perceptible crisis, in the shape of boils, fever, or diarrhœa, was thought much more needful to a cure, than it is now. A great many boils were made by eating greasy, bad food, and submitting to a treatment more forcible than wise or prudent. Diarrhœas were brought on by chilling the weakened skin continually in cold water—for both patients and practitioners had become hastily convinced that they could not have too much of a good thing;

then the food of most water cure patients was very improper; and the general notion that they must get sick before they could get well, and the immense quantities of water drank indiscriminately by all sorts of patients, made them sick, comforted them with crisis, but did not cure them. Much of this is changed now. Patients, as well as physicians, have got clearer ideas of what is needed in water cure. There is more care with regard to diet; greasy food is less used: there is more judgment in adapting treatment to reactive power; the treatment is milder; water drinking is practised with more discretion. People have learned that "the longest way round is the shortest way home:" hence we have more cures, and less crisis, than formerly.

About a tenth part of my patients have crisis—not more. Formerly, if one in ten escaped crisis, it was considered very bad practice. People are wiser now, and more patient under treatment, especially as they find that with proper direction, they can cure themselves at home. Some of the best cures I have known, have been made at home, with careful and long-continued treatment. Some of them were made by persons whom I have never seen, but who have consulted me by letter from time to time, and others I have seen once. The cost of these cures, which does not average more than ten dollars, is no trifling consideration to those who are in moderate circumstances, or who have spent all their living on physicians.

Many persons do not know how to manage when they have crisis. Boils should be kept constantly covered with several folds of wet linen, and wet sheet packing should be used, and very little food taken.

Critical diarrhœas and fever should be treated in the same way as if they were not crisis, for, after all, crisis is, like all diseases, only the action of the nervous energy, to expel morbid matter; and when caused by a skilful application of water cure, is indeed a blessing.

THE END.

INDEX.

ACUTE DISEASES....................32
Allopathy, credit due to................25
Apoplexy and Lightning..............105
Author's Medical Studies..............21
" Practice and Success.........29
" " Change in.......v
After Pains, cause and prevention of,...78

Baths, their temperature, &c...........14
Blanket pack...........................16
Blood-letting..........................27
Brain Fever............................41
Bilious Diarrhœa......................101
Blindness and Deafness...............105

Causes of Disease..................8—27
Case of the Author....................20
CHOLERA...............................94
" Cases of.......................95
" Domestic treatment of........99
Cholera Infantum......................52
Children, rules for management of......54
" diseases of...................49
Childbirth, speedy and painless........75
" water cure in..............76
" diseased...................51
Chicken Pox...........................60
CHRONIC DISEASES.....................44
Colds................................103
Colic................................103
CONSUMPTION..........................79
" symptoms of.............80
" causes of...............81
" cure in Author's case..20–89
" alleviated..............90
" cases cured..............92
Consultations...........................v
Crisis...............................105
Croup.................................33
Cutaneous Eruptions..................104

Delirium Tremens......................42
Diet..................................88
Diabetes and Prurigo..................73
Diseases curable by water..............11
DISEASES OF INFANCY..................49
Domestic practice of water cure........45
Douche................................15
Drugs, effects of...................8–28
Dripping Sheet........................15
Dyspepsia.............................47
" with great coldness...........46
Dysentery.........................42–43

Early experience of the Author........19
Earache..............................104

FEMALE DISEASES...................10–60
Female Physicians.....................17
Female Medical Education..............vi
Fever and Ague........................40
Food for Infants.......................55

GESTATION AND PARTURITION.........73
Gout and Rheumatism.................103

Health and Disease defined..............7
Homœopathy...........................26

Infant mortality...................49–83
" causes of............50–84
Infants, medication and treatment of....52
Idiot Child, case of....................56
Inflammation of the Lungs.............39
" of uterus..............67–71

Labor, treatment in....................75
Lungs, functions of the................81
" inflammation of............39–103

Malignant Typhus......................36
Malpractice........................43–66
Marriage, unfitness for.................50
Measles...............................59
MEDICAL PRACTICE.....................24
Medical Studies of the Author..........21
Menstruation, interrupted..............62

Nervous and Uterine disease...........63
Neuralgia.............................48

Obstetrics......................10–54–75

PRINCIPLES AND PROCESSES OF WATER CURE...........................7
Pathology, Theories of..................25
Parturition painless in health..........74
Pneumonia...........................103
Pork, effects of.....................53–88
Pregnancy, treatment in...............74
Prolapsus Uteri and Spinal Disease.....69

Rheumatism, inflammatory............42
" and Gout...............103
Rupture and Premature Delivery.......65

Salt-rheum..........................104
Scarlatina......................37–57–58
Scrofula..........................38–46
Sitz Bath.............................15
Shallow or half Bath..................15
Ship-fever............................36
Skin, functions of.....................86
" Diseases of...................104
Sleeping..............................87
Small-pox.............................34

Spinal Disease and Distortion..........46
Syphilis..............................72

Tic-doloreux..........................49
Typhus Fever......................36–40
Toothache............................104

Ulceration of the Womb...............71
Uterine Disease...................62–68
Uterus, inflammation of...........67–71

Varioloid.........................37–60
Vaccination, perils of................84
Ventilation...........................85

Water cure defined.....................8
" true philosophy of...........96
" authorities..................26
" effects of....................9
" economy of..................12
Water, qualities of...................13
Wet Sheet Pack........................16
Woman's sufferings....................18
Women, particular directions to.......61
Whooping Cough........................60

THE

PARENTS' GUIDE

FOR THE TRANSMISSION OF

DESIRED QUALITIES TO OFFSPRING,

AND

CHILDBIRTH MADE EASY.

BY MRS. HESTER PENDLETON.

STEREOTYPE EDITION.

NEW YORK:
FOWLERS AND WELLS, PUBLISHERS,
PHRENOLOGICAL CABINET, 131 NASSAU STREET.
SOLD BY BOOKSELLERS GENERALLY.
1850.

TABLE OF CONTENTS.

INTRODUCTION . . . . page 7–10

Origin of the work—Importance of the principles advocated—Diversity of disposition and character of different individuals—How to develope the faculties in the yet unborn—The necessity of human cultivation.

CHAPTER I.

IMPROVEMENT OF OFFSPRING 11–18

Means of perpetuating talent and virtue from parent to offspring—The elevation of the race—Talent and genius—The propagation of the mental and physical qualities—Inherited and educated qualities compared—Investigation of the natural laws of inheritance—Man's duty to improve the human species—Conduct of children the result of physical organization—The proper condition of parents while transmitting their own qualities—The first children of very young mothers deficient in intellect and stability—The effects of dissipation of parents inflicted on their children—Dr. Franklin—The mother of Washington—Ages of parents—Their effects on offspring—Napoleon's mother on the battle-field—The effect on her own mind transmitted to her son—Testimony of Mrs. E. W. Farnham.

CHAPTER II.

THE MOTHER'S DISPOSITION TRANSMITTED 19–26

Goethe's mother—Her peculiarities inherited by her son—The importance of attention to the mother from the father—Kind treatment—Lord Byron—The character and disposition of his parents—His inheritance, birth, and early education—Cuvier and his mother—His mental improvement in youth—Offspring of eminent men—The brain the organ of the mind—Its development and perfection—The strong are born of the strong.

CHAPTER III.

COMBINATION OF QUALITIES 27–33

Queen Elizabeth—Her extraordinary conduct—King James, the son of Mary, Queen of Scots, who married her first cousin, a youth of nineteen—The deteriorating effect of marriages between blood relations exemplified—Partial idiocy of King James—The cause—The private character of Marie Louise—Her strong propensities transmitted—The effects of the union of excessive animal propensities—The Emperor Nero a striking coincidence of the inheritance of perverted human nature—His parents were cousins—Pope Alexander VI.—His vices, their causes, and their results—Hereditary vices and virtues contrasted—Henry IV. and his ancestors.

CHAPTER IV.

FACTS AND ARGUMENTS 34–62

Jonathan Edwards—His parentage, birth, education, and life—Hereditary talent—The Arab's value of the blood and pedigree of his horse—Patrick Henry—His ancestry, birth, history, and genius—The constitution and character of Franklin's father—His superior judgment—The mother of Franklin—Number of children—Her age, etc—Interesting sketch—Lord Bacon—His parents—Their age at his birth—The government of the family—The inheritance of talent not the result of chance, but of immutable laws—Natural laws, and their application—The object of human inquiry—The writings of George and Andrew Combe—Different modes of education, and their effects—Milton—His parentage, ancestors, and descendants—His domestic life and experience—Importance of female education.

CHAPTER V.

CULTIVATED INTELLECT IN PARENTS 63-69

The parentage of Madame de Stael—Her superior talent inherited—State of the mother's mind transmitted—Personal observations—Deleterious effects on the wife of neglect by the husband—The temper of the mother during pregnancy inherited by her offspring—Connection between the mind and body.

CHAPTER VI.

MENTAL POWER AUGMENTED BY UNION 70-76

Character and qualities of Sir William Jones—His parentage and education—Exercise of the faculties—The mother of Guizot—Love of truth.

CHAPTER VII.

PRINCIPLES OF TRANSMISSION ILLUSTRATED 77-81

The Wesley family—John Wesley's marriage—Samuel Wesley—His industry and perseverance—His marriage, and the character of his wife—Doctor Doddridge—His superior natural, moral, and intellectual qualities—His parentage—The twentieth child—Industry—Circumstances of his birth—His early impressions—Important examples.

CHAPTER VIII.

THE ADVENT OF GENIUSES EXPLAINED BY CIRCUMSTANCES . 82-89

Robert Burns—His parents—Their care and influence on their son—The literary taste and character of the Scotch, as a people—John Knox—His character and influence—Thomas Carlyle, and his ancestry—His wit, and honesty—The influence of his mother on his character—Physical imbecility inherited—Shortsightedness—Sluggishness—Contrast—Economy—Activity—Cases and facts illustrated—Period of gestation—Acquisitiveness and secretiveness inherited.

CHAPTER IX.

THE CAUSES OF INSANITY 90-97

Excessive mental emotion—Prevention and cure of insanity—Causes of fatuity—Dean Swift—Employments and conditions in life produce lunatics and idiots—Facts—Pauperism—The causes—Idiots in England and Wales—The Indian race—Easy labor, and speedy delivery—Size of heads of male and female children—Spinal column—Bones of the pelvis—Tight lacing—Fresh air—Exercise—Cases contrasted—Duty of women—Death of children—Mental anguish—Its causes—A hard case—Physiological knowledge necessary—Reason—Experience.

CHAPTER X.

RESPONSIBILITY OF WOMAN 98-104

Influence and rights of woman—Mode of education—Treatment of children—Obedience—Cold water—Diet—Fruits—Luxurious living—Muscular action—Mother's anxiety—Error and crime—Music—Drawing—Recreation—Painting—Composition—The natural sciences—Chemistry—Geology—Botany—Perceptive and reflective organs should be exercised—The use and value of money—The economical mother—Home education.

CHAPTER XI.

PHYSICAL, MENTAL, AND MORAL POSITION OF WOMAN . . 105-111

The present age—Liberal education—Improvement and elevation of society—Ignorant and intelligent mothers compared—Rights and privileges of woman—Mary Woolstoncraft—Her influence—Roman women—Mrs. Jamieson's appeal—Our law makers—Dependence and sufferings of woman—Importance of her moral and intellectual culture.

CHAPTER XII.

AMERICAN WOMEN 112-118

The influence of pursuits on the rising generation—Delicacy of female youth in cities—Deterioration of the species—Female schools—Ignorance of the principles of physiology—Contracted chests—Beauty—Disease—Early decay of teeth—Sallowness of complexion—Stooping—The lungs—The blood—Sedentary habits—Round shoulders—Walking and gymnastic exercises—Matrimony—The ball room—Doctors, dentists, and druggists—National character formed by woman.

CHAPTER XIII.

CONCLUSION 119-127

Dependence of offspring on their parents—Fixed laws by which health is governed—The moral aspect of society—Woman's mission—She controls the destiny of her race—Her preparation and responsibility—The necessity of a proper direction of her mind.

APPENDIX.

MALFORMATIONS AND THEIR CAUSES 128-148

Effects of the mother's imagination—Cases and facts from Dr. Elliotson—The Chinese—Their imbecility—The Swiss—Crossing among individuals and nations—Improvement of progeny—Polygamy—Its effects—The ancients—Love and hate—Imperfections in offspring caused by early marriages—Ages of husband and wife—Nature's laws relative to marriages—Scrofula and other diseases inherited—Determination of the sexes of offspring—Mr. Combe's views—Causes of sterility and its cure—Facts—A warning—Sterility cured by change of temperament—A sea voyage—Abstemiousness a cause of fecundity—The Irish—East Indians—Functional derangement—Cultivated faculties transmitted—Dogs—Sir Anthony Carlisle.

CHILDBIRTH MADE EASY.

CHILDBIRTH WITHOUT PAIN 151-186

Pain in childbirth a morbid symptom—Dr. Combe's views—Dr. Graham's views—Mrs. Gove's Lectures to Ladies—Essay on Human Parturition—Chemistry—Professor Liebig's views—Children of the lower classes—Effects of fashion—The young wife—Beauty, grace, cheerfulness, and health—Child-bearing natural—Pain unnecessary—Cleanliness—Regimen of pregnant women—Influence of atmosphere in pregnancy—Exercise—Mrs. Wright's opinion.

WATER-CURE IN CHILDBIRTH.

A REMARKABLE CASE 186-208

Directions for using the bath in all its forms during pregnancy—Vegetable food—Effects on the child—Mortality of infants—Child-bearing—Importance of an acquaintance with physiology—Female midwives to administer to the wants of the mother during delivery—Inflammation and swelling of the breasts—Facts and examples—Clysters—Temperature of water for bathing—Sitting bath—Easy labor and speedy delivery—Male and female children—Birth of Dr. Johnson—Producing abortion or miscarriage—Effect on the mother—Facts—Hazarding the life of the mother—Madame Restell—Confession of a victim—Premature death—Momentous importance of the subjects treated in this work.

ADVERTISEMENT.

IN presenting this work to the public, we feel that we are doing mankind a GREAT GOOD. In fact, the whole subject is but imperfectly understood by the people generally, especially in so far as these laws are applicable to THEMSELVES. Farmers understand and apply the principle to its fullest extent, in the improvement of horses, hogs, sheep, and cattle, while but very few ever think of improving their OWN KIND. To a more complete development of the laws which govern ALL TRANSMISSION, this work is devoted. The importance of this subject is infinitely above that of all others within the comprehension of man, so far as relates to his PHYSICAL, and, per consequence, MORAL well-being.

S. R. WELLS.

PHRENOLOGICAL CABINET,
131 Nassau street, New York.

INTRODUCTION.

The theory which this work endeavors to establish, was not taken up suddenly and thrown out hastily, but is the result of long and mature reflection, and a well-grounded *induction from history, from observation, and from experience.*

The attention of the writer was early attracted to the subject, by observing the diversity of disposition and mental capacity among the companions of her youth. Some of them appeared to be so happily constituted, that the acquirement of knowledge and the conscientious performance of their social duties, afforded a constant source of pleasure and delight. In others, purity and goodness were so perfectly innate, that no bad example could affect, nor evil influence corrupt them: while others were so dull and stupid, that it was impossible to teach them any thing more than the mere rudiments of education. Some, again, were so obstinate and vicious, that no punishment could deter, nor counsel persuade them from evil courses. The question naturally suggests itself, "Why is this?" Surely it cannot be a mere matter of chance, that one child is born a knave or a fool, and another a prodigy of sense and goodness. And when those very children were observed to pass unchanged from youth to manhood—the path of the reckless, the selfish, and the sensual, marked by misery and ruin, while the quiet, diligent, reflective student, became the high-minded, useful, and honored member of society—the inquiry, "Why is this?" assumed still greater importance. The descent of hereditary qualities only answered the question in part; for the different dispositions and degrees of mental activity found in children of the same parents, again involved the subject in perplexity and doubt. To endeavor to solve this problem in nature, has constituted the life-work of the authoress: and if she has failed to elucidate the subject—if her observations were founded in error, or her conclusions not warranted, she hopes that the publication of her work will lead to the further investigation of this momentous subject—the transmission of intellectual and moral qualities from parents to offspring.

A deep conviction of the truth and importance of this theory, and the many benefits that would flow from a knowledge of its principles, and an obedience to its laws, renders the publication, in the estimation of the writer, a solemn duty; hoping that, thereby, the attention of her countrywomen will be directed to the subject, and their feelings enlisted in the great cause of humanity, the improvement of the human race. For, if they believe in this theory, and act upon that belief, they assuredly will accomplish the high mission assigned to them by the Creator, and also attain that degree of intellectual and moral perfection, for which they are by nature so eminently designed.

"Let a person of the most ordinary capacity," says a British writer, "once acquire a sincere and lasting interest in any thing capable of affording exercise to the understanding, and see how that *interest will call forth faculties never previously observed in him.* This is one reason why periods of skepticism, though they may produce extraordinary individuals, are seldom rich in the general stock of persons of talent. For, in an age of strong convictions, the second and third-rate of talents, being combined with earnestness, grow up and attain full development and fructify; but in an age of uncertainty, none but the first order of intellects are able to lay for themselves so firm and solid a foundation of what they believe to be truth, as they can build upon afterward in full self-reliance, and stake the repose of their consciences upon without anxiety. The people of second-rate talents *feel sure of nothing, therefore they care for nothing, and by an inevitable chain of consequences accomplish nothing.*"

The truth of the preceding observation is illustrated in the history of our own country. Columbus, from his knowledge of navigation, and from his study of the natural sciences, was led to believe that there was another continent on the other side of the globe. To discover the truth of this belief, he sacrificed all his worldly interests, and suffered extreme anxiety and distress, in wandering from court to court in Europe, in search of those capable of assisting him in his great undertaking. He was looked upon as an enthusiast, and his theory rejected, until he came before Isabella of Spain. Her strong mind and quick perception at once saw the probability of it, even after it had been coldly and sneeringly treated by the learned men and courtiers about the throne. Disregarding the selfish suggestions of the mean spirits of that age, she made the noble declaration: "I will assume the undertaking for my own crown of Castile, and I am ready to pawn my jewels to defray the expense of it, if the funds in the treasury should be found inadequate!"

Again, our pilgrim fathers, through a firm faith in the truths of the Protestant religion, were enabled to resign their home and country, and commit themselves and their families to the dangers of the mighty deep, an uncongenial clime, and a wilderness of savages. They were sustained through unparalleled sufferings and privations, by an elevating belief in the all-protecting power of the Almighty. A deep conviction of the equal and inalienable rights of man, impelled the descendants of the pilgrims to oppose tyranny and oppression, and assert and attain that independence, of which the present generation are enjoying the fruits. And there is a deep-rooted belief in the hearts of all the friends of humanity of the present age, that if our wise constitution were administered by heads as clear and hearts as pure and disinterested as those who framed it, we might look forward to no remote period, and behold all the civilized nations of the world remodeled, by the example of the prosperity, happiness, and virtue attained by an enlightened people, under a free government!

When we reflect upon the privileges we enjoy, and the liberal institutions conferred on us, by the diligent, self-denying, prudent habits and pious liberality of those who preceded us, is it not incumbent on us to do all in our power to promote the happiness and well-being of future generations? And how can this be done more effectually than by transmitting to them sound constitutions and virtuous inclinations? That this is practicable, the writer trusts in the following pages to show; and also, that it is a power and duty that devolves principally upon the mother, for the due performance of which she ought to be held responsible, at least by public opinion.

"Minds," says Madame Roland, "which have any claims to greatness, are capable of divesting themselves of all selfish considerations; they feel that they belong to the whole human race, and their views are directed to posterity alone." With such minds our country abounds; they only require to perceive the true interest of their offspring, to be enabled to devote the best energies of their lives to promote it. ——"I firmly believe," says the Rev. Timothy Flint, "that if this world is ever regenerated, it will be by the power and influence of woman."

TRANSMISSION

OF

INTELLECTUAL AND MORAL QUALITIES.

CHAPTER I.

IMPROVEMENT OF OFFSPRING.

Every century, since the revival of literature, appears to have been occupied in discovering and establishing some new and important truth. The power and application of steam in physics, and the discovery and confirmation of Phrenology in metaphysics, have been the principal objects of interest in the present century. The former has multiplied power to an incalculable extent, and almost annihilated time and space; while the latter has scarcely advanced further than to disclose to man the nature and extent of his sentiments, passions, and intellect. But to what great and important results this science is destined to lead, time only can unfold. It has, however, already made known to those who will see by its light, not only the certainty, but also the means of perpetuating talent and virtue from parent to offspring. This subject, possibly, will occupy the attention of the twentieth century; and so general is the belief in the omnipotence of education, that it may require a whole century to apply its truths to the practical elevation of the race. For there are many persons even in this enlightened age, who believe with Helvetius, that all men are born with equal mental capacities, and that education and circumstances develop genius or stifle it. "To which opinion," says Carlyle, "I should as soon agree as to this other, that an acorn might, by favorable or unfavorable influence of soil or climate, be nursed into a cabbage, or the cabbage-seed into an oak. Nevertheless, I, too, acknowledge the all but omnipotence of early culture and nurture ; thereby we have either a doddard dwarf bush, or high-towering, wide-shadowing tree ; either a sick, yellow cabbage, or an edible, luxuriant, green one." Talent or Genius—the God-like attribute of man, that Elijah-mantle falling upon so few of the sons of Adam—is generally considered as an accidental, though priceless gift of nature. So entirely has this condition been regarded the result of chance, or other uncontrollable cause, that the question, Can we by our own efforts obtain this blessing—shall our unborn infant possess the link, uniting mortal with immortal nature ? has never entered the mind of the parent, or become a subject of consideration.

"Yet," says that close observer, Dr. Good, in his "Book of Nature," "the variable talents of the mind are as certainly propagated as the various features of the body ; how, or by what means, we know not, but the fact is incontrovertible. Wit and dullness, genius and idiotism, run in direct lines from generation to generation ; hence the moral characters of families, of tribes, and of whole nations."

The learned writer could not fail to remark, and admit the numerous evidences that met him in all directions, of the result of a fixed law. But the *modus operandi* by which that law operated in transmitting peculiar qualities of mind from parent to offspring, he was, as yet, unable to point out.

Great pains have been taken by the biographers of eminent individuals to ascertain and point out at what school or college they were educated, under what able professor, and the particular course of study pursued.* Yet how unimportant are these facts, when we reflect, that a vast number of youth, of only common capacities, pass through the same college, under the same able professors, without having been raised above mediocrity ? The inference, then, is, that the biographer must go further back than education to elicit the true

* "He who can convince the world of the importance of the laws of hereditary descent, and induce mankind to act accordingly, will do more good to them, and contribute more to their improvement, than all institutions and all systems of education."—*Spurzheim's Education.*

cause which produced this pre-eminence in the subject of his memoir. To what great results might not such inquiry lead; what bounds could we set to the career of mental and physical improvement which it would open to the race of man? Looking back upon the discoveries of the last fifty years, and then beholding the great and important truths which have been developed and established by wisdom and science, who shall presume to prescribe bounds to the future investigations of human intellect? For has not the great and wise Creator given man his peculiar reasoning faculties for the purpose that universally, and as well *here as elsewhere*, he might acquire the direction of events, by discovering the *laws regulating their successions?*

It cannot be denied that if the same amount of knowledge and care which has been taken to improve the domestic animals, had been bestowed upon the human species, during the last century, there would not have been so great a number of immoral patients for the prisons, or the lunatic asylums, as there are at present. That the human species is as susceptible of improvement as domestic animals, who can deny? Then is it not strange that man, possessing so much information on this subject, and acknowledging the laws which govern such matters, should lose sight of those laws in perpetuating his own species? Yet, how extremely short-sighted is that individual, who, in forming a matrimonial connection, overlooks the important consideration of the quality of the physical and mental constitution which his children will be likely to inherit? And, also, that a great portion of the happiness or misery of his future life will depend upon the conduct of those children; and again, that their manifestations, whether good or evil, will be the effect of the mental and physical organization which they inherit.* The time is fast approaching when men will

* "The laws of hereditary descent should be attended to, not only with respect to organic life, but also to the manifestations of mind, since these depend upon the nervous system. There are many examples on record, of certain feelings, or intellectual powers, being inherited in whole families. Now, if it be ascertained that the hereditary condition of the brain is the cause, there is a great additional motive to be careful in the

feel the necessity of giving more attention to this subject; for Phrenology, the science which tests these matters, is rapidly spreading; consequently, the parent cannot hope much longer to receive the sympathy of the world for the perverse conduct of his child; on the contrary, the child will be commiserated for having inherited active animal propensities, accompanied by deficient moral and reflective organs.

Impressed with the importance of these views, the natural dispositions and capabilities of children, whether inherited or produced by favorable or unfavorable circumstances (operating on the parents previous to the birth), became to the writer a subject of the deepest interest. From observation, it appeared that the first children of very young mothers, whatever sprightliness they might evince from a high flow of animal spirits, were generally deficient in strength of intellect and stability of character. How, indeed, could it be otherwise, when the parents had spent the first years of married life in a career of dissipated amusements, in which the cultivation of the mind had been totally neglected—neither reading, rational conversation, nor reflection had been practiced to exer-

choice of a partner in marriage. No person of sense can be indifferent about having selfish or benevolent, stupid or intelligent children.

"An objection may be made against the doctrine of hereditary effects resulting from the laws of propagation, viz., that in large families there are individuals of very different capacities.

"This observation shows at least that the children are born with different dispositions, and it proves nothing against the laws of propagation. The young ones of animals that propagate indiscriminately, are very different; but when the races are pure, and all conditions attended to, the nature of the young can be determined beforehand. As long as the races of mankind are mixed, their progeny must vary extremely. But let persons of determinate dispositions breed in and in, and the races will become distinct. Moreover, the condition of the mother is commonly less valued than it ought to be. It is, however, observed, that boys commonly resemble their mother, and girls their father; and that men of great talents generally descend from intelligent mothers. But as long as eminent men are marrying to partners of inferior capacities, the qualities of the offspring must be uncertain. The Arabs seem to understand the great importance of females, since they do not allow to sell females to foreigners, and note the nobility of their horse after the females."—*Spurzheim's Education.*

cise and strengthen it? What wonder, then, that the minds of their offspring should resemble the first-born of Jacob, the luckless Reuben, who, "unstable as water, was doomed never to excel?"

In biography, it may also be observed, that those men most conspicuous for native strength of mind, were not generally the first-born of their parents. Dr. Franklin was the fifteenth child of his father and the eighth of his mother; Benjamin West was the tenth child of his parents; the mother of Dr. Samuel Johnson was past forty at the period of his birth; and the mother of Washington was twenty-eight years of age when her illustrious son was born. We might also cite the names of Lord Bacon, Fenelon, Sir William Jones, and Baron Cuvier, who were born after their parents had attained the full maturity of their mental and physical powers.

The world is greatly indebted to the "Constitution of Man," by George Combe, for the first clear views and forcible illustrations on the hereditary transmission of qualities. Mr. Combe, however, draws one conclusion, which admits of much doubt, as to its truth and justness. He assumes that the particular turn or tone of mind is given at the moment of conception. This opinion is in direct opposition to the experience of many strong-minded, observing mothers, who have recognized in their children the same sentiments in which they indulged, and the peculiar habits which they had practiced, during the whole period of their pregnancy. To such testimony, the most ingenious hypothesis must give way; and from such evidence it must be inferred, that the brain of the unborn child is powerfully influenced by the thoughts and sentiments of its mother; and that the particular organs which her habits and pursuits bring into the greatest activity, become most prominently developed in the brain of her child.(*a*) Hence, it ought to be an object of the first importance with every woman about to become a mother, to exercise her mental perceptions, reasoning faculties, and moral sentiments, to their full extent—to cultivate kind feelings and noble aspirations—to indulge in no pursuits unworthy of a rational immortal being—and to ascertain and live in accordance with the laws instituted by the Creator for the preservation of health—so that her child may be perfect in mental, moral, and physical organization.*

In the life of Napoleon, we learn that his mother was, for some months previous to his birth, sharing the fortunes of war with her husband, in constant peril and danger, and passed much of her time on horseback:—any person accustomed to this mode of riding, must acknowledge that it causes exciting, aspiring emotions. What conveys to the mind of man a greater consciousness of power than to be raised, as it were, above earth, and direct at will an animal so much his superior in physical strength? There we can have the causes that produced a mind like Napoleon's. The active and health-inspiring habits of his mother gave him a strong constitution and great physical powers of endurance, while the excitement induced by constant exposure to danger and peril conduced to an activity of intellect highly favorable in producing corresponding qualities in the mind of her unborn child. And behold, the first manifestations of the young Napoleon were pride, an indomitable spirit, a passion for warlike pursuits; these being innate and constantly exercised, increased to such a degree, that nothing short of the subjugation of a world could bound his ambition.†

* "The innate constitution, which depends upon both parents, and the state of the mother during pregnancy, is the basis of all future development."—*Spurzheim's Education.*

† We almost universally, in looking at any state of society, take it as we find it, without inquiring into the causes why it is as it is. If men and women are moral and intelligent, we accept them so, and are gratified; if they are ignorant and immoral, we lament over their condition, without ever allowing our minds to revert to the cause why they are thus. Historians, in giving the character of any age, describe men as they are, as political and civil revolutions have made them, as great national calamities or enterprises have made them, as indolence or industry have made them, as vice or virtue have made them; but, except in rare instances, they never describe men *as women have made them.* This, the primary source of individual and of national character, is left untouched. True, we are sometimes informed, in regard to a character conspicuous for moral or intellectual greatness, that he "owed much to his mother."

In our own country, we have a venerable example of a mother being honored by a whole nation for the good work she had done, in rearing a

The authoress is perfectly aware that the above theory is not new, and that it has been advanced by many writers, in a general way, from Tacitus down to the present time. Sir James Mackintosh, in speaking of the great genius of Count

great man, to be also a good one. No republican can pass the tomb of Washington's mother without feeling the heart warm with gratitude toward her. See how much has sprung from this single example of female influence. Had Washington inherited the same talents with less moral purpose; had his better feelings not been trained and stimulated by the action of a highly moral and intellectual mind upon them, he might have proved himself equally well skilled in the field, and able in council, but where would have been the philanthropy, benevolence, and justice, that hushed the voice of ambition the moment a people's freedom was won, and made him reject with indignation the glitter of an offered crown? Where would have been that love of his fellow-men that drew him from the retirement he so much coveted and enjoyed, and made him willingly resume the toils of public life, which led him to spare no efforts to place around the freedom of his country every guard that could protect it from the inroads of the ambitious and unprincipled?

"Contrast this son and mother with two other individuals, bearing the same relation to each other, who, like these, have long since gone to the final home of man. This mother, highly intellectual, highly spirited, highly intelligent and accomplished, but destitute of those high moral qualities which win our love, though linked with humbler powers of mind: this mother transmitted to her son all the powers of her intellect, and the intense spirit of her character, but she had no moral excellence to implant them; she had none to cherish in his childhood. Out at a military review but a few days before his birth—in camp during many months previous—surrounded with, and enjoying all the pomp and circumstance of war—familiarized with, and reconciled to its horrors and anguish—it is no wonder that her son was born with an appetite for blood; no wonder that, during his life, the Continent of Europe was made one vast altar, on which human sacrifice was offered to the ambition of a Napoleon.

"Have such facts no interest for female minds? Do we see nothing in them to arouse our noblest ambition—to stir the soul to noble execution? Shall the voice of ages appeal to us in vain? Shall reason continue to urge her claim upon us only to be denied? Shall duty plead in vain with us? Have the happiness of our children and of society no weight in our minds, compared with the follies of fashion, and the momentary pursuit of pleasure? Are our patriotism and philanthropy worthless, as they are asserted to be? If not, let us prove it by showing that we can cast away trifles when they interfere with the discharge of our duty. If not, let us show that we are women, worthy of being the mothers of a free nation."—*Mrs. E. W. Farnam.*

D'Alban, says, "His mother, though in an humble station, was a woman of superior mind. All great men have had able mothers." Biography furnishes sufficient examples to prove the truth of this opinion. Those examples, however, require to be brought forward and forced upon general observation, for this theory is a theory that will require manifold and striking facts to establish it, as it will have to contend with the pride and prejudice of the unreflecting. (*b*)

CHAPTER II.

DISPOSITION OF THE MOTHER INHERITED BY HER OFFSPRING.

It will be seen, in the following extract from "Falk's Life of Goethe," how frequently the result of this theory has been observed; yet it appears to have been observed as a mere phenomenon of nature, and dismissed with an idle exclamation of wonder. Hence, the principles which might have been deduced from it, for the improvement of future generations, have been overlooked.

"It has often been remarked, that great and eminent men receive from their mothers, even before they see the light, half the mental disposition and other peculiarities of character by which they are afterward distinguished." "Thus, in Goethe's character, we find a most sensitive shrinking from all intense impressions, which by every means, and under every circumstance of his life, he sought to ward off from himself. We find the same peculiarities in his mother, as we shall see from the following curious and characteristic traits. They were related to me by a female friend who was extremely intimate with her at Frankfort.

"Goethe's mother, whenever she hired a servant, used to make the following condition: You are not to tell me any thing horrible, afflicting, or agitating, whether it happened in my own house, in the town, or in the neighborhood. I desire, once for all, that I may hear nothing of the kind. If it concerns me, I shall know it soon enough; if it does not concern me, I have nothing whatever to do with it. Even if there should be a fire in the street in which I live, I am to know nothing of it till it is absolutely necessary that I should."

After relating many other striking peculiarities (more amiable than the above) of the mind and character of Goethe's mother, in which her son exactly resembled her, Falk adds: "Those who were at all acquainted with Goethe's person and manners, will instantly agree with me, that much of this amiable temper, and of this vein of *naive* humor, which nothing in life or death could subdue, flowed in full tide from her veins into his. We shall give further proof of this hereafter from the history of his early years, as well as of his more serious moods, from the latter."

If such facts as this had been more generally observed and carefully reported, principles might have been deduced from them of vital importance to mankind, and that which at present is advanced as a theory, might have long since been established as a truth.

Yet it may be said, Is not this an absurd theory, in giving so much power to the mother, and considering the father of so little importance? But if it be an absurdity, it has been practiced to the full extent heretofore, in the opposite direction, without having been noticed. The father, however, is of the utmost importance; for does not his conduct influence the thoughts and feelings of his wife? And can he not, by the softening influence of kindness and affection, mould her to his will, or to whatever her natural capability will admit? We often see children inheriting not only the form and features, but the intellect, also, of the father. And this most frequently occurs in families where the husband is in the habit of spending much of his time in the society of his wife; treating her with delicacy and respect; calling into exercise the highest attributes of her nature, and is enshrined in her heart as the model of all excellence and goodness. Possibly, her ardent desire that her children should resemble their father, in part, produces the effect.

So, also, may the evil dispositions inherited from the parents be accounted for. The bad passions of the wife may be roused into activity by the injustice, cruelty, or neglect of her husband; so that her unborn child may be afflicted by their baneful influence. That this was the case with Lord Byron, no unprejudiced mind can doubt, who is acquainted with the history and character of his parents. With that of his father, we will not sully these pages; but of his mother, Dr. Madden says: "Little is known of the early history of Mrs. Byron, but quite enough of the extraordinary violence of her temper, and its effects upon her health after any sudden explosion of her choler, to warrant the belief that some cerebral disease occasioned that degree of excitability which is quite unparalleled in the history of any lady of sane mind." On one occasion, we are told by Moore, that "at the Edinburgh Theatre she was so affected by the performance, that she fell into violent fits, and was carried out of the theatre screaming loudly." Madden also says, "that Byron was the child of passion, born in bitterness,

'And nurtured in convulsions.'

"All the elements of domestic discord were let loose upon his youth—a home without a tie to bind his affections to its hearth—a mother disqualified by the frenzied violence of her temper for the offices of a parent; and if he would escape from the recollection of that violence, no father's fondness to fall back upon, and no virtue coupled with his memory to make the contemplation a pleasure to his child."

From Dr. Madden's account of Mrs. Byron, it would seem that Lord Byron inherited the poetic temperament from his mother; and in the following brief description of some of his innate characteristics, there can be clearly traced a combination of the vices of both his parents.* "Never," says Macaulay, "had any writer so vast a command of the whole

* Yet that these could have been modified and subdued by a wise education and careful moral culture, no one will doubt. Perhaps the most striking illustration of the all but omnipotence of early culture is shown in the lives and characters of Rev. Timothy Dwight and Aaron Burr. These gentlemen were cousins; their mothers were the daughters of President Edwards, and are said to have inherited much of the uncommon powers of their father; from which it may be inferred, that the great mental capability of their sons was also inherited; and, that the difference in their moral characters arose from the circumstance that the former grew up under the judicious care of an affectionate and pious mother, while the latter lost both of his parents in infancy. This also shows the power of the mother in shaping the future character of her child.

eloquence of scorn, misanthropy, and despair. That Marah was never dry. No art could sweeten, no draughts could exhaust its perennial waters of bitterness. Never was there such variety in monotony as that of Byron. From maniac laughter to piercing lamentation, there was not a single note of human anguish of which he was not master. Year after year, and month after month, he continued to repeat, that to be wretched is the destiny of all; that to be eminently wretched, is the destiny of the eminent; that all the desires by which we are cursed lead alike to misery—if they are not gratified, to the misery of disappointment; if they are gratified, to the misery of satiety. His principal heroes are men who have arrived by different roads to the same goal of despair, who are sick of life, who are at war with society, who are supported in their anguish only by an unconquerable pride, resembling that of Prometheus on the rock, or Satan in the burning marl; who can master their agonies by the force of their will; who, to the last, defy the whole powers of earth and heaven. He always described himself as a man of the same kind, with his favorite creations; as a man whose heart had been withered, whose capacity for happiness was gone, and could not be restored; but whose invincible spirit dared the worst that could befall him here or hereafter."

Macaulay also says, that "from the poetry of Lord Byron his youthful admirers drew a system of ethics, compounded of misanthropy and voluptuousness; a system in which the two great commandments were, to hate your neighbor and to love your neighbor's wife." Here, again, were manifested the violent and bitter temper of his mother, and the sensual propensities of his father. The enthusiastic admirers of Lord Byron will perhaps consider this an unjust and unreasonable view of the character of the poet, and an attack on the sacred attributes of genius itself. But let us beg of them not to confound the glare of an ignis-fatuus, shining only to delude, with the heavenward aspirations of a Milton or a Cowper, whose aim was to exalt, to enlighten, and to spiritualize mankind.

An invaluable moral for the instruction of youth is to be

drawn from the abrupt, fitful, and desponding life of Lord Byron, when placed in opposition to the long, happy, and useful one of William Wilberforce. And if "the philosophy of history is experience teaching by example," then is it not the duty of the mother to point out these examples to her children? Showing them how poor a gift is intellect, even the most transcendent, when unaccompanied by moral sentiments, and how happy the life, and how honored the memory of that being, who, with a self-denying, Christian spirit, seeks to glorify his Creator by doing good to his creatures.

In the following extract from an article in the Foreign Quarterly, on the Life and Works of Baron Cuvier, we find the fact also noticed, that great men have generally been the sons of women of superior understanding. "His parents were not in easy circumstances, his father being a half-pay officer, who, after forty years' service, was unable to afford to his son more than the common advantages of a provincial school education. At fifty years of age he had married a young and accomplished woman, who became the mother of George Cuvier, and by whom his early years were guarded with affectionate and judicious care. Her more than parental solicitude for his mental improvement justifies us in adding the instance of Cuvier to the many examples of distinguished men who, perhaps, owed a considerable share of their greatness to the attainments and character of a mother of superior understanding. History presents us with numerous instances of this nature; and they seem the more curious when contrasted with an equally well-established fact, that the children of very eminent men have seldom been distinguished for ability, and have frequently proved either feeble in mind, or of precocious talents, and a fragile, unenduring frame. In many families rendered illustrious by one great name, the father and grandfather of the distinguished member of the family were men of good understandings, without being brilliant;* but after the

* This was the case in the family of Dr. Franklin. If, however, the theory we have advanced be correct, it requires no hypothesis, in this instance, to explain why, "after the great man, the line immediately and sensibly declined." For, if Dr. Franklin had married into a family as

great man, the line has immediately and sensibly declined. The physiological hypothesis may be, that the offspring of men devoted to the pursuit of fame in arduous paths, are necessarily of imperfect organization; or that there is some law which, permitting an ascending scale of intellect to render families eminent in a generation, checks the vain aspirations after perpetuity of influence, by withdrawing the gift when it has reached a certain elevation, leaving the proud edifice of their fame, which once they flattered themselves would reach to the heavens, a mere unfinished monument. However this may be, Cuvier's mother was worthy to bear such a son. She watched over his infirm infancy with the tenderest care, and she saw and directed the development of his wonderful faculties. "The joys of parents," says Bacon, "are secret;" and great, although it may have been unexpressed and inexpressible, must have been the joy of such a mother watching such a son. He was singularly diligent and thoughtful, and when no more than ten years old, was not only a delighted reader of Buffon, but faithfully copied all the plates, and colored them according to the directions which he had read. Accustomed as we are to speak of Cuvier as the great interpreter of nature, it is a pleasure to read that his affection for this admirable parent was cherished by him to the latest period of his life; and that nothing gave the great philosopher and harassed minister more delight, than when some friendly hand had placed in his apartment the flowers which his mother had taught him in his youthful days to love.

It is truly astonishing how rapidly mental philosophy has advanced, since it has been decided that the brain is the organ of the mind. And this decision is of more recent date than many persons probably imagine. Even Dr. Lawrence found it necessary to demonstrate this fact in his lectures on the Natural History of Man, delivered in 1828, in London. The mental philosopher now has something tangible and useful on which to exercise his reflections. Accordingly, he finds the

conspicuous for native strength of understanding as that of his own father's and mother's, it is more than probable that his immediate descendants would not have been added to the general rule above noticed.

talents of individuals to increase in the ratio of their perfection in this organ, from the most imperfect in the idiot, to the most perfect in the man of transcendent genius. "And as certain knowledge obtained through some of its convolutions," says a medical writer, "is perfect in some persons, it follows that an individual having a brain perfectly developed and symmetrically formed in all its parts, would be capable of, and might acquire, perfect knowledge in all its departments." Of the truth of this remark, Cuvier is an example: "For," continues the reviewer, "his vast and diversified undertakings prove that he possessed a brain of the most perfect organization, as much as its ample developments, and the depth of its convolutions, and the absolute weight of its cerebral lobes. His habits of life show that his superiority to other men arose from the most diligent employment of his time, of every possible interval that could be taken from public business, from social duties, and from needful rest. But so limited was the time that he could absolutely command, that we see beyond dispute, that no mere plodding industry could have effected what he performed, and that the rapidity of his mental operations was no less wonderful than their power." Thus we learn that Cuvier possessed a fine nervous temperament, and a superior organized brain; and this it was that marked him from the crowd of aimless and undistinguished men, enabled him to unfold to an admiring world the more profound mysteries of nature, ensured to him personal safety in the political convulsions through which he passed, and conferred immortality on his name. Hence the importance of the inquiry, How, and by what means, can such qualities be perpetuated? And this question is of more importance to parents than is generally suspected. For, a child possessing the above temperament and organization, if properly cultivated and directed, will become a quiet observer of nature, reflective and studious, himself a delightful companion, and an object of interesting contemplation, as one of the most perfect works of a beneficent Creator. Whereas, a child of the opposite temperament and organization, which is the *vital* and *animal*, is perfectly restless and selfish, ever seeking his own gratification in opposition to every principle of justice and duty, is difficult to govern or to instruct; and of this class are those "who bring the gray hairs of their parents with sorrow to the grave." "Meantime," says Kepler, "*the strong are born of the strong, and the good of the good.* What we find in nature ill prepared, let us endeavor to correct."

CHAPTER III.

PROOF OF COMBINATION OF QUALITIES.

It is to the theory which we have attempted to illustrate in the preceding pages, that we must have recourse, to account for and explain the singular combination of talent and error which is exhibited in the biography of many eminent individuals. Among these we notice, in strong relief, the character of that most eccentric of monarchs, James I., of England, and VI., of Scotland. Various causes, not necessary to be enumerated here, have combined to produce much misconception in regard to the true character of this personage. We annex a sketch from a master hand, forcible, graphic, and true ; one who has rarely, if ever, been equaled in this species of portraiture.

Macaulay, in tracing the struggle for political and religious liberty of the sixteenth century, thus speaks of Elizabeth, and her successor, James. " The conduct of the extraordinary woman who then governed England, is an admirable study for politicians who live in unquiet times. It shows how thoroughly she understood the people whom she ruled, and the crisis in which she was called to act. What she held, she held firmly ; what she gave, she gave graciously. She saw that it was necessary to make a concession to the nation, and she made it—not grudgingly—not tardily—not as a matter of bargain and sale—not, in a word, as Charles the First would have made it—but promptly and cordially. Before a bill could be framed, or an address presented, she applied a remedy to the evil of which the nation complained. She expressed, in the warmest terms, her gratitude to her faithful Commons for detecting abuses which interested persons had concealed from her. If her successors had inherited her wisdom with her crown, Charles the First might have died of old age, and James the Second would never have seen St. Germains.

"She died, and her kingdom passed to one who was, in his own opinion, the greatest master of kingcraft that ever lived; who was, in truth, one of those kings whom God seems to send for the express purpose of hastening revolutions. Of all the enemies of liberty whom England has produced, he was at once the most harmless and the most provoking. His office resembled that of the man who, in a Spanish bull-fight, goads the torpid savage to fury by shaking a red rag in the air, and now and then throwing a dart sharp enough to sting, but too small to injure. The policy of wise tyrants has always been, to cover their violent acts with popular forms. James was always obtruding his despotic theories on his subjects without the slightest necessity. His foolish talk exasperated them infinitely more than forced loans or benevolences would have done. Yet, in practice, no king held his prerogatives less tenaciously. He neither gave way gracefully to the advancing spirit of liberty, nor took vigorous measures to stop it; but retreated before it with ludicrous haste, blustering and insulting as he retreated. The English people had been governed for nearly a hundred and fifty years by princes who, whatever might have been their frailties or vices, had all possessed great force of character, and who, whether loved or hated, had always been feared. Now, at length, for the first time since the day when the sceptre of Henry the Fourth dropped from the hand of his lethargic grandson, England had a king whom she despised.

"The follies and vices of the man increased the contempt which was produced by the feeble policy of the sovereign. The indecorous gallantries of the court, the habits of gross intoxication in which even the ladies indulged, were alone sufficient to disgust a people whose manners were beginning to be strongly tinctured with austerity. But these were trifles. Crimes of the most frightful kind had been discovered; others were suspected. The strange story of the Gowries was not forgotten. The ignominious fondness of the king for his minions—the perjuries, the sorceries, the poisonings, which his chief favorites had planned within the walls of his palace—the pardon which, in direct violation of his duty and of his word, he had granted to the mysterious threats of a murderer—made him an object of loathing to many of his subjects." "This was not all. The most ridiculous weaknesses seemed to meet in the wretched Solomon of Whitehall—pedantry, buffoonry, garrulity, low curiosity, the most contemptible cowardice. Nature and education had done their best to produce a finished specimen of all that a king ought not to be." And this king was the son of Mary, Queen of Scots, who, in the twenty-third year of her age, married her first cousin, a youth of nineteen.

This marriage was not the dictate of state policy, but a transitory passion produced in the queen by the outward graces of Darnley. The alliance, according to Mr. Combe, promised any thing except intellectual or moral offspring.* Keith gives the following account of Mary's youthful husband. "He was one of the tallest and handsomest young men of the age; he had a comely face and a pleasant countenance; a most dexterous horseman, and exceedingly well skilled in all gentle exercises; prompt and ready for all games and sports; much given to the diversions of hawking and hunting, to horse-racing and music, especially playing on the lute; he could speak and write well, and was bountiful and liberal enough. To balance these good natural qualifications, he was much addicted to intemperance, to base and unmanly pleasures; he was haughty and proud, and so very weak in mind as to be a prey to all that came near him; he

* "When two parties marry very young, the eldest of their children generally inherit a less favorable development of the moral and intellectual organs than those produced in more mature age. The animal organs in the human race are, in general, most vigorous in early life, and this energy appears to cause them to be most readily transmitted to offspring." Mr. Combe also shows the deteriorating effects of marriages between blood relations, which is now too well established to be doubted. Yet, regardless of the importance of this knowledge, it is a common practice of the novel-writer to create a passion between youthful cousins, and then have the folly to call their union a happy consummation of the story.

was inconstant, credulous, and facile—unable to abide by any resolution—capable of being imposed upon by designing men; and could conceal no secret, let it tend ever so much to his own welfare or detriment."

The beauty, grace, and accomplishments of Mary, have been dwelt upon by the historian and the novelist; but, from her conduct in life, it cannot be inferred that she possessed either strength of understanding or purity of heart. For proof of this, we refer the reader to the notes on this subject in Hume's History of England. After examining these statements, the unprejudiced mind must ascribe the strong tendency to sensuality in James to both his parents; while his partial idiocy and nervous trembling at the sight of naked steel, was caused, doubtless, by the terror which his mother experienced at the brutal murder of Rizzio in her presence, a few months previous to his birth.*

Yet is it not humiliating to reflect, that from a union of two young persons, the aim and end of whose existence appeared to be the gratification of their selfish passions, should proceed a race of kings who were to involve their country in revolution and bloodshed for nearly a century? Let us not, however, question the mysterious ways of Providence; for who can tell how much the present prosperity of this country is indebted to the weak and wicked race of the Stuarts, whose licentiousness and folly so disgusted the most virtuous and high-minded portion of their subjects, that many of them, to escape from the effects of it, emigrated to America? And to their intellectual, moral, and energetic posterity, is to be mainly attributed the present prosperity and happiness of the country.†

* "So palpable, indeed, is the connection between the mother's state and the constitution of the future child, that the philosopher, Hobbes, unhesitatingly ascribed his own excessive timidity and nervous sensibility to the fright in which his mother lived before he was born, on account of the threatened invasion of the Spanish Armada, and which affected her to such a pitch on the news of its actual approach, as to bring on premature birth."—*Combe on Infancy*, p. 65.

† Those who have doubts on this subject, and also upon the transmission of moral qualities, should inform themselves respecting the state of

In approaching our own times, another remarkable case presents itself—the son of Napoleon. The private character of both Maria Louisa and her son afford a lamentable instance of the direct descent of strong propensities and weak intellect, unaccompanied by moral sentiments. The scandalous chronicle of the court of Parma, and the well-known habits of the Duke of Reichstadt, furnish sufficient evidence that the mother's nature prevailed in the offspring; and that the father's anticipations of the future greatness of the new-born heir to his monarchy never could have been realized.

Napoleon was once told, "Sire, the education of your son should be watched over with great attention; he must be educated so that he may replace you."* "Replace me?" he answered: "I could not replace myself; I am the child of circumstances." True; and he might have added, the child of a very different mother, whose energetic mind was affected by circumstances very dissimilar from those which operated on the mother of the young King of Rome. Maria Louisa was of an inert, lymphatic temperament; her habits indolent, luxurious, and sensual; and in every respect the opposite of Letitia Romilini, the mother of Napoleon. "The circumstances," says Dr. Combe, "in which the brightest order of

society in New South Wales, a community of the same Anglo-Saxon origin as this country, but whose progenitors were of a very different moral character from the "Pilgrim Fathers." Hence the difference between the present state of society in the two countries.

* A very different opinion of the power of education is held by Dr. James Johnson, who says, "To expect a good crop of science or literature from some intellects, is about as hopeless as to expect olives to thrive on the craggy summit of Ben Nevis, or the pineapple to expand amid the glaciers of Grinderwalde. Yet, from these sterile regions of mind, the hapless pedagogue is expected, by parents, to turn out Miltons, Lockes, and Newtons, with as much facility as a gardener raises brocoli or cauliflower from the rich alluvial grounds about Fulham! It is in vain for poor Syntax to urge in excuse, that

'Non ex aliquovis ligno fit Mercurius.'

This is only adding insult to injury, in the eyes of parents, who consider that any hint of imperfection in the offspring, is, by innuendo, a reproach cast upon themselves."

minds most frequently appear, are, where the father is healthy and active, and the mother unites an energetic character with vigorous bodily health, or with some *high and sustaining excitement animating all her mental and bodily functions.* The mother of Bonaparte was of this description ; and the mothers of most of the celebrated men will be found to have been more or less distinguished for similar characteristics ; and accordingly, how often, in the biographies of men of genius, do we remark, that it was the mother who first perceived and fanned the flame that burst into after brightness ?"

The union of two, each having an excess of the propensities, will result in an increased malignity of evil passions in their descendants. Such is the record of that distinguished family of ancient Rome, which ended in the monster Nero. Julia, the daughter of Augustus Cæsar, and the great-grandmother of Nero, was a woman of dissolute conduct, libidinous passions, and abandoned infamy. Her daughter, Agrippina, possessed an uncontrollable and violent temper, and was insatiably ambitious of power. For her own aggrandizement, she was ever ready to sacrifice the interests, or even the lives of her children. Her only redeemable quality was chastity ; and, although Germanicus, "the worthiest son of the worthiest parents," was her husband, her children appear to have inherited her fierce disposition. Caligula, that emperor of Rome who wished the Roman people had but one neck, that he might, at a blow, destroy the whole race, was one of them, and Agrippina, of infamous memory, the mother of Nero, was another. The paternal grandfather of Nero was Lucius Domitius Ænobarbus, a man of impetuous temper, violent, proud, extravagant, and cruel. The life of his son, Cneius Domitius, was a series of evil deeds ; he married his cousin, Agrippina, and used to remark, "that from himself and Agrippina nothing good or valuable could come." They were the parents of Nero, whose name is now another word for the most savage cruelty.

Again, at a more recent period, we find a family in which the vices of the parents assumed an increased degree of malignity in the offspring—the Borgia family, of whom Pope

Alexander VI., and his infamous son and daughter, Cæsar and Lucrezia, were members, whose vices and crimes surpassed, in atrocity, all those who preceded them.

They are thus spoken of by a writer of the present day: "The unholy trio—Pope Alexander VI., who had gained the chair of St. Peter by the most unblushing simony, his daughter Lucrezia, and his son Cæsar—was a choice assemblage, who had assumed a right to indulge in all the odious want of faith of miserable modern intriguers, as well as in all the odious excesses and nameless vices of a Nero and a Tiberius: indeed, it is doubtful whether the worst character in Suetonius would not have paused awhile before he associated with Cæsar Borgia."

The lives of Catherine de Medici, the talented, the profligate, the cruel, and her equally sensual and vicious sons, are as forcible examples of the descent of hereditary vices, as that of Henry IV. of France, and his ancestors, are of hereditary virtues.

The illustrious Margaret, queen of Navarre, and her equally strong-minded and virtuous husband, Henry d'Albert, were the grand-parents of Henry IV., the most beloved and honored of all the French monarchs. His mother, Jane d'Albert, ranks high among women distinguished for their great and good qualities. She possessed a strong and vigorous understanding, a cultivated mind, and an acquaintance with the languages. She left several compositions, both in prose and verse. D'Aubine, speaking of Jane, queen of Navarre, says, "She possessed a manly mind, an elevated capacity, and a magnanimity of soul proof against all the storms of adversity." De Thou concurs in these eulogiums on her talents and greatness of mind. A son and daughter survived her; the former, the celebrated Henry IV., was the most amiable and illustrious of the French monarchs; the latter, Catherine of Navarre, emulated the example of her mother, and preserved a prudent and exemplary conduct in the midst of a corrupt court, and was tenderly esteemed by her brother.

CHAPTER IV.

APPEAL TO FACTS.

THESE views, however, can be carried out and demonstrated by facts of a more agreeable nature than the preceding, and more creditable to humanity; facts which clearly point out the certainty and manner of perpetuating desirable, intellectual, and moral qualities. The history of our own country affords innumerable examples in proof of this. Probably the most extensive one may be found in the family of President Edwards.

"The number of great men," says his biographer, one of his descendants, "who have produced great and permanent changes in the character and condition of mankind, and stamped their own image on the mind of succeeding generations, is comparatively small; and even of that small number, the great body have been indebted for their superior efficiency, at least in part, to extraneous circumstances, while very few can ascribe it to the simple strength of their own intellect. Yet, here and there an individual can be found, who, by his mere mental energy, has changed the course of human thought and feeling, and led mankind onward in that new and better path which he had opened to their view.

"Such an individual was Jonathan Edwards. Born in an obscure colony in the midst of a wilderness, and educated at a seminary just commencing its existence; passing the better part of his life as the pastor of a frontier village, and the residue as an Indian missionary in an humble hamlet, he discovered and unfolded a system of the Divine moral government so new, so clear, so full, that while at its first disclosure it needed no aid from its friends, and feared no opposition from its enemies, it has at length constrained a reluctant world to bow in homage to its truth.

"The Reverend Timothy Edwards, the father of President Edwards, was born at Hartford, May 14, 1669, and pursued his studies, preparatory to his admission to college, under the Rev. Mr. Glover, of Springfield, a gentleman distinguished for his classical attainments. In 1687, he entered Harvard College, at that time the only seminary in the colonies, and received the two degrees of Bachelor and Master of Arts, on the same day, July 4th, 1691, one in the morning, the other in the afternoon: an uncommon mark of respect paid to his extraordinary proficiency in learning. After the usual course of theological study, at that time more thorough than it was during the latter half of the following century, he was ordained to the Gospel ministry in the east parish of Windsor, in Connecticut, in May, 1694. Six months after his ordination, and in the twenty-sixth year of his age, Mr. Edwards was married to Esther Stoddard, daughter of the Rev. Solomon Stoddard, aged twenty-two.

"The management not only of his domestic concerns, but of his property generally, was intrusted to the care of Mrs. Edwards, who discharged the duties of a wife and mother with singular fidelity and success. *In strength of character she resembled her father*, and, like him, she left behind her, in the place where she resided for seventy-six years, that 'good name which is better than precious ointment.' On a visit to East Windsor, in 1823, I found a considerable number of persons advanced in years, who had been well acquainted with Mrs. Edwards; and two, upward of ninety, who had been pupils of her husband. From them I learned that she received a superior education in Boston, was tall, dignified, and commanding in her appearance, affable and gentle in her manners, and was regarded as surpassing her husband in native vigor of understanding. They all united in speaking of her as possessed of remarkable judgment and prudence, of an exact sense of propriety, of extensive information, of a thorough knowledge of the Scriptures and of theology, and of singular conscientiousness, piety, and excellence of character. By her careful attention to all his domestic concerns, her husband was left at full liberty to devote himself to the proper duties of his profession. Like many of the clergy of that early period in New England, he was well acquainted with Hebrew literature, and was regarded as a man of more than usual learning, but was particularly distinguished in the Greek and Latin classics. In addition to his other duties, he annually prepared a number of pupils for college, there being at that time no academies or public schools endowed for this purpose. One of my informants, who pursued his preparatory studies under him, told me, that on his admission to college, when the officers learned with whom he had studied, they remarked to him, that there was no need of examining Mr. Edwards' scholars.

"He was, for that period, unusually liberal and enlightened with regard to the education of his children; preparing not only his son, but each of his daughters, also, for college. In a letter bearing date August 3, 1711, while absent on the expedition to Canada, he wishes that Jonathan and the girls may continue to prosecute the study of Latin; and in another of August 7, that he continue to recite his Latin to his elder sisters. When his daughters were of the proper age, he sent them to Boston to finish their education. Both he and Mrs. Edwards were exemplary in their care of their religious instruction, and as the reward of their parental fidelity, were permitted to see the fruits of piety in them all during their youth."

Such were the parents of President Edwards; and their virtues were not wanting in his posterity, for he married a woman of superior mind and attainments, and his descendants, and those of his sisters, are distinguished for talent and virtue among the literati of the Eastern States. And many of them, down to the seventh generation, experience the ennobling emotions of hereditary excellence, and feel a purer pride in the contemplation of the wisdom and virtue of their ancestors, than the European, who can trace back his genealogy from century to century, and boast of having the blood of kings and conquerors in his veins.

If, in biography generally, the same care had been taken to ascertain and describe the characters of the *parents* of great men, the *sources* of talent and genius would not so long have remained doubtful. The general indifference, however, of man to this subject is truly surprising, when we consider the importance which he gives to the pedigree of his horse and dog. The Newmarket jockey, when he has a fine horse to run or to dispose of, does not merely show by whom he was trained, and his manner of training, but produces a long and well-authenticated pedigree. And, in this particular, he is greatly inferior to the untutored son of the Desert, the otherwise ignorant Arab, whose greatest anxiety is to obtain purity of descent, in this, his most valuable treasure; well knowing, through the experience of ages, that the high qualities of which the noble animal is capable, are only to be looked for where this condition has been strictly observed.

Patrick Henry is another distinguished instance in proof of mental and moral qualities being hereditary. The families of both his parents were eminent for talent and virtue; but it would appear that the peculiar powers of oratory for which he was so remarkable, were derived from the maternal line.

"He was," says Mr. Wirt, "the orator of nature, and such a one as nature might not blush to avow. If the reader shall still demand how he acquired those wonderful powers of speaking which have been assigned to him, we can only answer, that they were the gift of Heaven—the birthright of genius."

"It has been said of Mr. Henry, with inimitable felicity, that 'he was SHAKSPEARE and GARRICK combined!' Let the reader, then, imagine the wonderful talents of those two men united in the same individual, and transferred from the scenes of fiction to the business of real life, and he will have formed some conception of the eloquence of Patrick Henry. In a word, he was one of those perfect prodigies of nature, of whom very few have been produced since the foundation of the earth was laid."

"Mrs. Henry, the widow of Colonel Syme, as we have seen, and the mother of Patrick Henry, was a native of Hanover county, and of the family of the Winstons. She possessed, in an eminent degree, the mild and benevolent disposition, the undeviating probity, the correct understanding, and easy elocution by which that ancient family has been so long distinguished. Her brother William, the brother of the present Judge Winston, is said to have been highly endowed with that peculiar cast of eloquence for which Mr. Henry became, afterward, so justly celebrated. Of this gentleman, I have an anecdote from a correspondent, which I shall give in his own words: 'I have often heard my father, who was intimately acquainted with this William Winston, say, that he was the greatest orator whom he ever heard, Patrick Henry excepted; that during the last French and Indian war, and soon after Braddock's defeat, when the militia were marched to the frontier of Virginia against the enemy, this William Winston was the lieutenant of a company; that the men, who were indifferently clothed, without tents, and exposed to the rigor and inclemency of the weather, discovered great aversion to the service, and were anxious, and even clamorous to return to their families, when this William Winston, mounting a stump, addressed them with such keenness of invective, and declaimed with such force of eloquence, on liberty and patriotism, that when he concluded, the general cry was, "Let us march on; lead us against the enemy!" and they were now willing, nay, anxious to encounter all those difficulties and dangers which, but a few moments before, had almost produced a mutiny.'"

"Patrick Henry, the second son of John and Sarah Henry, and one of nine children, was born on the 29th of May, 1736, at the family seat, called Studly, in the county of Hanover, and colony of Virginia. His parents, though not rich, were in easy circumstances, and, in point of personal character, were among the most respectable inhabitants of the colony."

"His father, Colonel John Henry, was a native of Aberdeen, in Scotland. He was, it is said, a first cousin of David Henry, who was the brother-in-law and successor of Edward Cave, in the publication of that celebrated work, the Gentlemen's Magazine, and himself the author of several literary tracts: John Henry is also said to have been a nephew, in the maternal line, to the great historian, Dr. William Robertson. He came over to Virginia, in quest of fortune, some time prior to the year 1730, and the tradition is, that he enjoyed the friendship and patronage of Mr. Dinwiddie, afterward the governor of the colony. By this gentleman, it is reported, that he was introduced to the elder Colonel Syme, of Hanover, in whose family it is certain that he became domesticated during the life of that gentleman; after his death, he intermarried with his widow, and resided on the estate which he had left. It is considered as a fair proof of the personal merit of Mr. John Henry, that in those days, when offices were bestowed with peculiar caution, he was the colonel of his regiment, the principal surveyor of the county, and for many years the presiding magistrate of the county court. His surviving acquaintances concur in stating that he was a man of liberal education; that he possessed a plain, but solid understanding; and lived a life of the most irreproachable integrity and exemplary piety."

"Thus much," continues Mr. Wirt, "I have been able to collect of the parentage and family of Mr. Henry; and this, I presume, will be thought quite sufficient, in relation to a man who owed no part of his greatness to the lustre of his pedigree, but was in truth the sole founder of his own fortunes." Yet, according to the new mental philosophy, the pedigree of Mr. Henry was most illustrious; inasmuch as the aristocracy of talent and virtue, the true nobility of nature, is superior to that of wealth and blood.

The following beautiful description of Mr. Henry in private life, displays a striking contrast with the pursuits and habits of the present generation; whose every effort appears to be directed to the acquisition of wealth, of political power, or the gratification of the selfish sentiments in some of their protean forms.

"Whatever difference of opinion may exist as to the other parts of his character, in this the concurrence is universal—that there never was a man better constituted than Mr. Henry to enjoy and adorn the retirement on which he had now entered. Nothing can be more amiable, nothing more interesting and attaching, than those pictures which have been furnished from every quarter, without one dissenting stroke of the pencil, of this great and virtuous man in the bosom of private life. Mr. Jefferson says, that 'he was the best-humored companion in the world.' His disposition was, indeed, all sweetness; his affections were warm, kind, and social; his patience invincible; his temper ever unclouded, cheerful, and serene; his manners plain, open, familiar, and simple; his conversation easy, ingenuous, and unaffected, full of entertainment, full of instruction, and irradiated with all those light and softer graces, which his genius threw, without effort, over the most common subjects. It is said that there stood in the court, before his door, a large walnut tree, under whose shade it was his delight to pass his summer evenings, surrounded by his affectionate and happy family, and by a circle of neighbors who loved him almost to idolatry. Here he would disport himself with all the careless gayety of infancy. Here, too, he would sometimes warm the bosoms of the old, and strike fire from the eyes of his younger hearers, by recounting the tales of other times; sketching, with the boldness of a master's hand, those great historic incidents in which he had borne a part; and by drawing to the life, and placing before his audience, in colors as fresh and strong as those of nature, the many illustrious men in every quarter of the continent with whom he had acted a part on the public stage. Here, too, he would discourse with all the wisdom and all the eloquence of a Grecian sage, of the various duties and offices of life; and pour forth those lessons of practical utility with which long experience and observation had stored his mind. Many were the visitors from a distance, old and young, who came on a kind of pious pilgrimage to the retreat of the veteran patriot, and found him thus delightfully and usefully employed—the old to gaze upon him with long-remembered affection and ancient gratitude—the young, the ardent, the emulous, to behold and admire, with swimming eyes, the champion of other days, and to look with a sigh of regret upon that height of glory which they could never hope to reach.

Blessed be the shade of that venerable tree—ever hallowed the spot which his genius has consecrated!"

The life of Dr. Franklin, by Jared Sparks, contains a full account of his ancestors, both in the paternal and maternal line. His mother was the *youngest* of nine children of Peter Folger, a man of talent, worth, and consideration; whose numerous descendants sustained a high character for strength of mind, versatility of talent, probity, and honor; while not only his father, but also his father's brothers, were remarkable for strength of understanding and excellence of character. Dr. Franklin gives the following description of his parents:

"I suppose you may like to know what kind of a man my father was. He had an excellent constitution, was of a middle stature, well set, and very strong. He could draw prettily, and was skilled a little in music. His voice was sonorous and agreeable, so that when he played on his violin, and sung withal, as he was accustomed to do after the business of the day was over, it was extremely agreeable to hear. He had some knowledge of mechanics, and, on occasion, was very handy with other tradesmen's tools. But his great excellence was his sound understanding, and his solid judgment in prudential matters, both in private and public affairs. It is true he was never employed in the latter, the numerous family he had to educate, and the straitness of his circumstances, keeping him close to his trade; but I remember well his being frequently visited by leading men, who consulted him for his opinion in public affairs, and those of the church he belonged to; and who showed great respect for his judgment and advice.

"He was also much consulted by private persons about their affairs, when any difficulty occurred, and frequently chosen an arbiter between contending parties. At his table he liked to have, as often as he could, some sensible friend or neighbor to converse with, and always took care to start some ingenious or useful topic for discourse, which might tend to improve the minds of his children. By this means he turned our attention to what was good, just, and prudent, in the conduct of life; and little or no notice was ever taken of what related to the victuals on the table; whether it was well or ill dressed, in or out of season, of good or bad flavor, preferable to this or that other kind of thing; so that I was brought up in such a perfect inattention to those matters, as to be quite indifferent what kind of food was set before me. Indeed, I am so unobservant of it, that to this day I can scarce tell, a few hours after dinner, of what dishes it consisted. This has been a great convenience to me in traveling, where my companions have been sometimes very unhappy for want of a suitable gratification of their more delicate, because better-instructed tastes and appetites.

"My mother had likewise an excellent constitution; she suckled all her ten children. I never knew either my father or mother to have any sickness but that of which they died; he at eighty-nine, and she at eighty-five years of age. They lie buried together at Boston, where I some years since placed a marble over their grave, with this inscription:

"JOSIAH FRANKLIN,
and
ABIAH, his wife,
Lie here interred.
They lived lovingly together in wedlock,
fifty-five years;
And, without an estate, or any gainful employment,
By constant labor and honest industry
(With God's blessing),
Maintained a large family comfortably;
And brought up thirteen children and seven grandchildren
Respectably
From this instance, reader,
Be encouraged to diligence in thy calling,
And distrust not Providence.
He was a pious and prudent man,
She a discreet and virtuous woman.
Their youngest son,
In filial regard to their memory,
Places this stone."

The following beautiful and touching account of the mother of the "first of men," furnishes further evidence of the direct descent of superior intellectual and moral qualities.

It is much to be regretted that the two principal biographies of Washington contain so few particulars respecting his ancestors. It is principally from sources independent of those two works, that we learn the character of his parents. The annexed extract, rich in its instruction to the young mother, is copied from Mrs. Hale's Magazine of September, 1831.

THE MOTHER OF WASHINGTON.

"The character of woman becomes distinguished much oftener by the reflection of her great and good qualities, in the conduct of those men with whom she is particularly connected or associated, than by the exhibition of any extraordinary achievements in her own person. In the parental relations, particularly, the talents of the female are the transmitted inheritance of her sons; and this seems a wise dispensation of Providence, by which the endowments of the sexes are equalized, and both alike made to participate in the glories of their common nature. Certain it is, that far the greatest number of eminent men have owed their superiority and success to the genius, example, and care of their mothers. These reflections need not make women proud; but they should make mothers emulous to train their children to be useful and good; for by laying such a foundation of excellence in early life, the richest hopes for maturity may be rationally entertained.

"The mother of our illustrious Washington furnishes an example of female excellence, and *its reward,* which is unequaled; and yet the model has been hitherto little known. This neglect has not arisen from any indifference of the American people to the virtues of their patriots; but simply that at the time of the Revolution, the public history of the events was paramount to any private relations; and the novel, rapid, and successful experiment of our national character has left little opportunity for domestic and individual history. But a different sentiment is beginning to prevail; the public mind is well-nigh wearied with the monotony of Fourth of July orations; and it is time to turn from the great and brilliant theatre of action, and the well-known and glorious performers, to examine the movements behind the scenes, and the humble and unheeded, but effective assistants that then proposed the astonishing exhibition.

" For the succeeding sketch we are indebted to George W. P. Custis, Esq. (grandson of Mrs. Washington, the wife of General Washington), of Virginia.

" The mother of Washington was descended from the very respectable family of Ball, who settled as English colonists on the banks of the Potomac. Bred in those domestic and independent habits which graced Virginia matrons in the old days of Virginia, this lady, by the death of her husband, became involved in the cares of a young family, at a period when those cares seem more especially to claim the aid and control of the stronger sex. It was left for this eminent woman, by a method the most rare—by an education and discipline the most peculiar and imposing—to form, in the youth-time of her son, those great and essential qualities which gave lustre to the glories of his after life. If the school savored the more of the Spartan than the Persian character, it was a fitter school to form a hero, destined to be the ornament of the age in which he flourished, and a standard of excellence for ages yet to come.

" It was remarked by the ancients, that the mother always gave the tone to the character of the child; and we may be permitted to say, that since the days of old renown, a mother has not lived better fitted to give the tone and character of real greatness to her child, than she whose remarkable life and actions this reminiscence will endeavor to illustrate.

" At the time of his father's death, George Washington was only twelve years of age. He has been heard to say, that he knew little of his father except the remembrance of his person, and of his parental fondness. To his mother's forming care he himself ascribed the origin of his fortunes and his fame.

" The home of Mrs. Washington, of which she was always mistress, was a pattern of order. There the levity and indulgence common to youth was tempered by a deference and well-regulated restraint, which, while it neither suppressed nor condemned any rational enjoyment usual in the spring-time of life, prescribed those enjoyments within the bounds of moderation and propriety. Thus, the chief was taught the duty of obedience, which prepared him to command. Still, the mother held in reserve an authority which never departed from her, not even when her son had become the most illustrious of men. It seemed to say, 'I am your *mother*—the being who gave you life—the guide who directed your steps when they needed a guardian; my maternal affection drew forth your love; my authority constrained your spirit; whatever may be your success or your renown, next to your God, your reverence is due to me!' Nor did the chief dissent from these truths; but to the last moments of his venerable parent, yielded to her will the most dutiful and implicit obedience, and felt for her person and character the highest respect, and the most enthusiastic attachment. The late Lawrence Washington, Esq., of Chotank, one of the associates of the juvenile years of the chief, and remembered by him in his will, thus describes the home of his mother:

"'I was often there with George, his playmate, schoolmate, and young man's companion. Of the mother I was ten times more afraid than I ever was of my own parents; she awed me in the midst of her kindness, for she was indeed truly kind. And even now, when time has whitened my locks, and I am the grand-parent of the second generation, I could not behold that majestic woman without feelings it is impossible to describe. Whoever has seen the awe-inspiring air and manner so characteristic in the father of his country, will remember the matron as she appeared when the presiding genius of her well-ordered household, commanding and being obeyed.'

"Such were the domestic influences under which the mind of Washington was formed; and that he not only profited, but fully appreciated their excellence and the character of his mother, his behavior at all times testified. Upon his appointment to the command in chief of the American armies, previously to his joining the forces at Cambridge, he removed his mother from her country residence to the village of Fredericksburg, a situation remote from danger, and contiguous to her friends and relations.

"It was there the matron remained during nearly the whole of the trying period of the Revolution, directly in the way of the news, as it passed from north to south: one carrier would bring intelligence of success to our arms; another, 'swiftly coursing at his heels,' the saddening reverse of disaster and defeat. While thus ebbed and flowed the fortunes of our cause, the mother, trusting to the wisdom and protection of Divine Providence, preserved the even tenor of her life, affording an example to those matrons whose sons were alike engaged in the arduous contest; and showing that unavailing anxieties, however belonging to nature, were unworthy of mothers whose sons were combating for the inestimable rights of man, and the freedom and happiness of the world.

"When the comforting and glorious intelligence arrived of the passage of the Delaware (December, '76), an event which restored our hopes from the very brink of despair, a number of her friends waited upon the mother, with congratulations. She received them with kindness; observed that it was most pleasurable news, and that George appeared to have deserved well of his country for such signal services; and continued, in reply to the congratulation of patriots (most of whom held letters in their hands, from which they read extracts), 'But, my good sirs, here is too much flattery—still, George will not forget the lessons I early taught him—he will not forget *himself*, though he is the subject of so much praise!'

"Here let me remark upon the absurdity of an idea which, from some strange cause or other, has been suggested, though certainly never believed, that the mother was disposed to favor the royal cause. Such a surmise has not the slightest foundation in truth. Like many others, whose days of enthusiasm were in the wane, the lady doubted the prospects of success in the beginning of the war, and long, during its continuance, feared that our means would be found inadequate to a successful contest with so formidable a power as Britain; and our soldiers, brave, but undisciplined, and ill-provided, be unequal to cope with the veteran and well-appointed troops of the king. Doubts like these were by no means confined to a female, but were both entertained and expressed by the staunchest of patriots, and most determined of men. But when the mother, who had been removed to the county of Frederick, on the invasion of Virginia, in 1781, was informed by express of the surrender of Cornwallis, she raised her hands to heaven, and exclaimed, 'Thank God! war will now be ended, and peace, independence, and happiness bless our country.'

"During the war, and, indeed, during her useful life, up to the advanced age of eighty-two, until within three years of her death (when an afflictive disease prevented exertion), the mother set a most valuable example, in the management of her domestic concerns, carrying her keys, bustling in her household affairs, providing for her family, and living and moving in all the pride of independence. She was not actuated by the *ambition for show which pervades lesser minds*, and the peculiar plainness and dignity of her manners became in nowise altered when the sun of glory arose upon her house. There are some of the aged inhabitants of Fredericksburg who well remember the matron as, seated in an old-fashioned open chaise, she was in the habit of visiting, almost daily, her little farm in the vicinity of the town. When there, she would ride about her fields, giving her orders, and seeing that they were obeyed.

"Her great industry, with the well-regulated economy of all her concerns, enabled the matron to dispense considerable charities to the poor, although her own circumstances were always far from rich. All manner of domestic economies, so useful in those times of privation and trouble, met her zealous attention; while every thing about her household bore marks of her care and management, and very many things the impress of her own hands. In a very humble dwelling, and suffering under an excruciating disease (cancer of the breast), thus lived this mother of the first of men, preserving unchanged her peculiar nobleness and independence of character.

"She was continually visited and solaced by her children, and numerous grand-children, particularly her daughter, Mrs. Lewis. To the repeated and earnest solicitations of this lady, that she would remove to her house and pass the remainder of her days; to the pressing entreaties of her son, that she would make Mount Vernon the home of her age, the matron replied, 'I thank you for your affectionate and dutiful offers, but my wants are but few in this world, and I feel perfectly competent to take care of myself.' Her son-in-law, Colonel Fielding Lewis, proposed to relieve her of the direction of her affairs: she observed, 'Do you, Fielding, keep my books in order, for your eyesight is better than mine; but leave the executive management to me.'

"One weakness alone attached to this lofty-minded and intrepid woman, and that proceeded from a most affecting cause—she was afraid of lightning. In early life, she had a female friend killed by her side, while sitting at table; the knife and fork in the hands of the unfortunate girl were melted by the electric fluid. The matron never recovered from the fright and shock occasioned by this distressing accident. On the approach of a thunder-cloud, she would retire to her chamber, and not leave it again till the storm had passed away.

"She was always pious, but in her latter days her devotions were performed in private. She was in the habit of repairing every day to a secluded spot, formed by rocks and trees near her dwelling, where, abstracted from the world and worldly things, she communed with her Creator in humiliation and prayer.

"After an absence of nearly seven years, it was, at length, on the return of the combined armies from Yorktown, permitted to the mother again to see and embrace her illustrious son. So soon as he had dismounted, in the midst of a numerous and brilliant suite, he sent to apprise her of his arrival, and to know when it would be her pleasure to receive him. And now mark the force of early education and habits, and the superiority of the Spartan over the Persian school, in this interview of the great Washington with his admirable parent and instructor. No pageantry of war proclaimed his coming, no trumpets sounded, no banners waved. Alone, and on foot, the marshal of France, the general-in-chief of the combined armies of France and America, the deliverer of his country, the hero of the age, repaired to pay his humble duty to her whom he venerated as the author of his being, the founder of his fortune and his fame. For, full well he knew that the matron would not be moved by all the pride that glory ever gave, nor by all the 'pomp and circumstance' of power.

"The lady was alone, her aged hands employed in the works of domestic industry, when the good news was announced, and it was further told that the victor chief was in waiting at the threshold. She welcomed him with a warm embrace, and by the well-remembered and endearing name of his childhood; inquiring as to his health, she remarked the lines which mighty cares and many trials had made on his manly countenance, spoke much of old times and old friends, but of his glory—*not one word!*

"Meantime, in the village of Fredericksburg, all was joy and revelry; the town was crowded with the officers of the French and American armies, and with gentlemen from all the country around, who hastened to welcome the conquerors of Cornwallis. The citizens made arrangements for a splendid ball, to which the mother of Washington was specially invited. She observed, that although her dancing days were *pretty well over*, she should feel happy in contributing to the general festivity, and consented to attend.

"The foreign officers were anxious to see the mother of their chief. They had heard indistinct rumors respecting her remarkable life and character, but forming their judgments from European examples, they were prepared to expect in the mother that glare and show which would have been attached to the parents of the great in the Old World. How were they surprised, when the matron, leaning on the arm of her son, entered the room! She was arrayed in the very plain, yet becoming, garb worn by the Virginia lady of the olden time. Her address, always dignified and imposing, was courteous, though reserved. She received the complimentary attentions which were profusely paid her, without evincing the slightest elevation, and at an early hour, wishing the company much enjoyment of their pleasures, retired, observing that it was time for old people to be at home.

"The foreign officers were amazed to behold one whom so

many causes contributed to elevate, preserving the even tenor of her life, while such a blaze of glory shone upon her name and offspring. The European world furnished no examples of such magnanimity. Names of ancient lore were heard to escape from their lips, and they observed, that 'if such were the matrons of America, it was not wonderful the sons were illustrious.'

"It was on this festival occasion that General Washington danced a minuet with Mrs. Willis. It closed his dancing days. The minuet was much in vogue at that period, and was peculiarly calculated for the display of the splendid figure of the chief, and his natural grace and elegance of air and manner. The gallant Frenchmen who were present, of which fine people it may be said, that dancing forms one of the elements of their existence, so much admired the American performance, as to admit that a Parisian education could not have improved it. As the evening advanced, the commander-in-chief, yielding to the gayety of the scene, went down some dozen couple, in the contra-dance, with great spirit and satisfaction.

"The Marquis de Lafayette repaired to Fredericksburg, previous to his departure for Europe, in the fall of 1784, to pay his parting respects to the mother, and to ask her blessing.

"Conducted by one of her grandsons, he approached the house, when the young gentleman observed, 'There, sir, is my grandmother.' Lafayette beheld, working in the garden, clad in domestic-made clothes, and her gray head covered by a plain straw hat, the *mother* of 'his hero!' The lady saluted him kindly, observing, 'Ah, marquis! you see an old woman—but come, I can make you welcome to my poor dwelling, without the parade of changing my dress.'

"Much as Lafayette had seen and heard of the matron before, at this interesting interview he was charmed and struck with wonder. When he considered her great age, the transcendent elevation of her son, who, surpassing all rivals in the race of glory, 'bore the palm alone,' and at the same time discovered no change in her plain, yet dignified life and manners, he became assured that the Roman matron could flourish in the modern day.

"The marquis spoke of the happy effects of the Revolution, and the goodly prospect which opened upon independent America, stated his speedy departure for his native land, paid the tribute of his heart, his love and admiration of her illustrious son, and concluded by asking her blessing. She blessed him—and to the encomiums which he had lavished upon his hero and paternal chief, the matron replied in these words: '*I am not surprised at what George has done, for he was always a very good boy.*'

"Immediately after the organization of the present government, the chief magistrate repaired to Fredericksburg, to pay his humble duty to his mother, preparatory to his departure for New York. An affecting scene ensued. The son feelingly remarked the ravages which a torturing disease had made upon the aged frame of his mother, and thus addressed her:

"'The people, madam, have been pleased, with the most flattering unanimity, to elect me to the chief magistracy of the United States; but before I can assume the functions of my office, I have come to bid you an affectionate farewell. So soon as the public business, which must necessarily be encountered in arranging a new government, can be disposed of, I shall hasten to Virginia, and—'

"Here the matron interrupted him: 'You will see me no more. My great age, and the disease which is fast approaching my vitals, warn me that I shall not be long of this world. I trust in God I am somewhat prepared for a better. But go, George, fulfill the high destinies which heaven appears to assign you; go, my son, and may that heaven's and your mother's blessing be with you always.'

"The president was deeply affected. His head rested upon the shoulder of his parent, whose aged arm feebly yet fondly encircled his neck. That brow, on which fame had wreathed the purest laurel virtue ever gave to created man, relaxed from its lofty bearing. That look, which could have awed a Roman senate in its Fabrician day, was bent in filial tenderness upon the time-worn features of the venerable matron.

"The great man wept. A thousand recollections crowded upon his mind, as memory, retracing scenes long past, carried him back to the paternal mansion, and the days of his youth; and there, the centre of attraction, was his mother, whose care, instructions, and discipline had prepared him to reach the topmost height of laudable ambition; yet how were his glories forgotten while he gazed upon her whom, wasted by time and malady, he must soon part with to meet no more.

"The matron's predictions were true. The disease which so long had preyed upon her frame completed its triumph, and she expired at the age of eighty-five, rejoicing in the consciousness of a life well spent, and confiding in the promises of immortality to the humble believer.

"In her person, Mrs. Washington was of middle size, and finely formed; her features pleasing, yet strongly marked. It is not the happiness of the writer to remember her, having only seen her with infant eyes. The sister of the chief he perfectly well remembers. She was a most majestic woman, and so strikingly like the brother, that it was a matter of frolic to throw a cloak around her, and place a military hat upon her head, and such was the perfect resemblance, that, had she appeared on her brother's steed, battalions would have presented arms, and senates risen to do homage to the chief.

"In her latter days, the mother often spoke of her own *good boy*, of the merits of his early life, of his love and dutifulness to herself; but of the deliverer of his country, the chief magistrate of the great republic, she never spoke. Call you this insensibility, or want of ambition? Oh, no! her ambition had been gratified to overflowing. She had taught him to be *good;* that he became *great* when the opportunity presented, was a consequence, not a cause.

"Thus lived and died this distinguished woman. Had she been a Roman dame, statues would have been erected to her memory in the capital, and we should have read in classic pages the story of her virtues.

"When another century shall have elapsed, and the nations of the earth, as well as our descendants, shall have learned the true value of liberty, the name of our hero will gather a glory it has never yet been invested with; and then will youth and age, maid and matron, aged and bearded men, with pilgrim step, repair to the *now neglected grave* of the mother of Washington."

Lord Bacon is universally admitted to have possessed one of the most powerful intellects of any man who has appeared upon the earth. Both his parents were remarkable for soundness of judgment and highly cultivated intellectual powers; qualities which had descended to them through several generations. They also belonged to that class of society from which have emanated such men as Milton, Sir Thomas More, Lord Burleigh, Oliver Cromwell, John Hampden, and a host of other great minds.

Sir Anthony Cook, the maternal grandfather of Lord Bacon, became eminent in the whole circle of the arts, being a thorough master of the Latin and Greek languages, an exact critic and philologist, and equally skilled in poetry, history, and the mathematics. He was at the same time adorned with singular piety and goodness, preferring contemplation to active life. He managed his family with such prudence and discretion, that Lord Seymour, standing by one day when this gentleman chid his son, said, "Some men govern their families with more skill than others do kingdoms," and thereupon commended him to the government of his nephew, Edward VI. Such the majesty of his looks and gait, that awe governed; such the reason and sweetness, that love obliged all his family—a family equally afraid to displease so *good* a head, and to offend so *great*. He had five daughters, whose education he superintended himself; and thinking that *women are as capable of learning as men*, he instilled that into his daughters at night, which he had taught the prince during the day. If he was great and happy in himself, he was greater and happier in his daughters. "His first care was to give them a true sense of religion, and his next to inure them to submission, modesty, and obedience.

"Their book and pen were their recreation; the music and dancing-school, the court and city, their accomplishment; the needle in the closet, and housewifery in the hall and kitchen, their business. They all married splendidly and happily; and in their marriage they were guided more by the reason of their father than by his will, and were directed rather by his counsel than led by his authority." "Their classical acquirements," says Macaulay, "made them conspicuous even among the women of fashion of that age. Anne, the mother of Francis Bacon, was distinguished both as a linguist and as a theologian. She corresponded in Greek with Bishop Jewel, and translated his *Apologia* from the Latin so correctly, that neither he nor Archbishop Parker could suggest a single alteration. She also translated a series of sermons on Fate and Free-will, from the Tuscan of Bernardo Ochino." "Her parental care of her two sons, Anthony and Francis, two of the most extraordinary men of her time, or, indeed, of any time, is, possibly, the best test of her powers, which was deeply felt by Francis, who, in his will, says: 'For my burial, I desire that it may be in St. Michael's church, near St. Alban's—there was my mother buried.' In Birch's Memoirs of the Reign of Queen Elizabeth, the extraordinary vigilance used by Lady Anne in superintending their conduct long after they were adults, may be seen."

"Sir Nicholas Bacon," continues Macaulay, "was no ordinary man; but the fame of the father was thrown into shade by that of the son." "Sir Nicholas Bacon," says Lloyd, "was a man full of wit and wisdom. He had the deepest reach of any man at the council-table; the knottiest head to pierce into difficulties; the most comprehensive judgment to surmount the merits of a case; the strongest memory to recollect all the circumstances at one view; the greatest patience to debate and consider, and the clearest reason to urge any thing that came in his way in the courts of chancery. His favor was eminent with his mistress, and his alliance strong with her statesmen. He was lord keeper of the great seal during the time of Elizabeth. He was, in a word, father of his country, and of Sir Francis Bacon."

With these unquestioned truths before us, it requires neither a physiological nor a metaphysical hypothesis to account for the great mental abilities of Lord Bacon. But we see, beyond a doubt, that those abilities were a legitimate inheritance, and owed their superior strength to the *not common occurrence* of the union of great intellectual culture and attainments in *both* of his parents. Let us here revert to what seems more than a coincidence, and strongly in support of the argument of a transmission of the experience and acquirements of the parents. The biographer of Sir Nicholas Bacon, the father of the philosopher, informs us, that by his first marriage he had six children; those, and the mother who bore them, passed into oblivion, leaving no trace except the record "They were." Sir Nicholas again married, and we presume his mature judgment made a wiser choice. He obtained Anne, one of the highly educated daughters of Sir Anthony Cook, before mentioned, and mark the result: Anthony and Francis, two of the most extraordinary men of their time, or of any time, were the issue of this fortunate union; the latter born when the father had attained the mature age of fifty, and the mother thirty-two, the prime of womanhood. And when we note the circumstance that the fathers of Dr. Franklin, Dr. Johnson, Sir William Jones, Cuvier, Fenelon, and many other eminent men, were about the same age, and also that their mothers were in the meridian of life, surely such facts ought not to be looked upon as mere coincidences, but rather the result of some certain law of nature. When we reflect that order and law pervade all nature, both animate and inanimate, from the geometrical lines in the flake of snow, to the striated formation of the earth we inhabit—from the three millions of animalculæ contained in a single drop of water, to man, the most perfect work of the Creator—is it not the height of presumption to suppose that the mind of a Bacon, or an idiot, a Melancthon, or an Alexander VI., was the result of chance, or produced by some unaccountable freak of nature, independent of the immutable principles of *cause* and *effect*?*

* The following paragraph, from a late review, recognizes the great truth, that the object of human inquiry should be the knowledge of *law*,

"It is quite true," as Locke has said, "that the human mind (as well as its material organ, the brain) is devoid of innate ideas, and like a blank sheet of paper, at birth. All ideas, all knowledge, must be subsequently acquired through the medium of the senses and reflection. But it does not follow that, because all the sheets are blank, they are all equally well calculated for *acquiring* knowledge. Far from it. Some of them are like thick Bath post, others like thin foolscap; and many of them resemble common blotting paper, incapable of retaining or exhibiting any distinct or legible impression. The mind and its organ being, in fact, a '*rudis indigestaque moles.*' This part of the subject, in fine, may be summed up in a very few words, though it has occasioned interminable discussions among metaphysicians. *The qualities of our minds, or of the material organs of our minds, are hereditary, or born with us.*"*

Admitting the truth of this opinion, and then referring to the facts last noticed, the legitimate conclusion arrived at is,

and its application to a class of phenomena, hitherto assumed to have had an arbitrary origin.

"It would be well if the public were accustomed to define, and if each of us were to keep clearly before our minds throughout life, the distinction between learning and true wisdom. What should be the object of knowledge? What is it, that we should seek to know it? Is it words, or even things? Neither; it is *causation*—the order in which events have occurred that may occur again. It is in the discovery of principles and processes that we are chiefly interested. The past is nothing to us; but *in the laws that govern the past we may read the future.* The knowledge of these is the true end of philosophy; but of this philosophers have been too generally unmindful. One man compiles dictionaries; another catalogues the stars; a third describes new or unobserved plants or animals; a fourth collects rare specimens of minerals or fossils; all useful and honorable employments, but only useful as subsidiary to the grand inquiry, beyond these—the laws of mind and matter by which the world is governed. The recent discovery of a new planet will immortalize the names of M. Leverrier and Mr. Adams; but the fact of one planet more or less in the solar system is of absolute insignificance, compared with the knowledge of that universal principle of gravitation which supplied the data for calculating the path of the new planet, before its exact place on a particular night had been pointed out in the heavens."

* Johnson's Economy of Health.

that early marriages cannot be too much deprecated, for reasons analogous throughout all organized nature, and well known to the physiologist and the moralist. Those who are unacquainted with these reasons will find them clearly elucidated in the writings of George and Andrew Combe.

If, however, fathers would more generally follow the example of Sir Anthony Cook, and pay greater attention to the education of their daughters, giving them solid and useful attainments, rather than light and showy accomplishments, and extend their education to a later period in life, the evil of early marriages would be very materially lessened; and the good effects of marriages entered into at a mature age, would be seen in the mental, moral, and physical improvement of succeeding generations.

Elizabeth, of England, and Mary, of Scotland, are striking examples of the effects of the two preceding modes of education on the life and conduct of women of equal natural abilities, and similar conditions. The youth of Elizabeth was passed in retirement, study, and contemplation. "The literary instruction," says Mackintosh, "which she had received from Roger Ascham, had familiarized her mind, in her sixteenth year, with the two ancient languages. Latin she acquired from the complete perusal of Cicero and Livy, the greatest prose writers of Rome. She compared the philosophical works of Plato with the abridgments of a Grecian philosophy by which Cicero instructed and delighted his fellow-citizens; and she would be taught by Ascham how much the orations of Demosthenes, which she read under his eye, surpassed those of the great masters of Roman eloquence. She is mentioned by her preceptor as at the head of the lettered ladies of England, excelling even Lady Jane Grey and Margaret Roper." Thus, at the age of twenty-five, with a mind expanded by knowledge, and a heart softened by adversity, she was called to the throne; and her reign was the most prosperous, distinguished, and happy, of any that preceded or followed it.

The youth of Mary, Queen of Scots, on the contrary, until her nineteenth year, was passed in the gay, frivolous, and licentious court of Catharine de Medicis. Her education was confined to personal accomplishments, which had the effect, as intended by her mother-in-law, of rendering her trifling, selfish, and sensual; and we behold her, at the age of twenty-five, the deserted wife of her third husband, flying from her justly incensed and scandalized subjects, to seek protection and aid from a kinswoman whose counsel she had rejected, whose womanly feelings she had wantonly outraged, and on whose good name her violent death, according to popular opinion, was destined to throw an indelible stain. Yet, we cannot but perceive the injustice of this opinion, when we reflect upon the high estimation in which the patriotic act of Brutus is held for sacrificing his two sons to the political liberty of his country. A higher and holier cause—that of religious liberty and the reformation—called for the death of Mary. Nineteen years of imprisonment had not served to subdue her intriguing spirit; she had become the rallying-point for the Catholics, who had perpetrated the massacre of St. Bartholomew, and were deluging Europe in innocent blood; hence, her restoration would have served as a signal for relighting the fires of Smithfield; and while her death-warrant was drawn up and subscribed by the clergy and laity in power, the whole odium of its execution is unjustly thrown upon Elizabeth.

That the inspired author of Paradise Lost inherited the qualities of his mind from his parents, cannot be doubted; for Mitford says, "His mother was a woman of incomparable virtue and goodness, and exemplary in her liberality to the poor.* And his father was a person of superior and accom-

* "If there be in the character, not only sense and soundness, but virtue of a high order, then, however little appearance there may be of talent, a certain portion of wisdom may be relied upon most implicitly; for the correspondencies of wisdom and goodness are manifold; and that they will accompany each other, is to be inferred, not only because men's wisdom makes them good, but also because their goodness makes them wise. Questions of right and wrong are a perpetual exercise of the faculties of those who are solicitous as to the right or wrong of what they do or see; and a deep interest of the heart in those questions carries with it a deeper cultivation of the understanding than can be easily effected by any other excitement to intellectual activity."—*Taylor's Statesman*, p. 30.

plished mind, and was greatly distinguished for musical tal ents. He saw the early promises of genius in his son, and encouraged them by a careful and liberal education."

Milton, however, did not repay this obligation to his parents, by carefully and liberally educating his own offspring. Johnson says, " What we know of Milton's character in domestic relations is, that he was severe and arbitrary. His family consisted of women ; and there appears in his books something like a Turkish contempt for females, as subordinate and inferior beings. That his own daughters might not break the ranks, he suffered them to be depressed by a mean and penurious education."

Milton had children only by his first wife, Mary, Ann, and Deborah. Ann, though deformed, married a master-builder, and died of her first child. Mary died single. Deborah married Abraham Clark, a weaver of Spitalfields. She had seven sons and three daughters ; but none of them had any children, except her son Caleb, and her daughter Elizabeth. Caleb went to Fort St. George, in the East Indies, and had two sons, of whom nothing is now known. Elizabeth married Thomas Foster, a weaver, in Spitalfields, and had seven children, who all died. She kept a petty grocer's or chandler's shop, first in Halloway, and afterward in Cock Lane, near Shoreditch Church. She knew little of her grandfather, and that little was not good. She told of his harshness to his daughters, and his refusal to have them taught to write. In 1750, April 4, "Comus" was played for her benefit. She had so little acquaintance with diversion or gayety, that she did not know what was intended, when a benefit was offered her.

Thus we see what ignorance, poverty, and degradation Milton entailed on his posterity, by his contemptuous opinion of females, and by not educating his daughters ; thereby enabling them to sustain their proper place in society as the daughters of a man who was by birth a gentleman, by education a learned scholar, and by nature one of the greatest poets the world ever produced.

It is, however, very probable, and much more grateful to

our feelings to conclude, that the daughters of Milton were incapable of receiving a superior education, rather than it should have arisen from a want of parental care in the poet. That they were undutiful and unkind, careless of their father when blind, and deserted him in his old age, we have the authority of Milton himself. Therefore, it is very possible that his contemptuous opinion of females grew out of the *stupidity, dullness*, and *undutiful conduct* of his own wife and daughters. This inference, at least, appears legitimate, from the following extracts from his life and writings:

"In his thirty-fifth year, Milton married Mary, the daughter of Mr. Powell, a justice of the peace in Oxfordshire. After an absence of little more than a month, he brought his bride to town with him, and hoped, as Johnson observes, to enjoy the advantages of conjugal life; but spare diet, and hard study, and a house full of pupils, did not suit the young and gay daughter of a cavalier. She had been brought up in a very different society; so, after having lived for a month a philosophic life, after having been used at home to a great house, and much company and joviality, her friends, possibly at her own desire, made earnest suit to have her company for the remaining part of the summer, which was granted upon a promise of her return at Michaelmas. When Michaelmas came, the lady had no inclination to quit the hospitality and delight of her father's mansion for the austerer habits and seclusion of the poet's study."

"Milton sent repeated letters to her, which were all unanswered; and a messenger, who was dispatched to urge her return, was dismissed with contempt. He resolved immediately to repudiate her, on the ground of disobedience; and, to support the propriety and lawfulness of his conduct, he published 'The Doctrine and Discipline of Divorce.'"

"There is one passage in this treatise in which Milton clearly points to himself, and to the presumed causes of his unhappiness: 'The soberest and best-governed men,' he says, 'are least practiced in these affairs; and who knows not that the *bashful muteness of a virgin may oftentimes hide all the unloveliness and natural sloth which is really unfit for conversa tion?* Nor is there that freedom of access granted or presumed, as may suffice to a perfect discerning, until too late; when any indisposition is suspected, what more usual than the persuasions of friends, that acquaintance, as it increases, will mend all? And lastly, is it not strange that many who have spent their *youth chastely, are, in some things, not so quick-sighted, while they haste too eagerly to light the nuptial torch?* Nor is it, therefore, for a modest error, that a man should forfeit so great a happiness, and no charitable means to relieve him. Since they who have lived most loosely, by reason of their bold accustomings, prove most successful in their matches, because their wild affections, unsettling at will, have been so many divorces to teach them experience. Whereas the sober man, honoring the appearance of modesty, and hoping well of every social virtue under that veil, may easily chance to meet with a mind to all other due conversation inaccessible, and to the more estimable and superior purposes of matrimony useless—and almost lifeless; and what a solace, what a fit help such a consort would be through the whole life of a man, is less pain to conjecture than to have experience.' He speaks, again, of a 'mute and spiritless mate;' and again, 'if he shall find *himself bound fast to an image of earth and phlegm,* with whom he looked to be the copartner of a sweet and gladsome society.'"

"These observations will, I think," continues Mitford, "put us in possession of his wife's 'fair defects,' and the causes of the separation." They also establish the fact, that she was of decided lymphatic temperament(*e*); of which the physiologist says, "If the temperament of the mother be lymphatic, the tendency of nature is to transmit this quality, with all its concomitant *heaviness, dullness, aud inertness, to the offspring;* and those individuals are incapable, in the struggle of life, of making head against difficulties and opposition, and are, generally, unfortunate. One of the great causes why men of talents frequently leave no gifted posterity is, that they form alliances with women of low temperament, in whose inert systems their vivacity is extinguished; and, on the other hand, the cause why men of genius often descend from fathers in whom no trace of ethereal qualities can be discovered, is, that those men were the fortunate husbands of women of high temperament and fine cerebral combinations, who transmitted these qualities to their offspring."

The prosperity and happiness which a wise education insures to woman, and through her to posterity, is illustrated in the different destinies of the daughters of Milton and those of Sir Anthony Cook, of whom there is a further account in the life of Lord Burleigh.

"For the *improvement of his children*, as well as his domestic happiness, Burleigh was chiefly indebted to his wife, the daughter of Sir Anthony Cook, a lady highly distinguished for her mental accomplishments." "The plan of female education, which the example of Sir Thomas More had rendered popular, continued to be pursued among the superior classes of the community.* Sir Anthony Cook bestowed the most careful education on his five daughters, and all of them rewarded his exertions, by becoming not only proficients in literature, but *distinguished for their excellent demeanor as mothers of families.* Lady Burleigh was adorned with every quality which could excite love and esteem; and many instances are recorded of her piety and beneficence. She had accompanied her husband through all the vicissitudes of his fortune, and an affectionate union of forty-three years rendered the loss of her the severest calamity of his life."

* It is from this cause, doubtless, that the seventeenth and eighteenth centuries were so prolific in men of talent and genius; for in the posterity of those well-educated women will be found the names of the great and good men of whom England is so justly proud.

CHAPTER V.

THE EFFECT OF CULTIVATED INTELLECT IN PARENTS ON THEIR CHILDREN.

THE daughter of Neckar is another brilliant example of the direct influence of cultivated intellect in both parents. Madame De Stael Holstein was the grand-daughter of a Swiss clergyman, a man of superior mind and attainments, who bestowed on his daughter an intellectual and moral cultivation rare in that age and country. The youthful girl accompanied Madame Vermenue to Paris, in the singular capacity of Latin teacher to her son; there she became known and appreciated for her taste and acquirements. Her fine qualities inspired the historian Gibbon with a tender passion, which, however, does not appear to have been reciprocated; for, in 1765, she became the wife of the great, though much abused, financier. Her heart, says her biographer, was not less carefully cultivated than her head; and on her husband's elevation to power, she used his influence and fortune only for purposes of benevolence. She had many associates among men of letters, particularly Thomas, Buffon, and Marmontel, and is the author of several literary productions.

Distinguished authors have pronounced Madame De Stael the first female writer of any age or country. It is certain that, since Rousseau or Voltaire, no French author has displayed equal energy and variety. Remarkable for her quick perception of character, and her brilliant conversational powers, she elicited the admiration of her hearers, by her ingenuity and acuteness in metaphysical speculations. These attributes were undoubtedly derived from her mother; while from her father she inherited a masculine understanding and a great fondness for political discussion. "She is, perhaps," says an English writer, "the only woman who can claim admission to an equality with the first order of manly talent.

She was one whom listening senates would have admired, as though it had been a Burke, a Chatham, a Fox, or a Mirabeau. She was one whom legislators might consult with profit. She was one whose voice and pen were feared, and because feared, unrelentingly persecuted by the absolute master of the mightiest empire that the world has witnessed since the days of Charlemagne."

The two following extracts, from different authors, show how little the talents of Madame De Stael were the result of education. "In her childhood, she was bandied about between opposite systems. Her mother was a pedantic disciplinarian ; her father, the celebrated Neckar, was, in the other extreme, indulgent. Under the rule of the former, she was crammed with learning, to the injury of her health ; and when the authority of the latter prevailed, she was, for some years, suffered to be idle, feed her imagination, write pastorals, and plain romances. With an exuberant buoyancy of childish spirit, she was scarcely ever a child in intellect. One of the games of her childhood was to compose tragedies, and make puppets to act them. Before twelve, she conversed with the intelligence of a grown person, with such men as Grimm and Marmontel. At fifteen, she wrote remarks on the *Esprit des Lois ;* at sixteen, she composed a long anonymous letter to her father on the subject of his *Compt. Rendu ;* and Raynal had so high an opinion of her powers, that he wished her to write for his work a paper on the Edict of Nantz." "Her lively spirit found much more satisfaction in the society of her father than in that of her mother. His character, in fact, was much more like her own, and he better understood how to act on her mind. His affection for her was mingled with a father's pride, and she was enthusiastically fond of him, while her respect for him bordered on veneration. Neckar, however, never encouraged her to write, as he disliked female writers, and had forbidden his wife to occupy herself in that way, because the idea of disturbing her pursuits when he entered her chamber was disagreeable to him. To escape a similar prohibition, his daughter, who early began to write, accustomed herself to bear interruption without impatience, and to write standing, so that she might not appear to be disturbed in a serious occupation by his approach."

Madame De Stael's passion for writing would, therefore, appear to be innate, and the result of the mother's disposition and habits previous to her birth. If so, we may infer that the want of this habit in the American mother has given rise to the accusation, that the daughters of America exhibit little or no bias for literature. This is, perhaps, true as far as their attempts have been directed to the useful and enduring. Yet, the pages of our light periodicals have brought forward, within a few years, a host of votaries for fame—students of nature in the closet, possessing brilliant imaginations and refined tastes. But how small a portion of this fair company have devoted their energies in a way to produce an abiding impression on the rising generation, or to suggest one train of thought useful or improving! It may be answered, that the public taste requires of the caterers this constant abuse of the mind and imagination, in constructing wonderful, absurd, and fanciful stories, which are too frequently as devoid of truth and nature, as of any sound principle of action. It should, however, be remembered, that this species of composition requires but little reflection or study, and is liable to produce in the reader a distaste for the more solid and substantial fruits of observation and experience.

Some European writer has said, that the papers of the Spectator had done more to improve the morals and manners of the English, than all the preaching of a hundred years had done previously. If this observation be correct, the inference is, that there is a vast field of usefulness open to the essayist. And who is more fitted by nature for this office than woman? Her nice moral perception is eminently calculated to detect evil influences, and her sympathetic and benevolent nature to discover and apply the antidote. I would, therefore, suggest, for the further consideration of my countrywomen, the good effects that might result from essays written in the manner of the papers of the Spectator; the aim of which should be to inculcate pure principles of virtue and integrity—to enforce on the attention of parents the necessity of a more thorough moral and physical training for youth—to warn the young and inexperienced of the dangers to their health, happiness, and peace of mind, by which they are constantly surrounded, and to cultivate in them a distaste for ostentation, display, and mere sensual pleasures.

It is therefore highly probable, that if the women of this country would give up many of the vain and idle pursuits which now occupy so much time and attention, and devote that time to self-culture, particularly to writing on useful and improving subjects, the latter portion of the nineteenth century would be as prolific in men of genius in America, as the same part of the eighteenth century was of this class in England.(*e*)

There is a large class of women who are so entirely engrossed by their own selfish pursuits and pleasures, that they are much averse to having children. And it may be observed, that those unwelcome children are generally pitiable specimens of humanity. There is a beautiful superstition among the Irish, that those children who are received from the Almighty as blessings, prove to be so; and that those who are not received as such, turn out the contrary. This belief, doubtless, was the result of observation and experience; for a child whose birth has been looked forward to with pleasure, has had the advantage of the exercise of the superior organs of the parents—and vice versa. This view of the subject can, perhaps, be best illustrated by an example.

The lovely Louisa M——, noted by the writer, among her intimate friends, as remarkable for her good sense and kindness of disposition, married, at the age of twenty-five, a man of superior abilities, enjoying the advantages of an ample fortune and the best society. Their residence was charmingly situated, overlooking a noble river, great extent and variety of country, and surrounded by many beautiful objects of nature. The interior arrangements comprehended all that was desirable in the way of literature and the arts; noted, also, as the abode of hospitality and the kindliest feelings. Thus situated, their children were born under the most happy influences—were beautiful, bright, and some of them highly talented. At the age of thirty-eight, the mother ceased bearing children, and felt happy at the thought of being at length free from the confinement attending the cares of infancy. This state of things continued a few years, but was unexpectedly changed by symptoms of pregnancy. This was a most unwelcome prospect for one who had entered into the dissipation of fashionable life, and was determined, in future, to enjoy and not suffer. Various means were resorted to, to avoid the approaching calamity, but were unsuccessful. After much discontent and repining, a girl was born, inheriting a large portion of the unhappy, repining, and bitter temper, which possessed the mother for months previous to her birth.

The attepmt to violate the laws of the Creator, in this instance, has been most signally punished ; for in the perverse, rebellious spirit, and cloudy brow of her unhappy daughter, the mother now recognizes the temper in which she so imprudently indulged during her pregnancy.

On no other principle than that on which this theory is founded, can the great diversity of character found in children of the same parents be accounted for.

A family in which the authoress was extremely intimate, presents members as dissimilar as it is possible to conceive. The parents have passed through many strange vicissitudes, and their children, born under different states of mind and circumstances, show the effect of them in the strongest light. The father was a man of talent, but had, until the age of forty, made pleasure his pursuit, and lived only for himself. At that period, having inherited a fine estate, which he wished to transmit to his posterity, he reformed and married.

Although a highly educated man, Mr. A—— appeared to possess no knowledge whatever of the conditions necessary to be fulfilled in order to insure a healthy and strong-minded progeny, (*d*) and was guided in his choice more by the animal propensities and selfish sentiments, than by enlightened intellect. His dissipated life having brought him in contact with women of loose morals, had induced a mistrust of those who lived much in society ; he therefore chose what he termed an unsophisticated child of nature—but, in fact, an immature, half-educated girl of sixteen. Immediately after his marriage he retired to his estate, remotely situated, the neighborhood of which contained very few inhabitants with whom his refined and cultivated taste could assimilate. His active temperament and versatility of talent, however, found sufficient excitement in improving his newly acquired property, in frequent excursions to the metropolis, and in anticipating the birth of an heir, whom his ardent imagination invested with the beauty and grace of its mother, and the talents and enthusiasm of its father—to whose dawning intellect he proposed devoting his leisure hours, his scholastic lore, and his knowledge of the world.

But, alas ! all those bright anticipations were doomed to bitter disappointment. For his youthful wife, having few tastes and pursuits in common with her husband, was necessarily left much alone ; her mental faculties being little exercised, her physical system immature, the brain of her child was imperfectly developed, and his system weakly organized ; hence, the efforts of his father to bestow upon him a liberal education were fruitless ; and after years of anxiety, vexation, and mortification, the unhappy father was constrained to admit the mental imbecility of his son.

Not wishing to identify this family, I must pass over a number of its members whose dispositions and characters were strongly marked by the circumstances and sentiments that preceded their births. I would, however, remark, that a number of them are daughters, who, instead of inheriting the beauty and grace of their mother, are decidedly plain in person and not agreeable in manners. This discordance in nature can only be accounted for by the unhappy frame of mind induced by the disagreeable situation of the mother, who was, in her country residence, cut off from all social intercourse, and neglected by her husband ; causes, it must be admitted, sufficient to destroy the equanimity of any temper, and to produce a fretful and repining state of mind ; and those unharmonious feelings appear to have been transferred, not only to the dispositions, but to the countenances also of her children.*

Mr. A——, at length growing weary of the monotony of country life, sold his estate and returned to the city. This was a most fortunate event for the children born afterward. For having become the inmate of an intellectual and highly educated family, whose house was frequented by much good society, the mind of Mrs. A—— expanded and strengthened; all her faculties being called into harmonious exercise, her physical system having acquired maturity, she became almost a different woman, and her children born subsequently were superior in every respect to those who preceded them.

One of the last of these children appeared, even from infancy, to be most delightfully constituted; was a source of joy and hope to his parents, an object of affection and pride to his brothers and sisters, and perfectly happy in himself. Nor did the bright promises of his childhood and youth disappoint his friends; for his parents gave him a careful intellectual and moral education, and now, arrived at manhood, he reflects honor on all connected with him, and is a source of pleasure and happiness to all who know him.

* The Margravine of Anspach observes, that "when a female is likely to become a mother, she ought to be doubly careful of her temper; and in particular, to indulge in no ideas that are not cheerful, and no sentiments that are not kind. Such is the connection between mind and body, that the features of the face are moulded commonly into an expression of the internal disposition; and is it not natural to think that an infant, before it is born, may be affected by the temper of its mother?"—(*Memoirs, Vol. II., Chap. VIII.*)

CHAPTER VI.

STRENGTH IMPROVED BY COMBINATION.

From the vast body of evidence not yet adduced, I will select a few more examples, showing the degree in which mental strength accumulates when united in the parents, and transmitted to them by preceding generations. Sir William Jones, the most profound scholar of his time, was a striking example in proof of transmitted talents; and so perfectly innate were those talents, that, at the age of fifteen, his teacher, Dr. Thackeray, said, that "he was a boy of so active a mind, that if he were left naked and friendless on Salisbury Plain, he would, nevertheless, find the road to fame and riches."

The following warm-hearted tribute of affection and respect, from the pen of the Bishop of Cologne, bears testimony to the early indications of superior qualities of both the head and heart of Sir William Jones. "I knew him," he writes, "from the early age of eight or nine, and he was always an *uncommon boy*. Great abilities and great particularity of thinking, fondness for writing verses and plays of various kinds, and a degree of integrity and manly courage, of which I remember many instances, distinguished him even at that period. I loved and revered him, and though one or two years older than he was, was always instructed by him from my earliest age. In a word, I can only say of this amiable and wonderful man, that he had more virtues and less faults than I ever yet saw in any human being; and that the goodness of his head, admirble as it was, was exceeded by that of his heart. I have never ceased to admire him from the moment I first saw him; and my esteem for his great qualities, and regret for his loss, will only end with my life."

"His father was the celebrated philosopher and mathematician, William Jones, who so eminently distinguished himself in the commencement of the last century. He was born in the year 1680, in Anglesey. His parents were yeomen, or little frmers, on that island, and he there received the best education which they were able to afford ; but the industrious exertion of vigorous intellectual power supplied the defects of inadequate instruction, and laid the foundation of his future fame and fortune. From his earliest years, Mr. Jones discovered a propensity to mathematical studies, and having cultivated them with assiduity, he began his career in life by teaching mathematics on board of a man of war, and in this situation he attracted the notice and obtained the friendship of Lord Anson. In his twenty-second year, Mr. Jones published a treatise on the art of navigation, which was received with great approbation. He was present at the capture of Vigo in 1702, and having joined his comrades in quest of pillage, he eagerly fixed upon a bookseller's shop as the object of his depredation ; but finding in it no literary treasures, which was the sole plunder that he coveted, he contented himself with a pair of scissors, which he frequently exhibited to his friends as a trophy of his military success, relating the adventure by which he gained it. He returned with the fleet to England, and immediately afterward established himself as a teacher of mathematics in London, where, at the age of twenty-six, he published his Synopsis Palmariorma Matheoses, a decisive proof of his early and consummate proficiency in his favorite science."

"The private character of Mr. Jones was respectable, his manners were agreeable and inviting ; and these qualities not only contributed to enlarge the circle of his friends, whom his established reputation for science had attracted, but also to secure their attachment to him."

"Among others who honored him with their esteem, I am authorized to mention the great and virtuous Lord Hardwicke. Mr. Jones attended him as a companion on the circuit, when he was chief justice ; and this nobleman, when he afterward held the great seal, availed himself of the opportunity to testify his regard for the merit and character of his friend, by conferring upon him the office of secretary for the peace. He was also introduced to the friendship of Lord Parker (afterward president of the Royal Society), which terminated only with his death; and, among other distinguished characters in the annals of science and literature, the names of Sir Isaac Newton, Halley, Mead, and Samuel Johnson, may be enumerated as the intimate friends of Mr. Jones. By Sir Isaac Newton, he was treated with particular regard and confidence, and prepared, with his assent, the very elegant edition of small tracts, on the higher mathematics, in a mode which obtained the approbation, and increased the esteem of the author for him."

"After the retirement of Lord Macclesfield to Sherborne Castle, Mr. Jones resided with his lordship as a member of his family, and instructed him in the sciences. In this situation he had the misfortune to lose the greatest part of his property, the accumulation of industry and economy, by the failure of a banker; but the friendship of Lord Macclesfield diminished the weight of the loss, by procuring for him a sinecure place of considerable emolument. The same nobleman, who was then teller of the exchequer, made him an offer of a more lucrative situation; but he declined the acceptance of it, as it would have imposed on him the obligation of more official attendance than was agreeable to his temper, or compatible with his attachment to scientific pursuits."

"In this retreat he became acquainted with Miss Mary Nix, the youngest daughter of George Nix, a cabinet-maker in London, who, although of low extraction, had raised himself to eminence in his profession, and, from the honest and pleasant frankness of his conversation, was admitted to the tables of the great, and to the intimacy of Lord Macclesfield. The acquaintance of Mr. Jones with Miss Nix terminated in marriage, and from this union sprang three children, the youngest of whom, the late Sir William Jones,* was born in London, on

* This is another instance in proof that maturity of age in the parents, is favorable to the development and activity of the higher mental and

the eve of the festival of St. Michael, in the year 1746; and a few days after his birth was baptized by the Christian name of his father. The first son, George, died in his infancy, and the second child, a daughter, Mary, who was born in 1736, married Mr. Rainsford, a merchant, retired from business in opulent circumstances."

"Mr. Jones survived the birth of his son William but three years. He was attacked with a disorder which the sagacity of Dr. Mead, who attended him with the anxiety of an affectionate friend, immediately discovered to be a polypus in the heart, and wholly incurable. This alarming secret was communicated to Mrs. Jones, who, from an affectionate but mistaken motive, could never be induced to discover it to her husband, and, on one occasion, displayed a remarkable instance of self-command and address in the concealment of it. A well-meaning friend, who knew his dangerous situation, had written to him a long letter of condolence, replete with philosophic axioms on the brevity of life. Mrs. Jones, who opened the letter, discovered the purport of it at a glance, and being desired by her husband to read it, composed, in a moment, another letter so clearly and rapidly, that he had no suspicion of the deception; and this she did in a style so cheerful and entertaining, that it greatly exhilarated him. He died soon after, in July, 1749, leaving behind him a great reputation and moderate property."

"The care of the education of William now devolved upon his mother, who, in many respects, was eminently qualified for the task. Her character, as delineated by her husband with somewhat of mathematical precision, is this: 'That she was virtuous without blemish—generous without extravagance—frugal, but not niggardly—cheerful, but not giddy—close, but not sullen—ingenious, but not conceited—of spirit,

moral organs in the offspring. Mr. Jones was sixty-three years of age when his youngest son was born. It is, however, to be regretted, that there is no account of the age of his wife at that period; but that she was middle-aged, may be inferred from the fact that her second child was born ten years previous to her last, the illustrious Sir William Jones.

but not passionate—in her friendship trusty—to her parents dutiful—and to her husband ever faithful, loving, and obedient.' She had, by nature, a strong understanding, which was improved by his conversation and instruction. Under his tuition she became a considerable proficient in algebra ; and, with a view to qualify herself for the office of preceptor to her sister's son, who was destined to a maritime profession, made herself perfect in trigonometry and the theory of navigation. Mrs. Jones, after the death of her husband, was urgently and repeatedly solicited by the Countess of Macclesfield to remain at Sherborne Castle ; but, having formed a plan for the education of her son, with an unalterable determination to pursue it, and being apprehensive that her residence at Sherborne might interfere with the execution of it, she declined accepting the friendly invitation of the countess, who never ceased to retain the most affectionate regard for her."

"In the plan adopted by Mrs. Jones for the instruction of her son, she proposed to reject the severity of discipline, and to lead his mind insensibly to knowledge and exertion by exciting his curiosity, and directing it to useful objects. To his incessant importunities for information on casual topics of conversation, which she watchfully stimulated, she constantly replied, '*Read, and you will know*'—a maxim to the observance of which he always acknowledged himself indebted for his future attainments. By this method, his desire to learn became as eager as her wish to teach ; and such was her talent for instruction, and his facility in retaining it, that in his fourth year he was able to read, distinctly and rapidly, any English book. She particularly attended, at the same time, to the cultivation of his memory, by making him learn and repeat some of the popular speeches of Shakspeare, and the best of Gay's fables. His faculties gained strength by exercise, and during his school vacations the sedulity of a fond parent was without intermission exerted to improve his knowledge of his own language. She also taught him the rudiments of drawing, in which she excelled."

"If, from the subsequent eminence of Sir William Jones,"

observes the biographer, "any general conclusion should be eagerly drawn in favor of early tuition, we must not forget to advert to the *uncommon talents, both of the pupil and the teacher.*"

The following extract not only corroborates the truth of the transmission of mental and moral qualities, but, with the preceding, bears testimony to the power and influence which a strong-minded mother has in forming the character of her son.

"The mother of Mr. Guizot was left a widow with two sons, the elder of whom had only begun his seventh year when her husband was led to the block. She showed herself worthy of the excellent and honorable man who had been separated from her, and of the examples of *goodness and greatness she found written in the history of her own family;* for she then commenced the austere practice of those severe and painful duties which her friends saw her so religiously accomplish, amid all the trials and dangers by which her path was beset during her passage through this life. Notwithstanding the public interest which was felt for her at Nismes and the neighborhood, and the public anxiety for the fate of her sons, she tore herself away from all these mitigations of her sorrows, and proceeded to Geneva, because she felt that the education of her sons required this sacrifice at her hands."

"From his first entrance into these schools, the young Francis took an honorable and even distinguished rank, and the most brilliant success crowned his assiduity and perseverance. It would be puerile, when writing the memoirs of such a man as Guizot, to render an account of all the academic honors conferred upon him as the reward for diligence and progress; but when he left the classes in 1815, success had been so marked and transcendent, that his professors did not hesitate to predict for him a brilliant career."

"Having accomplished the object she proposed by her residence at Geneva, Madame Guizot returned with her sons to Languedoc, there to fulfill, on her part, those filial duties to her then aged parents, which she knew so well how to perform. Her son left the maternal home soon afterward, and proceeded to Paris to study the principles of law and justice. On quitting his beloved parent, he took with him, however, her stern and inflexible love of truth and virtue, and had no other object in residing at Paris but to prepare for the future and important duties of an active life."

CHAPTER VII.

TRANSMISSION OF QUALITIES.

THERE is not, perhaps, a more forcible illustration of the truth of the transmission of qualities to be found in history, than that presented by the Wesley family. The same deep devotional feeling, the same active, energetic intellect, and the same readiness to sacrifice worldly interest for conscience' sake, may be traced back through four generations.

The conspicuous place given to the mother of the founder of the Methodists, in the biography of her son, is worthy of observation ; so, also, is the important part which she acted in her family, and the care which she bestowed on the moral training of her three highly-talented sons. In many biographies, the mother of the great man is not even mentioned—in those of Charles Fox and Edward Burke, for instance. In the latter, however, it is observed as a remarkable coincidence, that Pitt, Fox, and Burke, were all younger sons. "Coincidences," it might also be said, "are mere finger-posts, pointing to where things lie of which we remain ignorant." And when as much attention has been devoted to mental as to physical science, coincidences will become more rare, and the laws will be recognized by which similar results are produced. It may, however, require, yet, ages of observation and experience to confirm this simple truth—that the children born in the full maturity of the physical and mental constitution of the parents, are superior in every respect to those who preceded that condition.

"The founder of the Methodists," says Mr. Southey, "was emphatically of a good family, in the same sense wherein he himself would have used the term. Bartholomew Wesley, his great-grandfather, studied physic, as well as divinity, at the university—a practice not unusual at that time. He was ejected, by the act of uniformity, from the living of Allington, in Dorsetshire; and the medical knowledge which he had acquired from motives of charity, became then the means of his support. John, his son, was educated at New Inn Hall, Oxford, in the time of the Commonwealth; he was distinguished not only for his piety and diligence, but for his progress in the oriental tongues, by which he attracted the particular notice and esteem of the then vice-chancellor, John Owen, a man whom the Calvinistic dissenters still regarded as the greatest of their divines. If the government had continued in the Cromwell family, this patronage would have raised him to distinction. He obtained the living of Blandford, in his own county, and was ejected from it for non-conformity. Being thus adrift, he thought of emigrating to Maryland, or to Surinam, where the English were then intending to settle a colony; but reflection and advice determined him to take his lot in his native land. There, by continuing to preach, he became obnoxious to the laws, and was four times imprisoned: his spirits were broken by the loss of those he loved best, and by the evil days. He died at the early age of three or four and thirty; and such was the spirit of the times, that the Vicar of Preston, in which village he died, would not allow his body to be buried in the church. Bartholomew was then living; but the loss of this, his only son, soon brought his gray hairs with sorrow to the grave.

"This John Wesley married a woman of good stock, the niece of Thomas Fuller, the church historian—a man not more remarkable for wit and quaintness, than for the felicity with which he clothed fine thoughts in beautiful language. He left two sons, of whom Samuel, the younger, was only eight or nine years old at the time of his father's death. The circumstances of the father's life and sufferings, which have given him a place among the confessors of the non-conformists, were likely to influence the opinions of the son; but, happening to fall in with bigoted and ferocious men, he saw the worst parts of the dissenting character. Their defence of the execution of King Charles offended him. He separated from them, and, because of their intolerance, joined the church which had persecuted his father. This conduct, which was the result of feeling, was approved by his ripe judgment, and Samuel Wesley continued through life a zealous churchman. The feeling which urged him to this step must have been very powerful, and no common spirit was required to bear him through the difficulties which he brought upon himself; for, by withdrawing from the academy at which he had been placed, he so far offended his friends, that they lent him no further support; and, in the latter years of Charles II., there was little disposition to encourage proselytes who joined a church which the reigning family were endeavoring to subvert. But Samuel Wesley was made of good mould; he knew, and could depend upon, himself; he walked to Oxford, entered himself at Exeter College as a poor scholar, and began his studies there with no larger a fund than two pounds sixteen shillings, and no prospect of any future supply. From that time, till he graduated, a single crown was all the assistance he received from his friends. He composed exercises for those who had more money than learning, and he gave instruction to those who wished to profit by his lessons; and thus, by great industry and great frugality, he not only supported himself, but had accumulated the sum of ten pounds fifteen shillings when he went to London to be ordained. Having served a curacy there one year, and as chaplain during another on board a king's ship, he settled upon a curacy in the metropolis, and married Susannah, daughter of Dr. Annesley, one of the ejected ministers.

"No man was ever more suitably mated than the elder Wesley. The wife whom he chose was, like himself, the child of a man eminent among the non-conformists; and, like himself, in early youth she had chosen her own path. She had examined the controversy between the Dissenters and the Church of England, with conscientious diligence, and satisfied herself that the schismatics were in the wrong. The dispute, it must be remembered, related wholly to discipline; but her inquiries had not stopped there, and she had reasoned herself into Socinianism, from which she was reclaimed by her husband. She was an admirable woman, of highly-improved mind, and of a strong and masculine understanding—an obedient wife, an exemplary mother, and a fervent Christian."

A further account of this high-minded, excellent woman, and her equally talented and pious husband, may be found in Southey's life of her son, the first of the Methodists.

Dr. Doddridge was another remarkable instance of the direct descent of superior moral and intellectual qualities. His family, on the paternal side, through successive generations, produced lawyers, judges, and divines, of eminent talent and true piety. His mother was the daughter of the Rev. John Bourman, a native of Prague, in Bohemia, who, in consequence of religious persecution, was placed in a situation where there was no alternative but to abjure the Protestant faith, or to secure religious freedom by emigration. "This latter painful expedient he had the virtue and resolution to embrace, although it imposed the loss of his early associations, separated him from the friends of his youth, and deprived him of a considerable estate when he was beginning to enjoy it, being then just of age." "After having spent a considerable time in Gotha, in Saxony, and in the neighboring states, he came to England about the year 1646, with ample testimonials from many of the principal German divines; and, in consequence of these recommendations, was so fortunate as to be appointed to the mastership of a grammar school, at Kensington, upon Thames—a situation affording that opportunity for useful retirement that was congenial to his feelings, and where he died about the year 1668, leaving an only daughter, then of very tender age."

"This orphan was married to Daniel Doddridge, before alluded to, and bore him *twenty* children. Such, however, was the fatality which reigned in this large family, that, at the birth of the *twentieth*, there was only one other child, a daughter, surviving. This last child, who became Dr. Doddridge, was, from the circumstances of his birth—his mother having been in the utmost peril for a period of thirty-six hours—so destitute of every appearance of vitality, that the attendants felt convinced that it was actually dead, and put it aside accordingly; one of them, however, soon afterward, chancing to cast a glance upon the infant, fancied that she perceived a feeble heaving of the chest, and, moved with pity, took upon herself the apparently futile task of its resuscitation. The pious care was providentially rewarded; for, while she continued to cherish it, a faint moaning became audible, evincing that the babe was indeed alive: and thus, apparently by an accident, was that voice called into action, on whose eloquent accents thousands afterward hung with hushed delight, while their hearts grew warm with the holy love of God!"

"This child was called Philip, after his uncle; and, as the last hope of his parents, who had probably mourned the loss of many sons, was tended with the most indulgent care. Nor were they deficient in more important duties, as Dr. Doddridge observes in a letter to Mr. Wilbraham, when alluding to the period of his infancy: 'I was brought up in the early knowledge of religion by my pious parents, who were, in their character, very worthy of their *birth* and education. I well remember that my mother taught me the history of the Old and New Testament before I could read, by the assistance of some blue Dutch tiles in the chimney-place of the room where we commonly sat; and the *wise* and *pious* reflections she made upon these stories, were the means of enforcing such good impressions on my heart as never afterward wore out.' "*

Among the numerous examples which might be brought forward to illustrate the theory of transmission and inheritance, particularly through the maternal line, are the lives of Bishop Hall, Rev. John Newton, Herbert, Hooker, and Philip Henry. Nor should we forget the examples contained in the Bible; especially those of Samuel and Timothy, the latter of whom "from a child had known the Holy Scriptures," inheriting "that unfeigned faith which had dwelt first in his grandmother Lois, and in his mother Eunice."

* Dr. Doddridge lost both his parents at the early age of thirteen years; it may, therefore, be inferred that his mental organization was particularly constituted to receive and to retain good impressions.

CHAPTER VIII

CIRCUMSTANCES EXPLAIN THE ADVENT OF GENIUSES.

GENIUS, when manifested in the poorer class, is regarded with wonder, and too generally supposed to be like the Nazarite locks of Sampson, an especial gift of heaven bestowed upon the individual, and not the result of a happy organization, the effect of kindly influences exercised at the commencement, and during the infancy of the possessor. Could the circumstances attendant on these advents be truly ascertained, the miracle would be explained, and the parent might hope, by surrounding his offspring with similar causes, to bestow upon them the power of exhibiting similar effects. Thus, the case of the poet Burns—whose mental efforts have been regarded with wonder and delight by the Saxon world generally, and whose powers, considering his origin, have been thought most wonderful—is liable to the following explanation :

" The mother of Burns was a native of the county of Ayr; her birth was humble, and her personal attractions moderate ; yet, in all other respects, she was a remarkable woman. She was blessed with singular equanimity of temper ; her religious feelings were deep and constant ; she loved a well-regulated household ; and it was frequently her pleasure to give wings to the weary hours of a checkered life by chanting old songs and ballads, of which she had a large store. In her looks she resembled her eldest son ; her eyes were bright and intelligent ; her perception of character quick and keen. She lived to a great age, rejoiced in the fame of the poet, and partook of the fruits of his genius."

The following extracts show the excellent character of the father of Burns, and the care which he bestowed on the education and moral culture of his children. " Amid all these toils and trials, William Burns remembered the worth of religious instruction, and the usefulness of education in the rearing of his children. The former task he took upon himself, and, in a little manual of devotion still extant, sought to soften the rigor of the Calvinistic creed into the gentler Arminian. He set, too, the example which he taught. He abstained from all profane swearing and vain discourse, and shunned all approach to levity of conversation or behavior. A week-day, in his house, wore the sobriety of a Sunday; nor did he fail in performing family worship in a way which enabled his son to give to the world that fine picture of devotion, the 'Cotter's Saturday Night.'"

"The education of Burns was not over when the school-doors were shut. The peasantry of Scotland turn their cottages into schools; and when a father takes his arm-chair by the evening fire, he seldom neglects to communicate to his children whatever knowledge he possesses himself. Nor is this knowledge very limited; it extends, generally, to the history of Europe, and to the literature of the island; but more particularly to the divinity, the poetry, and what may be called the traditionary history of Scotland. An intelligent peasant is intimate with all those skirmishes, sieges, combats, and quarrels, domestic or national, of which public writers take no account. Genealogies of the chief families are quite familiar to him. He has by heart, too, whole columns of songs and ballads; nay, long poems sometimes abide in his recollection; nor will he think his knowledge much, unless he knows a little about the lives and actions of the men who have done most honor to Scotland. In addition to what he has on his memory, we may mention what he has on the shelf. A common husbandman is frequently master of a little library: history, divinity, and poetry, but mostly the latter, compose his collection. Milton and Young are favorites; the flowery meditations of Hervey, the religious romance of the Pilgrim's Progress, are seldom absent; while, of Scottish books, Ramsay, Thomson, Ferguson, and now Burns, together with songs and ballad-books innumerable, are all huddled together, soiled with smoke, and frail and tattered by frequent use.

The household of William Burns was an example of what I have described; and there is some truth in the assertion, that, in true knowledge, the poet was, at nineteen, a better scholar than nine tenths of our young gentlemen when they leave school for the college."

The great number of literary and scientific men which Scotland has produced, when compared with her sister kingdoms, is, to many reflecting minds, matter of surprise and wonder. The preceding account of the general literary taste and acquirements of the people, together with the following opinion of one of the most original thinkers of the age, may furnish an explanation, and, at the same time, support the theory of transmission and inheritance contended for in these pages.

"A country where the entire population is, or even once has been, laid hold of, filled to the heart with an infinite religious idea, has made a step from which it cannot retrograde. Thought, conscience—the sense that man is denizen of a universe, creature of an eternity—has penetrated the remotest cottage, to the simplest heart. Beautiful and awful, the feeling of a heavenly behest, of duty God-commanded, overcanopies all life. There is an inspiration in such a people; one may say, in a more special sense, 'the inspiration of the Almighty giveth them understanding.' Honor to all the brave and true; everlasting honor to the brave old Knox, one of the truest of the true! That in the moment while he and his cause, amid civil broils, in convulsion and confusion, were still but struggling for life, he sent the schoolmaster forth to all corners, and said, 'Let the people be taught'—this is but one, and, indeed, an inevitable, and, comparatively, inconsiderable item in his great message to men. His message, in its true compass, was, 'Let men know that they are men, created by God, responsible to God; who work in any meanest moment of time what will last through eternity.' It is, verily, a great message. Not ploughing and hammering machines - not patent digesters (never so ornamental), to digest the produce of these—no, in no wise—born slaves neither to their fellow-men, nor of their appetites—but men! This great message Knox did deliver with a man's voice and strength, and he found a people to believe him. Of such an achievement, we say, were it to be made once only, the results are immense. Thought, in such a country, may change its form, but it cannot go out; the country has attained *majority*, thought, and a certain spiritual manhood, ready for all work that man can do, endures there. It may take many forms—the form of hard-fisted, money-getting industry, as in the vulgar Scotchman, the vulgar New Englander; but, as compact, developed force, and alertness of faculty, it is still there. It may utter itself as the colossal skepticism of a Hume (beneficent, this, too, though painful, wrestling, Titan-like, through doubt and inquiry, toward new belief); and again, in some better day, it may utter itself in the inspired melody of a Burns; in a word, it is, and continues in the voice and the work of a nation of hardy, endeavoring, considering men, with whatever that may bear in it, or unfold from it. The Scotch national character originates in many circumstances. first of all, is the Saxon stuff there was to work on; but next, and beyond all else except that, the Presbyterian Gospel of John Knox."

The writer of the preceding extract is another distinguished example of the transmission of superior moral and intellectual qualities. A late English publication contains the following brief sketch of the parents of Thomas Carlyle, so justly celebrated for the power and originality of his writings.

"Carlyle is a borderer. The village of Ecclefechan, in Annandale, has the honor of giving him birth. From our admiration of the genius of Carlyle, we lately made a pilgrimage to his native village, and learned a few particulars of his early history. His father, who was a creditable yeoman, in comfortable circumstances, was a man of a strong and original mind, of very superior intelligence for his opportunities and station in society, and much respected for his moral worth, and strict, though somewhat awkward, honesty.

"By the villagers he seems to have been regarded as quite an oracle; and they still relate many instances of his striking original observations and rich, sarcastic wit. His mother, who is still living, and can enjoy, with a parent's pride and pleasure, the celebrity of her distinguished son, is also a superior, sensible, and pious woman. To this excellent mother he owes much, for the pains and care with which she imbued his youthful mind with the principles of religion, and that love of truth and virtue which characterizes his writings; and her solicitude, we were informed, is well repaid by the more than filial affection of her son, who venerates her with a devotion approaching to idolatry."

The following extract, from Washington Irving's Life of Margaret Davidson, shows the direct descent of peculiar characteristics from mother to child:

"The narrative will be found almost as illustrative of the character of the mother as of the child. They were singularly identified in tastes, in feelings, and pursuits; tenderly entwined together by maternal and filial affection, they reflected an inexpressibly touching grace and interest upon each other by this holy relationship; and, to my mind, it would be marring one of the most beautiful and affecting groups in the history of modern literature, to sunder them.

"This maternal instruction, while it kept her apart from the world, and fostered a singular purity and innocence of thought, contributed greatly to enhance her imaginative powers; for the mother partook largely of the poetical temperament of the child. It was, in fact, one poetical spirit ministering to another."

Again, in Alexander Young's discourse on the life and character of Dr. Bowditch, he relates having visited the town where the doctor was born, and the testimony he there received in favor of the excellent character of his mother. "This testimony, in substance, is, that he was a likely, clever, thoughtful boy; learning came natural to him; he did not seem like other children, but much better; and that his mother was a beautiful, cheerful, good-natured woman. Her children took after her, and she had a peculiar way of guarding them against evil."

"These," continues Mr. Young, "I testify to be their very words, as I penciled them down at the time; and they show,

I think, very clearly, the influence of the mother's mind and heart upon the character of her son. Of that mother, in after-life and to its close, he often spoke in terms of the highest admiration and the strongest affection, and in his earnest manner would say, 'My mother loved me—idolized me—worshiped me.'"

The closest students of natural philosophy admit, that, notwithstanding the splendid discoveries already made in the natural sciences, there are unsolved problems enough in nature to task the ingenuity and industry of all future ages. It is not, however, sufficient that the inquirer into the hidden mysteries of nature rests satisfied when he has discovered that a certain effect is produced by a certain cause. Should he not investigate further, and endeavor to ascertain what produced the cause also? For example, a child is found to be short-sighted; he looks into its organ of vision, and there perceives a dilated *pupil,* occasioned by want of contractibility in the *iris,* or an unusual convexity of the *cornea,* or a great depth of the *aqueous* humor, either of which causes short-sightedness. But what caused these defects in the eye—whether congenital, or produced by habit—he has not yet been able to discover.

From the greater number of short-sighted persons found in cities than in the country, and from this defect being more common among students than those of active habits, it might be inferred that it was acquired by sedentary and studious pursuits, and by not sufficiently exercising and strengthening the organs of sight in youth. Short-sightedness is, however, frequently congenital, and inherited; but when it appears in a family for the first time, should not the cause be looked for in the habits of the mother? May not her sedentary pursuits, and close attention to minute and near objects, such as fine needle-work, embroidery, etc., have caused this defect in the organ of vision of her unborn child?

Two early friends of the authoress, of very dissimilar characters, married about the same time, and their children have partaken strongly of the peculiarities of their mothers; one of whom was of a dull, sluggish nature, and as much averse to mental as to personal activity. Her conscience appeared quite at ease if her fingers were employed, even in the most trifling occupation; and the less mental effort her work required, the more pleasing it was to her. While thus employed, she frequently beguiled the time by caroling sentimental songs and ballads. The phrenological developments of her eldest daughter correspond perfectly with the habits and pursuits of the mother during her pregnancy: tune large—domestic sentiments and animal propensities large—reflective organs moderate—perceptive ones small—quite deficient in the organ of weight, and very near-sighted. That the last two defects were caused by the personal inactivity of the mother, and by her sight being constantly confined to small and near objects, appears the more probable, as her last children's organs of weight and vision were perfect—she having removed to the country, and been obliged to perform the active duties of her family.

The other youthful mother was blessed with a most happy, joyous temper, and possessed of mental and personal activity in a high degree—passionately fond of dancing, walking, riding on horseback, and all other exercises requiring action, skill, and grace. She was a perfect economist of her time, allowing no portions of it to be wasted. Her household was regulated with order, neatness, and taste. By her habit of early rising, she was enabled to arrange all her domestic matters before breakfast; after which, she usually occupied herself with plain needle-work, while her husband read aloud the morning papers. She would then accompany him in a walk of three miles to his office; and on her return, devote the remainder of the morning to pursuits congenial to a highly-cultivated literary taste; and thus, on her husband's return to dinner, she had something new, interesting, and amusing, to read or relate to him. A portion of the afternoon was generally devoted to exercise in the open air; or, the weather not permitting, to a game of battle-door, or the graces at home; or to chess, reading, and needle-work. Born under such pleasant influences, the children were sprightly, active, and graceful—perfect emanations of joy—their perceptions quick, their sensibilities acute, their understanding vigorous—no lesson a task, no duty a burden. Their father was a man of sense and feeling, who perfectly understood the influence of the mother's mind, during the period of gestation, on the temper and disposition of her child; therefore, never allowed her feelings to be disturbed, irritated, or annoyed. Hence, the sweetness, docility, and tractability of their children; and hence their dissimilarity to those first mentioned, whose parents allowed no such influence, nor would give themselves any trouble or thought about the matter—and their children were perfect clods of dullness, ill-temper, and stupidity.

Another remarkable instance of the effect of the habits and pursuits of the mother on her offspring, came under the immediate observation of the writer.

Mrs. A—— was a melancholy instance of strength of mind perverted to selfish ends. Ambitious of power and influence, she was unscrupulous in the means by which they were obtained. Owing to her plausibility and pertinacity, she once was elected to an office of trust in a benevolent society, of which she was a member. This was a situation of great temptation to one in whose head the selfish sentiments predominated, as the event proved; for, at the expiration of the year, she was dismissed under the imputation of having appropriated a portion of the funds of the society to her own use. During the year in which she held this office, Mrs. A—— gave birth to a daughter, whose first manifestations were acquisitiveness and secretiveness in excess, or a propensity to theft. That the great development and activity of those organs in the head of the child were the effect of the dishonest practices of the mother, previous to her birth, there can be but little doubt. Such facts require no comment. The inference to be deduced from them is so palpable, that "he who runs may read."

CHAPTER IX.

INSANITY ACCOUNTED FOR PHRENOLOGICALLY.

INSANITY, the most dreadful of all the diseases to which mankind is subject, has been a cause of interminable discussion. Innumerable, also, have been the theories formed to account for it. That of Dr. Rush, which placed it in the blood, was, perhaps, nearer the truth than any other formed without the aid of Phrenology. When, however, we reflect upon the light which Phrenology throws on this subject, it is no longer a matter of astonishment that, without its aid, no definite conclusion ever was arrived at respecting the source of this dire disease.

Dr. Rush discovered that copious bleeding relieved the paroxysms of the insane, and, on dissecting those subjects, he always found indications of a high state of inflammation in the brain; from which he inferred that the disease had its source in the blood.

The phrenologists, on the contrary, show that insanity is caused by the over-exercise of some of the passions or sentiments of the mind; and that this undue action causes a determination of blood to some of its organs, leaving others in a state of complete apathy. This information, however, would be of little importance, did it not accompany a system of prevention and cure which generally proves successful. Experience shows, that by exciting other organs, and thereby withdrawing the excess of blood from those which are overcharged, the balance is restored, the mind recovers its tone, and resumes a healthful action. Thus, for instance, when acquisitiveness, cautiousness, combativeness, or destructiveness, the organs most frequently disordered, are manifested in excess, and derangement ensues, it becomes the duty of the friends of the sufferer to excite, as early as possible, the observing and reasoning faculties, by the stimulus of change of air and scene—of society and employment—of diet and habits. Recourse should also be had to the shower bath, and whatever else might add to the comfort and well-being of the sufferer. These are the remedies substituted by the phrenologist, for the cruel practices of the lonesome cell, the iron chain, the straight jacket, and the discipline of the prison.

The following statistical observations show the effect which different employments and conditions in life have in producing lunatics and idiots.

In 1829, Sir A..Halliday made a report of lunatics and idiots in England and Wales. The lunatics were 6800, and the idiots 5741 ; to which he adds, for places not returned, 1500—making in all, 14,000. The paupers of them are estimated at 11,000.

In twelve counties in England, where the population is employed in agriculture, the proportion of the insane is, to the general population, as one in 820, and the idiots are one to 490 ; while in twelve counties where the population is employed in trade and manufacturing, the insane are only as one to 1200.*

* "Fatuity, from old age, cannot be cured, but it may be prevented, by employing the mind in reading and conversation in the evening of life. Dr. Johnson ascribes the fatuity of Dean Swift to two causes; 1st, to a esolution made in his youth, that he would never wear spectacles, from the want of which he was unable to read in the decline of life; and, 2d, to his avarice, which led him to abscond from visitors, or deny himself to company, by which means he deprived himself of the only two methods by which new ideas are acquired, or old ones renovated. His mind, from these causes, languished from the want of exercise, and gradually collapsed into idiotism, in which state he spent the close of his life, in a hospital founded by himself for persons afflicted with the same disorder, of which he finally died."

"Country people, who have no relish for books, when they lose the ability of working, or of going abroad, from age or weakness, are very apt to become fatuitous, especially as they are too often deserted in their old age by the younger branches of their families, in consequence of which their minds become torpid from the want of society and conversation. Fatuity is more rare in cities than in country places, only because society and conversation can be had in them upon more easy terms; and it is less common in women than men, because they seldom survive their ability

In seven counties in North Wales there is one idiot to 120, and one lunatic to 850 inhabitants; these are agricultural counties. And, says an English writer, "There is a general impression that, in agricultural districts, where the people work hard, and where females are employed in labor, the violent exertion required in this occupation produces distortion of the body, and may very materially affect the growth and development of the brain, and even the form of the cranium, *in utero*. It is well known that females are obliged to work during the whole of their pregnancy, and there can be no doubt of the injury which such occupation must have on the offspring."

This opinion is very correct, but it leaves much that is important to the subject unsaid. Of the 14,000 idiots and lunatics in England and Wales, 11,000 are of the pauper class. In England, the paupers receive very little education, and in Wales, it is believed, still less; this may account for the increased number of idiots in the latter country. The agricultural peasantry, male and female, of those countries, are not called upon for any more mental effort than their fellow-laborer, the ox, or the ass. "If," says Mr. Combe, "we exercise our muscles too severely, or too long, we drain off the whole nervous energy of our bodies by our arms and legs, and the brain then becomes incapable of thinking, and the nerves incapable of feeling, so that dullness and stupidity seize on our mental powers." From this dullness and stupidity in the parents, proceed the undeveloped brain of the idiot child, or the unequally-balanced one of the lunatic.

The easy labor and speedy delivery of women of the lower classes and of the Indian race, have occasioned much discussion among physiologists. The true cause, I apprehend, will

to work, and because their employments are of such a nature as to admit of their being carried on at the fireside, and in a sedentary posture. The illustrious Dr. Franklin exhibited a striking instance of the influence of reading, writing, and conversation, in prolonging a sound and active state of all the faculties of the mind. In his eighty-fourth year, he discovered no one mark of the weakness and decay usually observed in the minds of persons at that advanced period of life."

be found in the want of size and development in the heads of their children.

In the statistical tables of Europe, lately published in Paris, it is shown that there are three male children still-born to two females. This result certainly cannot be the effect of chance, but must have some physical cause; and this cause, doubtless, is the superior size of the heads of male children. For it is well known that the human head, male and female, varies as materially in form and size at birth, as at maturity; and also, that difficult and protracted labor, when the presentation is natural, and there is no distortion of the pelvis,* is caused by the large and firm skull of the fœtus.

There is an editorial note in Croker's edition of Boswell's Johnson, which, with the aid of Phrenology, sheds much light on this subject. It is stated in the text that the mother of Johnson had, at his birth, a very difficult and dangerous labor, and that he was born almost dead. To which Croker adds, that Addison, Lord Lyttleton, Voltaire, and many other eminent men, were born almost dead. That this peculiarity should have attended the birth of so many gifted individuals, cannot be considered accidental, but rather an evidence of a

* Distortions of the spinal column, and the bones of the pelvis, are more common among females of the middling and higher classes, than is generally suspected. This dangerous condition of the system is frequently caused by tight lacing in early youth, when the bones are soft and yielding; the viscera of the abdominal region being pressed down on those unconsolidated bones, they give way under the unnatural weight, and distortion is the result. The writer is acquainted with a family of four sisters, born of healthy parents, of course inheriting good constitutions. The eldest was adopted, when quite young, by a rich relation, and educated at a fashionable boarding-school, where little attention was paid to the laws of health. Want of fresh air and exercise, the excitement of going too early into society, late hours, and tight lacing, soon undermined her constitution, and produced a lateral curvature of the spine. She nevertheless married young, and has had numerous offspring; but each parturition was attended with excruciating suffering and imminent peril; nor has she ever given birth to a living child. The three other sisters, whose education and habits were more in accordance with nature, have each a large family of healthy children, born without difficulty or danger.

more powerful organization, resulting from an unusual development of the brain, the organ of the mind.

The truth of the preceding views has been corroborated by much testimony, and was forcibly presented to my attention by the circumstances attending the birth of two children which came under my immediate observation. The mother of one of them was about eighteen years of age, of a phlegmatic temperament, indolent habits, and educated for display. She was occupied, during the whole period of her pregnancy, in paying and receiving visits of ceremony, in practicing music, embroidery, and other fashionable accomplishments, and in endeavoring to attain the reputation of a superior taste in dress; her reading was limited and confined to works of imagination. She had neither inclination nor comprehension for any thing more profound than is to be met with in the pages of the New York Mirror, or the Parlor Visitor. Her child was born at the full time, but so brief and easy was the labor, that neither physician nor nurse was present. It was plump and fat enough, but with a head diminutive in size and soft in quality.

Years have not altered those conditions; the child in intellect is below mediocrity, and the man will be the same. In the other instance, the mother was past forty years of age, of an energetic temperament, active habits, and self-educated. For some months previous to the birth of her fifth child, she had become a convert to the belief in the transmission of mental and moral qualities. To test the truth of this belief, she exercised her own mental powers to their full extent. She attended the lectures of the season, both literary and scientific; read much, but such works only as tend to exercise and strengthen the reasoning faculties, and improve the judgment—the domestic and foreign reviews, history, biography, etc. She was also engaged in the active duties of a large family, in which she found full scope for the exercise of the moral sentiments, but never allowed any thing to disturb the equanimity of her temper. When her time came, she was in labor two days; all her suffering, however, was forgotten at the birth of a son with a head of the finest form, firmest quality, and largest size—with the reflecting organs of a Bacon, and the moral ones of a Melancthon. A head, in short, on which nature had written, in characters too legible to be misunderstood, strength, power, and capability; and of whom it is already said, "He is the youngest of his family, but will soon become its head."

But it may be said, the number of women is small who would be willing to encounter the extra pains and perils of childbirth induced by the training of the last example. To such we can only say, that when they discover the minds of their children to be "unstable as water," with scarcely understanding enough to distinguish good from evil, and not firmness of character sufficient to pursue any steady course through life, in the anxiety and unhappiness which such conduct occasions, they must reap the punishment of their own want of moral and physical courage at the time when the exercise of those qualities would have transmitted them to their offspring. It is, however, my firm conviction, that if women would study the structure of their own bodies, and the functions of its different organs, and acquire some knowledge of the principles of obstetrics, they might escape a great portion of the present dangers and sufferings of childbirth; but in the present system of female education, that branch of knowledge which would enable them to raise a family of healthy children with success, appears to be most neglected. A friend of the authoress, of good understanding, active temperament, and sound constitution, married in middle life, and has had two fine boys; but, from her utter ignorance of the organic laws, lost them both. The birth of the first was attended by protracted and dangerous labor; the child was still-born, but was resuscitated, and was a remarkably healthy and promising infant. His sudden death at the age of thirteen months was attended by very distressing circumstances, under which the mother was sustained by the prospect of the birth of another child in seven or eight months. Meantime, the mental anguish occasioned by the death of the first child could only be alleviated by constant occupation of the mind. She therefore undertook an extensive course of historical reading, varied by the study of mental and moral philosophy, to which was added the physiological and moral training of youth. The subject, however, of the most importance at that time—a knowledge of the proper habits and course of life necessary to ensure a speedy and safe delivery, was forgotten. The sedentary habits induced by study, protracted her time beyond the natural period, and her constant mental exercise developed the brain of the child to an unusual degree; hence, the second labor was more difficult and dangerous than the first. The attendant physician believed, that "nature, in a healthy subject, was always able to do her own work;" therefore, rendered her no assistance except copious bleeding. Nature did, indeed, do her own work; but she was so long about it, that a beautiful male child, weighing twelve pounds, was killed in the process. The unfortunate mother was then congratulated on her escape with life, and was advised, if she valued life, to pray that she might never have any more children, for it was impossible for children with heads as large and as firm as hers, to be born alive. To which she answered, "that life to her had no charms without children, and that she was willing to undergo the same three days' suffering, and as much more as it was possible to survive, or even the Cæsarian operation, for the sake of a living child." She immediately procured some books on midwifery, from which she learned, that if she had, for six or eight weeks previously to the expiration of her time, taken much gentle exercise in the open air, lived very abstemiously, and strengthened her system by cold baths, nature would have been in a proper condition to have done her own work; or, if she required some assistance from her handmaid, art (which it was possible she might, as this child could not have been called a child of nature, in the same degree as that of the uneducated peasant or the untutored savage), it was more than probable that a vapor bath might have relaxed the muscles, prevented the cramps and chills, and facilitated the labor to a successful issue, and she might have rejoiced in the birth of a living child.

It is highly gratifying to the writer to add, that, since the publication of the first edition of this work, the lady just referred to has given birth to a third son, and, by pursuing a course dictated by reason and experience—that is, by attention to diet, exercise, air, and cold water bathing—she gave birth to a healthy living child after only two hours' not severe labor.

Such cases are truly encouraging, and should teach women the importance of investigating the laws of nature for themselves, instead of relying, with blind confidence, on the opinions and prejudices of past ages.

Reason, observation, experience, and every consideration bearing on this subject, unite in persuading mothers to study the laws of health that govern the condition of pregnancy, to appreciate their own responsibility in such cases, and not to commit so great an injustice to medical science as to expect it to retrieve their errors, and carry them safely through the process of parturition, independently of their previous wrong habits. It should, therefore, be engraved upon the mind of every mother, as with a point of steel, that the degree of suffering and danger present at the period of parturition, will depend entirely upon her mode of life and habits during the term of gestation.

CHAPTER X

RESPONSIBILITIES, INFLUENCE, AND RIGHTS OF WOMEN.

Much has been written by the wise and the good on the influence and responsibility of mothers, but without producing any permanent effects, if we are to judge from the present standard of morality among the youth of our country. Virtue, however, cannot be learned by listening to precepts; it requires a field of action and constant practice. Many of the works alluded to are written in such general terms, that few individuals can apply the principles which they inculcate to their own particular circumstances. An example, therefore, may carry to the mind of the mother a just conviction of the duty which she owes to society and to her country, to train her children in the paths of virtue, knowledge, and usefulness.

The writer is perfectly aware that much legislation respecting the rights of property of married women is required, before the mother can be held entirely responsible for the improvement of her offspring. Under the present laws, a married woman is not a morally responsible agent, neither has she any control over her own property, but is subject to the will and power of her husband, and is too frequently kept in a state of dependence and penury sufficient to repress all her energies, and to render her a nonentity in her own estimation, as well as that of her family. Let her entertain the most liberal and enlightened views with regard to the improvement of her children, and the society in her neighborhood, she has neither the power nor the means of carrying them into effect; but, under the iron rule of her husband, and his all-grasping spirit of acquisitiveness, is obliged to shrink down into the very depths of nothingness, or live in a constant state of contention and strife.

The subject of the rights of women has been much discussed of late, but without any beneficial effects, because the advocates felt no real interest in the subject, and because they overlook the laws of nature, which have assigned to woman her appropriate sphere in the domestic circle, and claim for her political privileges totally discordant to her nature, her habits, or her inclinations. Whereas, if her rights of property were established upon the true principles of equity and justice—if the property which she inherited could not be taken from her except for debts of her own contracting—if the laws protected that which she accumulated by her own efforts, and assigned to her a portion of that acquired by her husband, for the benefit of her family—knowing that she possessed the power and the means of educating her children, she then would fully appreciate her responsibility, and might be held accountable for their intelligence, virtue, and integrity.

There are many mothers who, if they possessed the means of rendering their homes attractive and interesting to their sons, might prevent them from seeking amusement and excitement abroad, and thereby falling into those sensual excesses which too frequently lead to a life of remorse and suffering, or to an early grave. The power and influence which a strong-minded mother has over the happiness and prosperity of her sons, is illustrated by the example of a friend of the writer.

Mrs. W——, a woman of much observation and reflection, married at the age of thirty, and in eight years became the mother of four healthy, promising boys.* Having the misfortune to lose her husband at that period, the responsibility of training and educating her sons devolved entirely upon herself. The importance of this duty she fully appreciated; for, having seen many of the sons of the companions of her youth grow up to be a disgrace to their families, she felt deeply anxious for the welfare of her own sons, and endeavored to avoid the causes which had betrayed into error and crime those unfortunate youths, whose unhappy fate she sincerely lamented. Believing that moral, not any more than physical

* It may be observed that women possessing a high degree of mental activity generally give birth to more male than female offspring.(*d*)

evil is inherent in human nature, or the result of chance, Mrs. W——, in looking back at the education and habits of those sons of her early friends, could clearly trace the causes of their errors and vices to the blind indulgence, or to the indifference, neglect, and ignorance of their parents. There appeared, however, two important errors in their physical and mental training, more prolific sources of evil than all others. These consisted in luxurious living, and a great amount of unoccupied time. The former, by developing and giving activity to the animal propensities, leads to sensuality and excess; while the latter produces a taste for amusement and excitement, and an erroneous estimation of the value of time.

Mrs. W——'s principal object, during the childhood of her sons, was to give them sound constitutions, accompanied by clear and active minds. The first she accomplished by a free use of cold water, fresh air, and exercise; and the last by a healthy and temperate diet, consisting chiefly of bread, milk, and fruits. She never exacted from her children a blind obedience to her commands, but endeavored to give them correct views and sound principles of action, based upon a thorough knowledge of the laws of their own system, in connection with external circumstances. For instance, in explaining the function of the physical organs, she showed them that there existed a great sympathy between the stomach and the brain; hence, if the former were overloaded, the latter became inert and torpid; the reasoning faculties being thus paralyzed, the human gourmand was reduced to a level with the brute. She also explained to them the reason why animal food was incompatible with the reflective and sedentary habits of a student; because it induced an excess of the vascular system, which produced an irritability and restlessness requiring a great amount of muscular action to carry off. She also taught them that they were not created immortal, and endowed with the divine attribute of reason, to become the mere slaves of sense, or of selfish interests; but that they had a higher mission to fulfill: that of rendering themselves worthy of a more perfect state hereafter—by subduing the sensual, and improving the spiritual portion of their nature—by studying the works of the Creator, as manifesting his wisdom and goodness in their beauty and harmony—and by promoting the improvement and happiness of their fellow-beings. This, she taught them, was the end, and ought to be the aim, of their existence. And to this noble end she guided and directed them, both by precept and example.

In conducting the studies of her children, Mrs. W—— endeavored to render them interesting and agreeable. In this she found little difficulty; for, by assisting them to understand that which they had to learn, their lessons became easy and pleasant. Nor did she allow them to burden their memories with words without ideas, but, by a little explanation, rendered them perfectly familiar with the subject of their studies; and, by constantly conversing with them respecting that which they had learned, fixed the important portions of it in their recollection, and thus rendered the knowledge acquired ready and practical.

In the study of history, this sensible mother did not deem it sufficient that her sons were acquainted with the chronological events in the history of a nation—the genealogy of its rulers—the turns of its different dynasties—or the political, civil, and religious revolutions through which it had passed. She taught them that the most important portion of the history of a nation consisted in its institutions and its laws—in its science, its literature, and its commerce; for therein were to be found the causes, direct or indirect, which modified the character of nations, and decided their destiny. Nor must they overlook the *apparently* minor influences which promote or retard the improvement and happiness of a nation—such as the social condition and moral estimation in which females are held in different countries; and the effects which those influences have in elevating or depressing the character of a people, as illustrated by the British and Ottoman empires. In this manner the study of history was rendered most instructive, and its noblest lessons inculcated.

Mrs. W—— avoided wearying the attention of her children by frequent change of study and occupation. To the useful branches generally included in the education of boys, she added music and drawing. The latter accomplishment gave delightful occupation to those hours of recreation which many children spend in worse than idleness—in acquiring bad habits. The best books of instruction were provided for them, and good models; including casts, drawings, and paintings. With these, the pupils required no other instruction except that given by their mother; who, not satisfied that her sons should become mere copyists, instructed them in the laws of perspective, the beautiful effects of light and shadow, the harmony of colors, and the rules of composition. Thus, by judicious management, this delightful creative art was rendered so agreeable to the children, that an hour spent in its pursuit was deemed a sufficient reward for proficiency in less pleasant studies.

Equal care and attention was bestowed upon geology, bota ny, and chemistry. In a small laboratory fitted up for experimenting in the latter science, the young people were frequently delighted by the curious phenomena evolved in interrogating nature—not, indeed, with new questions, but in compelling her to verify those already asked by masters in the science.

The exercise and recreation necessary for youth were obtained by music, dancing, battle-door, and chess; while exercise in the open air was amply supplied by frequent botanizing and mineralizing excursions into the country. In those health-inspiring excursions, much useful manufacturing and agricultural knowledge was also obtained. The perceptive and reflective organs of the children being thus exercised and strengthened, they were enabled to comprehend the beautiful operations of nature, to see her efforts aided and directed by her hand-maidens, art and science, and made subservient to the necessities of man. Thus trained and instructed, those young lads looked with eyes of understanding upon things of which the ignorant take no note; they found

"Tongues in trees, books in the running brook,
Sermons in stones, and good in every thing."

Blessed with such mental resources, they never will require that excitement which the idle and vacant mind seeks in the intoxicating bowl, nor ever be found in those haunts of dissipation and vice frequented by the neglected sons of the careless and ignorant mother—of whom, it requires not the spirit of prophecy to foretell, that long after they shall have become food for the worms, and their names consigned to oblivion, the others, the knowledge-seeking, the self-denying, and the virtuous, shall still be denizens of this beautiful world, in the full enjoyment of all its blessings, the reward of a life led in obedience to the divine laws, both moral and physical—and their names, after illuminating many a bright page of history, shall be handed down to future ages by a virtuous posterity.

When we contrast the past with the present, and reflect upon the great discoveries which are continually being made, both in the material and the immaterial world, does it not suggest a strong desire for "length of days," that we may see to what all these things tend? Doubtless, it is reserved for this nineteenth century to develop truths and principles of more importance to mankind than all preceding events, from the beginning of the world to the present time.

Those unacquainted with the true use and value of money may, perhaps, imagine that it would require a large income to educate a family in the manner stated in the preceding. The income of Mrs. W——, however, did not exceed the sum which many families spent annually in ornamental articles of dress and the luxuries of the table, or the amount which is frequently paid for one year's education of a young lady at a fashionable boarding-school. But, limited as her income was, Mrs. W—— was enabled with it to give each of her sons, as he grew up, a liberal education, and establish them in a profession. This she accomplished by living much within her income during the childhood of her sons, by order and economy in her household, and by great application and self-denial on her own part. Those precious hours of the day which many mothers trifle away in morning calls, in shopping, in embellishing their persons and houses, and endeavoring to make an appearance above their condition, Mrs.

W—— spent in improving the minds of her children, in a course of reading which kept her informed of the onward progress of society, and in acquiring suitable knowledge to enable her to discharge with success the duties of a mother, who wished to see her sons act a noble part in life.

CHAPTER XI.

PRESENT POSITION OF WOMAN, PHYSICALLY, MENTALLY, AND MORALLY.

THE present age appears eminently distinguished by the efforts made to elevate woman in the scale of intellect, and to extend to her the advantages of a more liberal education. It would not, perhaps, be wise to inquire too particularly into the matter, in order to ascertain if it be by the disinterested justice and humanity of man, or by her own efforts, that woman, at length, has a prospect of attaining that degree of moral and mental excellence for which she was originally designed by the Creator. It must, however, be acknowledged, that most of the works lately published, advocating these liberal principles, have been from the pens of women. "If," says one of the "lords of the creation," "women require more advantages and privileges, they must exert themselves to obtain them, for it is not our interest to move the subject." A short-sighted, selfish sentiment, and evinces as little observation as reflection. It perhaps may not be for the interest of the sensualist, or the mere man of pleasure, who has chosen a life of celibacy, to cultivate the moral and intellectual faculties of woman, thereby rendering her an unfit minister to his gross appetites. But, to him whose soul is pregnant with holy aspirations of immortality—whose heart swells with gratitude to the all-wise Creator, in contemplating the beauty and harmony of his works—how divine the thought, that he has called into being, and will leave behind him, when he passes from this earth, a virtuous and intelligent posterity, who will assist in bringing about, and partake in that blessed state of perfection and happiness in this world, which the past and present condition of man show he was formed to attain.

It is, therefore, minds whose views are not bounded by the present, and whose visions are not obscured by the thick film of selfishness, but rather illuminated by the effulgent rays of benevolence, that can perceive how nearly their interest is concerned in raising woman from the dark abyss of ignorance, sensuality, and oppression, and calling into exercise the highest attributes of her nature. Let the gray-headed father, to whose face the blush of shame often mantles for the vices and follies of his children, reflect, if it would not have been for his interest to have devoted a portion of his time and attention to cultivating and developing the mental and moral faculties of the wife of his youth, and thus obviated that portion of sensual organization which his children inherited from her; for action is the first principle of nature, and if the higher faculties are not exercised, the animal propensities become the most active, and are thus "most readily transmitted to offspring."

"There is a feeling very generally entertained by literary and scientific individuals, that only those physical and moral qualities need be looked for in a woman which render her a good mother and a domestic housekeeper, and that a cultivated mind is of little importance."* "But," continues Mr. Walker, "this is a great error, not merely because these men, being compelled by their professions to remain much at home, are obliged, from having no one to comprehend them, to think alone, but because uneducated women are sure to communicate lower mental faculties to their children."† This

* We often hear fathers say, "Education is of no use to women; I had much rather my daughters should know how to compound a good pudding than to solve a problem, or to cook a beef-steak properly, than to write an essay." They do not seem to be aware that they are speaking the language of the selfish sentiments, instead of enlightened intellect, and that they are not consulting the happiness and well-being of their daughters, but the gratification of their own animal desires.

† After the cold, calculating selfishness of the preceding, the following tender and benevolent sentiment, of the most amiable of French philosophers, D'Alembert, appears like an oasis in the desert. "Let us not confine ourselves merely to the advantages society might derive from the education of woman; let us go further, and have the justice and humanity not to deny them what may sweeten life for themselves as well as for us. How often have we experienced a power in mental culture and the exercise of our talents to withdraw us from our calamities, and to console us in our sorrows! Why, then, refuse to the more amiable half of the

author, however, appears rather inconsistent; for, after admitting the degenerating effects of uneducated mothers, he says of the mental system, "This species of beauty is less proper to woman—less feminine than the preceding. It is not the intellectual system, but the vital one (that is, the animal) which is, and ought to be, developed in women." The authoress is acquainted with two brothers of superior abilities, and highly-cultivated minds, whose children differ so widely from each other, that it gives rise to much speculation among their friends to account for it. It is generally attributed to the different modes of education and training which they have received; the true cause, however, is to be found in the different characters of their mothers. In one of them, the vital system predominates; in the other, the intellectual. The former, also, has a large back-head, which indicates a predominance of the sentiments and passions over intellect; hence the great pleasure she finds in social intercourse and fashionable life. To enjoy society, she left her children, when young, to the care of ignorant hirelings; and when they became old enough, they were sent to a boarding-school, from which they were frequently expelled for turbulent and disorderly conduct. For, having inherited the temperament and organization of their mother, study and reflection were to them extremely irksome. The eldest son destroyed himself by dissipation before the age of twenty-one; another has been sent on a whaling voyage; while the daughters have formed early and imprudent marriages, in direct opposition to the wishes of their parents. The mother, on the contrary, in whom the intellectual system obtained, found pleasure only in acquiring knowledge, and in imparting it to her children. Her extensive reading, and close observation of life, had early impressed upon her mind the power and influence which the mother holds over the future destiny of her child. They also disclosed to her the constant necessity of guiding and controlling the impetuosity and inexperience of youth. She would not allow her sons to be absent from her for a single day, but assisted in

species, destined to share with us the ills of existence, the solace best fitted to enable them to be endured?"

their education herself. She led them, by the most pleasant paths, up the rugged ascent—difficult, at first, and hard to climb; but, when surmounted, full of sweet sounds and pleasant prospects. The eldest son has finished his collegiate studies with honor to himself and to his family, and promises to become an ornament to his country, while his younger brothers are emulating his good conduct. Who could look upon that intelligent, diligent, self-sacrificing mother, and her bright and beautiful boys, observing with what pleasure and facility they acquire knowledge, and the delightful influences it sheds around them, and agree with Mr. Walker, that "the vital system ought to be most developed in woman?"

> "Truth crushed to earth will rise again;
> The eternal years of God are hers—
> But error, wounded, writhes in pain,
> And dies amid her worshipers."

The history and writings of Mary Wolstoncraft illustrate the truth of the preceding lines. There never was, perhaps, any writer on whom contumely and ridicule have been so lavishly heaped, for having dared to assert and maintain the rights and privileges of woman. Had those rights no foundation in nature, the writings of Mary Wolstoncraft would have been evanescent as the morning dew; but having been founded upon the everlasting rock of truth, like the beautiful rainbow, they hold out a bright promise for the future. How well that promise has been fulfilled, and how much her principles are esteemed by the liberal and enlightened of the present age, the following extract from the Westminster Review will show:

"This high-minded woman has created an influence which defies calculation; she produced that impulse toward the education and improvement of woman which succeeding writers have developed. No one can have entered a family where her writings, or those of her class, are cherished, without being struck with the effect, and the manifest superiority of the daughters, in point of sincerity, purity, and gracefulness of mind. The women of England, before her time, from all we can gather, were coarse, ignorant, and sensual: when not debased by actual vices, they were always so by ignorance and narrow-mindedness; and if they, by any chance, had received an education, it was rendered disgusting in them by its open prostitution to vanity; and men were justified in their dislike of 'clever women.' If a woman were not an insipid 'creature of fashion,' she was sure to be a 'well-dressed housekeeper.' The effect of women on society is readily felt; the softening of men's ruder natures, the triumph of delicacy and sentiment over sensuality, the paradise of home—these we owe to women, and we know of no more *infallible sign of man's intense vanity and narrow-mindedness, than his objection to the education of women.*"

"The empire of women," says another eloquent foreigner, "is not theirs because men have willed it, but because it is the will of nature. Miserable must be the age in which this empire is lost, and in which the judgments of women are counted as nothing, by men. Every people in the ancient world, that can be said to have had morals, has respected the sex—Sparta, Germany, Rome. At Rome, the exploits of the victorious generals were honored by the grateful voices of *women;* on every public calamity, *their* tears were a public offering to the gods. In either case, their vows and their sorrows were thus consecrated as the most solemn judgments of the state. It is to them that all the great revolutions of the republic are to be traced. By a woman, Rome acquired liberty—by a woman, the plebeians acquired the consulate—by a woman, when the city was trembling with the vindictive exile at its gates, it was saved from that destruction which no other influence could avert."

The following eloquent appeal in favor of the better education of women, is from the pen of the talented and philanthropic Mrs. Jamieson:

"In these days, when society is becoming every day more artificial and more complex, and marriage, as the gentlemen assure us, more and more expensive, hazardous, and inexpedient, women must find means to fill up the void in existence.

Men, our natural protectors, our law-givers, our masters, throw us upon our own resources; the qualities which they pretend to admire in us—the overflowing, the clinging affections of a warm heart—the household devotion—the submissive wish to please, that feels 'every vanity in fondness lost'—the tender, shrinking sensitiveness which Adam thought so charming in his Eve—to cultivate these, to make them, by artificial means, the staple of the womanly character, is it not to cultivate a taste for sunshine and roses, in those we send to spend their lives in the arctic zone? We have gone away from nature, and we must, if we can, substitute another nature.

"Art, literature, and science remain to us. Religion—which formerly opened the doors of nunneries and convents to forlorn women—now mingling her beautiful and soothing influence with resources which the prejudices of the world have yet left open to us, only in the assiduous employment of such faculties as we are permitted to exercise can we find health, and peace, and compensation for the wasted or repulsed impulses and energies more proper to our sex—more natural—perhaps more pleasing to God; but, trusting in his mercy, and using the means he has given, we must do the best we can for ourselves and for our sisterhood. The prejudices which would have shut us out from nobler consolation and occupations, have ceased, in great part, and will soon be remembered only as the rude, coarse barbarism of a by-gone age. Let us, then, have no more caricatures of methodistical, card-playing, and acrimonious old maids. Let us have no more of scandal, parrots, cats, or lap-dogs—or worse!—these never-failing subjects of derision with the vulgar and the frivolous, but the source of a thousand compassionate and melancholy feelings in those who can reflect! In the name of humanity and womanhood, let us have no more of them. Coleridge, who has said and written the most beautiful, the most tender, the most reverential things of woman—who understands better than any man, any poet, what I will call the metaphysics of love—Coleridge, as you will remember, has asserted that the perfection of a woman's character is to be characterless. 'Every man,' said he, 'would like to have an Ophelia or a Desdemona for his wife.' No doubt; the sentiment is truly a masculine one; and what was their fate? What would now be the fate of such unresisting and confiding angels! Is this the age of Arcadia? Do we live among Paladins and Sir Charles Grandisons? and are our weakness, and our innocence, and our ignorance, safeguards—or snares? Do we, indeed, find our account in being 'fine by defect, and beautifully weak?' No, no; women need, in these times, character beyond every thing else; the qualities which will enable them to endure and resist evil; the self-governed, the cultivated, active mind, to protect and to maintain ourselves. How many wretched women marry for a maintenance! How many wretched women sell themselves to dishonor, for bread! and there is small difference, if any, in the infamy and the misery! How many unmarried women live in heart-wearing dependence; if poor, in solitary penury—loveless, joyless, unendeared; if rich, in aimless, pitiless trifling! How many, strange to say, marry for the independence they dare not otherwise claim! But, the snare-paths open to us, the less fear that we should go astray.

"Surely it is dangerous, it is wicked, in these days, to follow the old saw, to bring up women to be 'happy wives and mothers;' that is to say, to let all her accomplishments, her sentiments, her views of life, take one direction, as if for woman there existed only one destiny, one hope, one blessing, one object, one passion in existence. Some people say it ought to be so, but we know it is not so; we know that hundreds, that thousands of women are not happy wives and mothers—are never either wives or mothers at all. The cultivation of the moral strength and the active energies of a woman's mind, together with the intellectual faculties and tastes, will not make a woman a less good, less happy wife and mother, and will enable her to find content and independence when denied love and happiness."

CHAPTER XII.

THE CHARACTER AMERICAN WOMEN GIVE TO THEIR COUNTRY.

M. De Tocqueville, in the second part of the Democracy of America, says, "Now that I am drawing to a close, after having found so much to commend in the Americans, if I were asked to what I attribute their greatness, I should say, to the superiority of their women." This, certainly, is well-merited and just praise; and it ought to have the effect of stimulating the American women to great efforts to sustain the high national character which they have thus attained abroad. These efforts, however, should be directed to the improvement of the rising generation, for by them will the reputation of the present age be either sustained or forfeited. When we reflect that every age and opinion is produced by that which preceded it, and is responsible only for that which follows it, is it not evident that the present generation must revert to the circumstances, culture, and training by which their own characters were formed, and then ask themselves, if the same causes are operating upon their children by which only similar characteristics can be produced? It is much to be feared that the answer will be in the negative; for it must be evident to the most superficial observer, that much more time and attention is devoted to the acquisition of accomplishments, to personal embellishments, and to fashionable amusements, at present than formerly. It is now universally admitted that these pursuits add neither to the improvement of the heart nor of the understanding; therefore, it is not at all probable that the superior women to whom De Tocqueville alludes were those only who were trained to make an agreeable figure in society, or who were conspicuous for elegance and taste. For, as his own countrywomen excel in such matters, it would be idle to suppose that, with his philosophical views of society this branch of female education comprehended much of that superiority to which he ascribes such great results in this country. Is it not important, then, to inquire what influence these pursuits are likely to have upon the rising generation? When we look at the fragile forms and pale complexions of the female youth of large cities, the effect which seems most to be apprehended is, the deterioration of the species.

The writer had occasion, a short time since, to visit a school for young ladies of some celebrity, in which the general appearance of the want of health was too obvious to be overlooked. A great uniformity of figure was also observed to pervade the whole school, from the assistant teacher down to the youngest pupil. This uniformity consisted in round shoulders and a slender waist. Is it not astonishing, after all that has been said and written on the subject of tight lacing by the physician and the physiologist, that the habit should so universally prevail? There is, however, one result of tight lacing which, if generally known, would tend very materially to eradicate the evil. It is, that "among the many evils enumerated by the Germans as attributable to tight lacing, is UGLY CHILDREN." When we look at the high shoulders and awkward figures, the pinched-up features and painful expression of countenance of the weakly-organized victims of tight lacing, we must admit that the observation of the German is founded in truth.

No object in nature is so disagreeable and painful to the physiologist, as the round shoulders and contracted chests of the youth of both sexes of the present generation. Disagreeable, because they violate symmetry and beauty; painful, because they are a certain evidence of a feeble organization, and the precursor of a life of disease and suffering. May not most of our pulmonary complaints—early decay of the teeth, and sallowness of complexion, which are generally attributed to climate—be traced to this wretched habit of stooping, which, when contracted in early childhood, saps to the foundation the sources of health and vitality.

It is evident, from the structure of that portion of the human figure in which the lungs are situated, that it was the intention of the Creator that they should have free and full space to perform their function—the vitalizing of the blood, by which a healthful action of body and mind is kept up. This position of stooping, therefore, while it contracts the lungs and impedes their action, leaves the system overcharged with sluggish humors. Hence the inertness, and predisposition to sedentary habits, of round-shouldered young people; who display a melancholy contrast to the gay and joyous spirit of the healthy youth, in whom the very sense of existence is a positive pleasure.

Now who is, or ought to be, accountable for all this mischief? Surely the mother. If, from a similar neglect in childhood, she transmits a feeble constitution to her children, is it not her duty to discover and apply the means to remedy the evil? First, by strengthening and improving the general health by proper exercise and diet. Secondly, by enforcing, with the most rigid discipline, if necessary, an upright position of the body in sitting and in walking. Yet how is this to be accomplished by the unreflecting mother, when she cannot even see that, in the form of the busts of her children, the order of nature is reversed? Instead of a broad, well-expanded chest, straight back, and sloping shoulders, they have a narrow, hollow chest, high shoulders, and a hemispherically-formed back; which configuration, if it involve no other consequence, is extremely inelegant and ungraceful. And if the mother could appreciate, and would prefer symmetry and gracefulness of person to the mere extrinsic embellishments of dress, one tenth part of the time and attention which she bestows upon the latter, might suffice, with a judicious course of gymnastic exercises, to attain the former.

So much has been said on the subject of beauty unadorned, that any thing further may appear trite and unnecessary. Yet may there not be some error in the popular opinion of what constitutes beauty? Many persons think it a mere chance gift of nature, unattainable by cultivation, and exclusively confined to outward perfection in form and feature. But how much more desirable and interesting is that species of beauty which emanates from the mind? The animated and ever-varying expression of countenance, that indicates a strong and active intellect, kind and sympathetic feelings, refined and delicate habits, which, when combined with the native charm of youth, give to the possessor an air of purity and loveliness that is almost celestial!

The object of this chapter, however, is, to show the effects which the present inordinate pursuit of accomplishments may have on the rising generation. In the following graphic description of a wise and observant physician,* the effects which they have already produced in England will be seen.

"Female education is more detrimental to health and happiness than that of the male. Its grasp, its aim, is at accomplishments rather than acquirements—at gilding rather than at gold—at such ornaments as may dazzle by their lustre, and consume themselves in a few years by the intensity of their own brightness, rather than those which radiate a steady light till the lamp of life is extinguished. They are most properly termed *accomplishments*, because they are designed to *accomplish* a certain object—MATRIMONY. That end, or rather beginning, obtained, they are about as useful to their owner as a rudder is to a sheer hulk moored head and stern in Portsmouth harbor—the lease of a house after the term is expired—or a pair of wooden shoes during a paroxysm of gout.

"The mania for *music* injures the health, and even curtails the lives of thousands and tens of thousands annually of the fair sex, by the sedentary habits which it enjoins, and the morbid sympathies which it engenders. The story of the sirens is no fable. It is verified to the letter!

000 'Their song is death, and makes *destruction* please.'

Visit the ball-room and the bazar, the park and the concert, the theatre and the temple; among the myriads of the young and beautiful, whom you see dancing or dressing, driving or chanting, laughing or praying, you will not find *one*—no, not ONE, in the enjoyment of health! No wonder, then, that the doctors, the dentists, and the druggists multiply almost as rapidly as the pianos, the harps, and the guitars.

* Dr. Johnson's Economy of Health.

"The length of time occupied by music renders it morally impossible to dedicate sufficient attention to the health of the body or the cultivation of the mind. The *consequence* is, that the corporeal functions languish and become impaired—a condition that is fearfully augmented by the peculiar effects which music has upon the nervous system. The nature and extent of these injuries are not generally known, even to the faculty, and cannot be detailed here. But one effect, of immense importance, will not be denied, namely, the length of time absorbed by music, and the *consequent* deficiency of time for the acquisition of useful knowledge in the system of female education. If some of that time which is now spent on the piano, the harp, and the guitar, were dedicated to the elements of science, or, at all events, to useful information, as modern languages, history, astronomy, geography, and even mathematics, there would be better wives and mothers, than where the mind is *left comparatively* an uncultivated blank, in order to pamper the single sense of hearing! Mrs. Somerville has stolen harmony from the heavens as well as St. Cecilia! The time spent at the piano leaves not sufficient space for the acquirement of that 'useful knowledge,' which strengthens the mind against the vicissitudes of fortune, and the *moral crosses to which female life is doomed;* nor for the healthful exercise of the body, by which the material fabric may be fortified against the thousand diseases continually assailing it. I would therefore recommend that one half of the time spent in music should be allotted to bodily exercise, and to the acquisition of useful and ornamental knowledge, embracing Natural Philosophy, and, in short, many of the sciences which man has monopolized to himself, but for which *woman is as fit as the 'lord of the creation!'*"

If the preceding are the consequences of the present mode of female education in England, where the vital system obtains, what must be its effects on the highly nervous temperament of our own fair countrywomen? The melancholy answer will be found in the number of young married women whose names swell the weekly bills of mortality.

It, however, would appear that the same mental activity and

love of the beautiful which impels to the inordinate pursuit of personal accomplishments, is the source of that all-absorbing passion for dress which is so conspicuous in our highways, by-ways, and saloons. There are, doubtless, many young ladies who would be much mortified were they obliged to confess the amount of time and attention which they devote to acquiring, devising, and forming mere ornamental articles of dress—time which, if spent in a judicious course of reading and reflection, would fill their minds with beautiful and graceful images, open to their view sources of pleasure and happiness of which they could form no previous conception, and render them impervious to the many vexations to which vanity and ostentation are subject. It would also make them agreeable companions for men of sense, and in various ways conduce to the benefit and well-being of their own families. For, their knowledge being extended, their judgments exercised and strengthened, they would better understand the method of rendering their homes pleasant and attractive to their fathers and brothers, and thus obviate the necessity for their seeking amusement and recreation at those sources of many evils, the theatre and the convivial board.

The American women, possibly, are not aware of the numerous privileges which they enjoy, and the evil influences from which they are exempt—influences to which a large class of the women of Europe are subject, particularly in France, where many of the wives and daughters of the trades-people are confined to the desk or the counter a great portion of their lives, while in this country they are allowed to remain in the hallowed precincts of domestic privacy. To this wise and humane policy, the Americans are doubtless indebted for their domestic comfort and happiness, as well as for the superior purity of the lives and manners of their women ; and so long as this state of things continues, the future prosperity and security of this republic may, with safety, be predicted.

But, in order to attain a great and good national character, give the women attainments rather than accomplishments. Point out to them their capabilities and responsibilities. Let them know that they are responsible for the moral character of the rising generation; and also, that it depends upon themselves whether they become the mothers of wise and virtuous, or foolish and vicious men. For, in the same degree as these qualities are *possessed and exercised by themselves, will their children inherit and practice them.*

Let the careless, indolent mother reflect well upon this, and feel assured that nothing great was ever attained with ease, and that the sons of such mothers are never heard of beyond their generation, except for evil. Let, also, the gay votary of fashion remember, that the loftiest, the most angel-like ambition, is the earnest desire to contribute to the rational happiness and moral improvement of others. If she can do this—if she can smooth the path of one fellow-traveler—if she can give one good impression, is it not better than all the triumphs that fashion, wealth, or power ever attain?

CHAPTER XIII.

CONCLUSION.

THE reader who has followed the author thus far, will have become convinced, before turning to this page, that her object is no trivial one—that having been clearly presented to the mind, it cannot be dismissed with apathy or neglect. Any female, having become convinced of the doctrines advanced in this work, has assumed a responsibility, and incurred an obligation to live up to them, from which nothing but death or absolute inability can ever absolve her. She is ever thereafter bound to the most faithful observance of them.

It has been the aim of the writer to convince her sex that influence, such as few of them have ever dreamed of, is appointed them in nature, and that this influence is of such a character that it lies at the very foundation of the prosperity and welfare of mankind.

To accomplish her object, she has chosen the mode best adapted to the great mass of female minds, viz., that of illustrating the positions taken by cases brought from private experience, from biography, and from history. She might have gone into abstract reasoning upon the several laws stated, and have equally sustained herself; for where facts illustrate general principles, reason and philosophy never fail. But she has adopted that manner of making the truth apparent, which, while it detracts nothing from its power, will present it to the female mind in a more fascinating garb than if clothed in mere philosophical argument. The facts which have been adduced, and the arguments which have been offered, are designed to establish the following principles:

First. That offspring are dependent on their parents for their mental and physical constitutions.

Second. That these may be modified by the will of the parents.

Third. That, in the transmission from parents to offspring, more depends on the mother than the father.

Fourth. That this is especially and strikingly true of the intellect and feelings.

Fifth. That every female, from the moment she is liable to become a mother, is solemnly responsible to her Maker, to her future offspring, and society, for the mind she will impart, and the moral and physical qualities she will transmit.

Sixth. That it is the duty of every female (one of the highest she is called upon to discharge) to spare no efforts that the circumstances which make up her condition during the period of gestation, shall be such as will be most favorable to the transmission of a sound organization and of a well-balanced mind.

And lastly. That if any faculty, or set of faculties, are in frequent and high exercise in the mother during this period, they will be inherited in increased strength and energy by her offspring.

The importance of these principles to mankind at large, cannot be too highly estimated. They lie at the very basis of all that we desire for man. They embrace the springs of human ability, motive, and action. They show that the complicated physical and mental machine called man, is no random result of fortuitous circumstances, but a being taking his origin under fixed laws; that all the diversities of moral and physical aspect which he presents, are but the results of those laws.

No truth is more important than this, and none meets with a colder reception at the hands of those who should prize it as a means by which they are to work out their moral and physical salvation. To say that health is governed by fixed laws, which, if understood and obeyed, would perfectly preserve it, is to announce a proposition which has, as yet, obtained but a very limited foothold in the popular mind. But to say that the degree of health and physical vigor generally, which a person shall enjoy through life, is to a great extent determined by the obedience or disobedience of his parents before his birth, is to say what seems still less capable of procuring present belief. To go still farther, and say that the mind, that many-toned instrument, which seems in no two of all the myriads of like creatures to be alike, has its inception and unconscious growth under such laws as would enable those who call it into being to modify or strengthen its various powers as they please, will, it is feared, be considered almost heretical. Yet such is the ground which truth bids us take, and to this point the writer must beg leave earnestly to urge the attention of her countrywomen. And here let us pause and look forward for a moment to the results to which this truth points.

With the moral aspect of society, such as we have been accustomed to witness in the present, and to contemplate in past ages, it will be difficult for the mind to anticipate the long reach of change and improvement which it places before us. That we can, even to any degree, in obedience to wishes and motives known and weighed by ourselves, modify the minds and dispositions of those who derive their being from us, is a truth which bursts through the gloom of our foul moral atmosphere, as the first star may be supposed to have dawned on the trembling watchers in the Ark. But to females their extent and importance are incomparable, for they place them upon their natural throne. Possessed of these, woman feels that she wields the moral sceptre of the world. If properly addressed to her, they *must* rouse her ambition, they *must* kindle her energies, they *must* prompt her to pursuits worthy of herself. By their own inherent force they will procure what she has so long been struggling for in dim bewilderment —a recognition of her dignity and true rights from the other sex. When acquaintance with these comes to be acknowledged as the chief duty, and the results of obedience to them as the greatest charm of woman, she will be recognized among men for what she really is. The young man who sees in his future wife the mother of his children in this sense, would soon learn to estimate, according to their true value, the various personal and mental charms of the individual to be chosen.

Hour-glass waist, pale face, languid movement, feebleness and fragility, would wear far other aspect to his eyes, when looked upon as the prospective curses which his offspring must inherit, than now, when they are the highest current proofs of elegance and refinement. Nor will the demand for reform in her moral nature be less loudly uttered. The laws illustrated in the preceding pages will sustain us in the assertion, that when a female has lived all her life in obedience to the dictates of propensity, and suffers herself to be in the same state of mind during the periods which precede her entrance upon the maternal office, it is almost as impossible that she should become the mother of highly moral and intellectual children, as that the African female should become the mother of the fair-haired, clear-skinned Saxon. The only chance is, that if the father possess a considerable predominance of the latter, they may possibly descend to the first children. Perhaps the reason why the earlier offspring of such marriages exhibit better qualities than those born at later periods, might be found in the fact, that the mother, while the first romance of affection is fresh around her, loses in part her consciousness of self, and for a time the strength of propensity fades away, in the generous emotions she bears toward her husband. He is her model; his feelings, thoughts, and desires have a greater influence over her mind than her own. But as time familiarizes her with him, and the practical duties of life call her selfish powers into action, she becomes again more intensely conscious of her own emotions; and these form, as it were, the mental mould in which the mind of her offspring is cast. We might adduce facts, too, which would show that females of common and coarse minds have given birth to one or two children, among a number, whose mental endowments have been very different from those of their other offspring, and the cause may generally be traced to the fact, that some circumstances have, at these particular periods, tended to call into strong exercise the higher faculties of their nature, and their fortunate children have inherited the happy consequences. Thus deep griefs, wounded affections, the loss of friends, or any misfortune which touches the tenderer feelings, and by consequence subdues the propensities, may be the cause why one child should be born into a family, whose mind and disposition are so wholly unlike those of its other members, as to be the standing marvel of friends and acquaintances. So there are cases of an opposite character, where unhappy circumstances tend to keep the animal portion of the mother's nature inflamed, and there is little opportunity for the exercise of the better emotions and intellect. A child born of an intellectual and amiable woman under such circumstances, would inherit the unnatural activity of the selfish faculties under which the mother labored, and exhibit a character so strikingly different from those of the parents, and brothers, and sisters, as to be, according to the homely, but expressive proverb, "the black sheep of the flock."

The self-denial and sacrifice of the maternal office are implied to the largest extent in the truths herein propounded. Woman is shown to have been sent on a noble mission. She is shown to have been intrusted with the accomplishment of duties so important that we tremble when we contemplate their magnitude, and her self-imposed incompetency. She has slumbered these many ages on her post, and wide-spread evil and suffering are the consequence. How shall we waken her! How shall we place her upon her guard, that she shall no longer linger in her path of duty? Only by shownig her the commission she bears. Let her be convinced that she has a definite and important one, which *can be fulfilled by no other than herself*, and I believe she has still that fidelity that would lead her to gigantic efforts. Clear away, then, all obstacles; bring woman into the inner temple of science, where she may receive her instructions clearly; occupy her no longer in the outer courts with gewgaws and trifles, but let her learn what is expected of her, and then, if she neglect the duty and deny the obligation, brand her with a curse deeper and bitterer than that under which the first murderer went forth, but not till then.

The laws illustrated by the facts before stated, will give additional force to every incentive to mental culture. Not only this, they show that a high state of intelligence is attainable by the great body of the sex.

If every mother can transmit better minds to her offspring by improving her own in intellectual pursuits, it will be granted that nature demands it of her, and that society can only be approximating its highest state of perfection, in proportion as the great body of females do this. Doubtless it would be Utopian to talk of the immediate commencement of these pursuits by communities of females, as it would be to anticipate the instantaneous spread of any new doctrines; but that does not invalidate the force of truth, nor show that, in a true state of society, it would not be practicable. We learn from what has gone before, that it is the natural duty of every woman to give the highest tone to her mind of which it is capable, by engaging in intellectual and ennobling pursuits; and we infer that it is, therefore, perfectly practicable in a well-ordered state of society. As female time is appropriated in this day, the naked suggestion, no doubt, seems more like the dream of an enthusiast than the decision of cool reason. An overwhelming majority of females, if urged to adopt it, would pronounce it impossible—some from a real or imagined necessity of devoting themselves wholly to the earnest and stirring pursuits of life; some from the pressure of social customs and fashion; and others (though this class, it is hoped, is small) from sheer disinclination. The loudest cry from all quarters would be, "There is no time." We have no time for reading, say ladies, except a newspaper or magazine article of an hour or two, or an occasional volume, which is hastily dismissed without a second thought. But ought this to be so? Is it any part of truth for woman thus *to deny* the requisitions of nature? Is it not, rather, a terrible falsity?—one fertile source of appalling sin and misery? Yet, even while we mourn over it, there is joy in the thought that, being a falsity, it must, in time, disappear. "Truth is mighty, and will prevail," are words that contain a never-failing consolation to the philanthropist. But the event which they announce needs to be hastened. Mighty as truth is, she is not superior to human impediments nor human aid. Each age throws down some of the barriers which its predecessors have erected, but unfortunately rears others of its own. Each has, therefore, its labor to perform. The present has taken a large contract—has made tremendous promises. It seems to form a crisis in the history of man, which he cannot pass until some new and mighty principles of renovation and improvement are put in operation. Among all the sources whence these can issue, woman stands first: all that follows her is curative, not preventive—expedient, not first principle.

How long, then, shall we wait in idleness, witnessing the failure of these experiments? How long shall we refuse to address ourselves to duty? Do we wait some great change in public opinion, which shall assign us a commission more worthy of our acceptance? Where shall we find it? What more solemn charge devolves upon any human being, than upon our sex, in the mental and moral culture of the young? Weigh it in all its bearings upon the happiness of the individuals who derive their being from us, and grow up under our charge—upon the interest which society has in our mode of training them—upon the evils which pernicious treatment will inflict on those who have to associate with them through life—and upon the miseries which, through them, we perpetuate to future generations; and where, in the whole range of human duties, can we find any demanding so high preparation, and such assiduous care and attention? The great demand of society now is, for enlightened and true women. It begins to be obvious that they have something to do besides dressing themselves fashionably, and studying how to amuse. In this country they have much—more than any where else on the globe. The experiment which humanity is here conducting in its own behalf, is one which engages the attention of the whole world—one on which the happiness of ages depends. It cannot afford to lose any of the aid which is its due—still less that which its mothers owe it.

Our sons and daughters will be *the people*, who are to sit as arbiters of the Republic. The freemen who, thirty years hence, will speak through the ballot-box on the policy of this great nation, must derive from us the powers which shall dictate their utterance. What shall they be? Shall we make them virtuous, enlightened, efficient? Have we any love of our country, and its noble institutions—of the generosity which offers to the wretched and oppressed of all nations a home and freedom? Do we love to dispense these blessings? Have we patriotism to make us willing to sacrifice the ease and indolence of ordinary life, for the discharge of high and arduous duty? Have we energy and moral purpose to forego the frivolities of fashionable life, and set ourselves zealously to work to accomplish this great good? "If I were asked," said a talented and distinguished foreigner, writing from our country, "on what I found my hope of the permanency of republican institutions, I would answer, 'On the intelligence and virtue of the women of the United States.' The destinies of the nation are in the hands of females." If the sun of liberty set here, we shall be responsible; and where shall we next look for its rise? Has not its every return been ushered in by devastation, misery, and death? Has not its every dawn shone over empires smoking with blood—its every evening been attended by convulsive agony and despair?

I beseech my countrywomen to think whether the boon that is intrusted to us be not worth preserving? Has it not been costly enough to endear it? Is it not attended with blessings enough to make us prize it? As we respect ourselves and love humanity, let us regard it in this light. Let us forbear trifling—let us forget, in part at least, individual and selfish desires—let us bury the affected, pining, and helpless female, and rise the high-souled, strong-purposed woman—capable of being swayed by motives larger than the contemptible motes, which, magnified into mountains, sweep through society, bowing it hither and thither like reeds before the mighty blast—capable of losing that supreme deference for the small self and the minute creatures which move in its immediate vicinity, and forming some just appreciation of the interests of the whole—capable, in short, of being engaged in purposes whose magnitude makes them worthy of us, as the one half of the intelligence which God has created.

Let no devotee of fashion, ease, or pleasure, turn away from this as an idle or misplaced exhortation. The woman in whose bosom it wakes no response is unworthy her sex. She deserves none of the elevated joys and honors which woman is sent here to achieve, and she will reap none. She will go through life bending under the load of her insignificant purposes—absorbed in wearing out the petty disappointments and vexations they procure, and go down at last with a consciousness, dimmed though it be, of having failed to perform the true and worthy thing for which she came. From such minds may the sex be early delivered. We have too many by thousands now. There is not room for them. Better space and their absence, than indolence and falsity with their presence. Our task would be sadly interrupted by idle spectators. Nature's field is no place for them. She has not provided for any such. But if, instead of remaining idle, they strew our ground with noxious weeds, and, not content with being themselves obstacles in the way of the industrious, plant others, those whose growth we cannot check, though they breathe the deadly poison of the Upas into the moral atmosphere around, then we must lift our hands and pray that such may depart. They cannot be too hasty in yielding to our request. But let the faithful strive—let those who take knowledge of what there is to be done labor patiently, never forgetting that they cannot fail when truth is their leader, and honesty their law. The good they seek will one day be found—the truth they are nourishing will one day leave their fainting arms, and walk strongly forth alone, blessing and blest of all men.

APPENDIX.

(*a*) The strongest evidence that the offspring is affected by the mind of the mother, is to be deduced from instances of malformation produced from sudden fright by a disagreeable object, and from marks occasioned by ungratified longings. This subject, however, has given rise to much contrariety of opinion among physicians.* But so much well-authenticated

* 'Many people are satisfied that mental impressions made upon the mother may affect the offspring. Others, as Mr. Lawrence, consider it needless to pursue 'a question on which all rational persons, well acquainted with the circumstances, are already unanimous. This belief,' he continues, 'in the power of the imagination, like the belief in witchcraft, is greater or less according to the progress of knowledge, which, in truth, differs greatly in different countries and heads. We know that many enlightened women are fully convinced of its absurdity, while *soi-disant* philosophers are found to support it.'†

So many extraordinary coincidences, however, both in the human and the brute subject, have come to my knowledge, that I do not hesitate to believe the common opinion to be well founded; and, since I declared, in my edition of 1820, my inclination to support the opinion, I find it has many supporters.‡ That neither all nor most malformations can be thus

† "We may, perhaps, be excused," says Dr. Fletcher, "from at once chiming in with the accustomed cant, that the emotions of the mother '*cannot possibly*' have any effect on its organism. We 'cannot possibly' explain, perhaps, what is the immediate process by which such vitiated secretions have this effect; nor shall we be able to do so till we know a little more of the *vis plastica* than its numerous appellations; but neither shall we be able, till then, to explain why this effect should be impossible. It is much easier, in these matters, to look shrewd and *incredulous-odi-ish*, than to give any good reason for our unbelief; and if the result of process, however well accredited, is not to be believed in till the nature of the process is satisfactorily explained, we must be content to suspend, for the present, our belief in our own existence."—(*Rudiments of Physiology, Part II., p.* 12.)

‡ Sir Everard Home (Phil. Trans., 1825. p. 75, sqq.), and, according to Burdach, who considers the occurrence of monstrosity from this cause to be an incontestible fact (§360), Stark, Schneider, Bechstein, Sachs, Balz, Klein, Carus, Brandis, Hoare, and Toone, have given examples in its favor. Baer, whose name will carry weight, relates the following fact:

proof of the effects of the mother's imagination on her offspring has been accumulated, that the most charitable construction which can be put upon the motives of those who advocate opposing opinions, is, that they hope, by convincing the mother that her apprehensions are groundless, and thus diverting her thoughts from the contemplation of the subject, to remove the exciting cause, and fortify her mind successfully against the sudden influence of disagreeable impressions. Yet, to disguise or pervert a truth in nature, appears like apologizing for a defective law of the Creator. Would it not be more philosophical to inquire for what wise purpose this law of nature was instituted, and how it can be made subservient to the best

explained—that pregnant women are frequently alarmed without such consequences, even when most dreaded—and that highly-ridiculous resemblances are fancied to preceding longings and alarms, which were forgotten, or may be well suspected to have never existed, is incontestible. But, in other matters, when a circumstance may proceed from many causes, we do not universally reject any one because it is frequently alleged without reason. A diarrhea will arise from ingesta wrong, in quality or quantity, from cold, cathartic substances, and also from emotion; and yet emotion has, every day, no such effect. The notion is of great antiquity, as it prevailed in the time of Jacob. How those who believe the divine authority of the Bible, can reconcile the success of Jacob's stratagem with their contempt for the vulgar belief, they best can tell."—(*Human Physiology, by Dr. Elliotson, p.* 1117.)*

"A pregnant woman was greatly alarmed at the sight of a lengthened flame in the direction of her native place; and as she was at a distance from this of fourteen leagues, it was long before she learned the place of the fire; and this protracted uncertainty probably acted forcibly upon her imagination, for she afterward declared she had the figure of the flame constantly before her eyes. Two or three months after the fire, she gave birth to a girl with a red patch on her forehead, pointed, and like an undulating flame. This still existed at the age of seven years. I relate this fact because I know all the particulars; for the individual was my own sister, and I heard her complain, before her delivery, that she had the flame continually before her eyes; so that we were not obliged, in this case, as in most others, to refer to the past in order to explain the anomaly.—(*Contribution to Burdach,* §359.)

* Dr. Elliotson gives a number of cases, not only of marks, but also of malformations and loss of limbs, which came under his own observation. Many persons, however, say the latter case is impossible, and ask what becomes of the lost limb? But they do not observe that the fright, or affecting cause, took place in the early period of gestation, before the limb was developed, and might, therefore, have arrested its growth. So, also, in the case of idiots, when caused by some highly-distressing mental agitation, which had the effect of arresting the growth of the brain of the fœtus. This inference, at least, appears probable from the cases on record.

interests of mankind? We know that all the cerebral organs were bestowed upon man for a highly useful and benevolent purpose; and that their use or abuse depends on the will of the possessor. So, doubtless, this power of the mind, or imagination of the mother on her offspring, was intended by Superior Wisdom for the improvement of the race; and its legitimate use is the influence of favorable circumstances, particularly such impressions as proceed from virtuous principles, and the exercise of highly cultivated mental powers; while its abuse is the result of indulgence in vicious propensities, or other unfavorable influences acting upon a feeble intellect, or an irritable temperament.

"The fact of the improvement of progeny," says Dr. Elliotson, "by the operation of favorable causes upon parents, is highly encouraging. Horace, in his invective ode against the vices of the Romans, says:

> 'Ætas parentum, pijor avis, tulit
> Nos nequiores, mox daturos
> Progenium vitiosiorem.'

"But, as happy circumstances will tend to the production of a better progeny, we have great encouragement to exert all our energies for the improvement of mankind, whatever distress we must feel for our disappointments in individuals of whom we had thought well, and for whom we have done much. Ordinarily, a certain amount only of improvement by education can be effected in an individual. He generally stops at last; and defies all efforts to advance him farther. Happily, he dies, with all his uneradicable prejudices. His offspring has them not, or not so fixed; and it would seem that the offspring is likely to be still better organized than the parent, through the good influences exerted upon the parent.

"In vegetables and brutes, whatever improvement is made by good management of external circumstances, there is a constant tendency to fall back to the original state. It is the same with us; and the neglect of the physical and mental means of improvement will cause an inferior progeny to be established. But, great as this influence is, and greatly as we ought to rely upon it, that of the breed is far stronger; and, though almost entirely neglected by individuals, should always guide marrying people. No one has spoken better, or more plainly on this point, than Burton, in his *Anatomy of Melancholy*.* It is thought that a good cross within the same nation is always desirable, but that a cross between two nations begets offspring superior to either. The importance of crossing an inferior nation with a better, is shown by the great improvement of the Persians, who were, originally, ugly and clumsy, ill-made and rough-skinned, by intermixing with the Georgians and Circassians, the two most beautiful nations in the world. 'There is hardly a man of rank in Persia who is not born of a Georgian or Circassian mother; and even the king himself is commonly sprung, on the female side, from one or the other of these countries.'† But when one nation is not surpassed in any particular quality by another, I doubt whether this quality is improved by the cross: the superior race cannot gain, but must lose. Unfortunately, few nations are not inferior in some things, and national crossing is therefore generally useful; for there is less chance of the same defects meeting in the two than when they marry among themselves. What is excellent in one nation, must be deteriorated by mixture with the low degree of the same in the other. Crossing among nations may be more advantageous, as being more decided, than crossing among individuals of the same nation; but, without care, it may be an evil."—*Human Physiology*, p. 1139.

The preceding facts and opinions are worthy the attentive consideration of those benevolent, but short-sighted individuals, who advocate the principles of amalgamation—a practice which, if adopted to any considerable extent, would result in depressing our moral character many degrees below the present standard. This evil, however, is perhaps less serious in a mental point of view than the baneful practice of intermarrying in an early and immature state, thereby transmitting the faculties imperfectly developed. This practice has

* Part I. Sec. II

† Lawrence's Lectures.

been attended with wide-spread and serious detriment to the human family, wherever it has been, for ages, sanctioned by custom: for example, the Chinese nation. All accounts of this singular people unite in describing the oldest existing nation of the earth as alike distinguished for imbecility of mind and the practice of early marriages; the common custom being to unite in wedlock at the age of twelve and thirteen years. Contrast their want of energy, powers of reflection, and abject state of servitude, with the Swiss people; that indomitable race, who have preserved their independence for five hundred years, surrounded by despotism. The native of the Cantons, obedient to the law of nature as well as that of his country, seeks the permission of the magistrate when about to unite himself in marriage; and his assent is only accorded when the parties are fitted by nature, age, and circumstances. The consequence of this wise legislation is a hardy and mature race, capable of every manly effort and endurance.

Some observations on the 1117th page of the work last quoted shows the importance which Dr. Elliotson gives to maturity and strength of constitution in the parents; and also elucidates a subject which, to many reflecting minds, appears dark and mysterious. That is the reason why persons of illegitimate birth generally manifest superior powers. The reasons given are well known, and carefully practiced by those desirous of obtaining a fine breed of horses, or other animals, and are in perfect accordance with the theory of transmission and inheritance.

(*b*) All sincere inquirers after truth are truly grateful for every step which has been cleared before them, and for every ray of light shed upon the subject of their inquiry. The following just view of polygamy, and its effects, contains a decided opinion and illustration in favor of the truth of this theory:

"The increasing wealth of the Hebrews, under the patriarchal government of Israel, which forwarded its temporal power, was, however, morally counteracted in its influence by polygamy, the fatal tendency of which was soon discovered in the domestic misery, distracting the family and imbittering the days of the fondest and best, as he was the most unfortunate of fathers. The jealousies of the sisters, Rachael and Leah, for supremacy in their husbands' affections, and the contentions of the sons of Bilhah, of Zilpah, produced those dark divisions which finally ended in the expulsion of Joseph. This event, though it seated the great-grandson of Sarah near the throne of the Pharaohs, eventually caused the future slavery, during four centuries, of the tribes of Israel, with all the struggles and crimes that ensued. It was polygamy, also, that relaxed the spiritual faith of the Israelites—it was the women of strange tribes, and the demoralizing offspring of such ties, that aided mainly to substitute a superstitious devotion to idols, for the pure theism and simple worship of their fathers.

"These many wives of one husband, these numerous servants of one master, these slaves to selfish and to sensual passions, these victims of uneasy sensations, became the future mothers of those ill-organized, stubborn generations, which, in spite of their prophets and their legislators, drew down the reprobation of the 'God of Abraham and of Isaac'—'How long will these people provoke me, and how long will it be ere they believe me, for all the signs I have shown among them?'

"Throughout the remainder of this eventful history, the Israelites, indeed, appear perpetually relapsing into rebellion against the visible majesty of their Creator, refusing faith to the evidences of their own senses; ready, under every temptation of discontent or of novelty, to desert, for the idols of other nations, or even for their own creations, the sanctuary of Jehovah. It was thus the violated law of nature reacted, in virtue of its own wisdom, and that the injustice committed by the selfishness of the master was avenged in its results by the wrongs, and the consequent perversion of his servant.

"The twelve sons which Jacob had by his four wives seem respectively to have partaken of the idiosyncrasy of their different mothers. Reuben, the eldest child of the meek and submissive, but unloved Leah, and Joseph and Benjamin, the offspring of the beautiful and too well-beloved Rachael, seem alone to have been worthy of the house from which they sprung.

"The envious brothers, who hated Joseph for his virtue, who meditated his murder, sold him to slavery, and nearly broke his father's heart by the tale of his destruction, were such sons and such brothers as oriental despotism produces down to the present day—where woman is still the servant, man the master; and where polygamy is the ruling institute of the land.

"The child of Jacob's first deep and legitimate love, the son of the wife of his choice, the well-born offspring of a well-organized mother, rose superior to the terrible destiny prepared for him by fraternal jealousies and family dissensions; and the betrayed and persecuted Joseph finally attained to the highest rank and consideration, in the most civilized nation of the earth—in that nation which was to enlighten future ages."*

(*c*) "Among the duties incumbent on the human race, in relation to marriage, one is, that the parties to it should not unite before a proper age. The civil law of Scotland allows females to marry at twelve, and males at fourteen; but the law of nature is widely different. The female frame does not, in general, arrive at its full vigor and perfection, in this climate, earlier than twenty-two, nor the male earlier than from twenty-four to twenty-six. Before these ages, maturity of physical strength and of mental vigor is not, in general, attained, and the individuals, with particular exceptions, are neither corporeally nor mentally prepared to become parents, nor to discharge, with advantage, the duties of heads of a domestic establishment. Their animal propensities are strong, and their moral and intellectual organs have not yet attained their full development. Children born of such young parents are inferior, in the size and qualities of their brains, to chil-

* Woman and her Master, vol. i., p. 56.

dren born of the same parents when arrived at maturity. Such children, having inferior brains, are inferior in dispositions and capacity. It is a common remark, that the eldest son of a rich family is, generally, not equal to his younger brothers in mental ability ; and this is ascribed to his having relied on his hereditary fortune for his subsistence, and not exerted himself in obtaining education ; but you will find that very generally, in such cases, the parents, or one of them, married in extreme youth, and the eldest child inherits the imperfections of their immature condition.

"The statement of the evidence and consequences of this law belongs to Physiology ; and I can only remark, that if the Creator has prescribed ages previous to which marriage is punished by him with evil consequences, we are bound to pay deference to His enactments ; and that civil and ecclesiastical laws, when standing in opposition to His, are not only absurd, but mischievous. Conscience is misled by these erroneous human enactments ; for a girl of fifteen has no idea that she sins, if her marriage be authorized by the law and the church. In spite, however, of the sanction of acts of Parliament, and of clerical benedictions, the Creator punishes severely if His laws be infringed. His punishments assume the following, among other forms :

"The parties being young, ignorant, inexperienced, and chiefly actuated by passion, often make unfortunate selections of partners, and entail lasting unhappiness on themselves.

"They transmit imperfect constitutions and inferior dispositions to their earliest-born children. And,

"They often involve themselves in pecuniary difficulties, in consequence of a sufficient provision not having been made before marriage.

"These punishments, being inflicted by the Creator, indicate that His law has been violated ; in other words, that marriage at a too early age is positively sinful.

"There ought not to be a very great disparity between the ages of the husband and wife. There is a physical and mental condition naturally attendant on each age, and persons whose organs are in corresponding conditions, sympathize in their feelings, judgments, and pursuits, and therefore form suitable companions for each other. When the ages are widely different, this sympathy is wanting, and the offspring also is injured. In such cases, it is generally the husband who transgresses; old men are fond of marrying young women. The children of such unions often suffer grievously from the disparity. The late Dr. Robert Macnish, in a letter addressed to me, gives the following illustration of this remark: 'I know,' says he, 'an *old* gentleman, who has been twice married. The children of his first marriage are strong, active, healthy people, and their children are the same. The offspring of his second marriage are very inferior, especially in an intellectual point of view; and the younger the children are, the more is this obvious. The girls are superior to the boys, both physically and intellectually. Indeed, their mother told me she had great difficulty in rearing her sons, but none with her daughters. The gentleman himself, at the time of his second marriage, was upward of sixty, and his wife about twenty-five. This shows, very clearly, that the boys have taken chiefly off the father, and the daughters off the mother.'

"Another natural law in regard to marriage is, that the parties should not be related to each other in blood. This law holds good in the transmission of all organized beings. Even vegetables are deteriorated, if the same stock be repeatedly planted on the same ground. In the case of the lower animals, a continued disregard of this law is almost universally admitted to be detrimental, and human nature affords no exception to the rule. It is written in our organization, and the consequences of its infringement may be discovered in the degeneracy, physical and mental, of many nobles and royal families, who have long and systematically set it at defiance. Kings of Portugal and Spain, for instance, occasionally apply to the Pope for permission to marry their nieces. The Pope grants the dispensation, and the marriage is celebrated with all the solemnities of religion. The blessing of Heaven is invoked on the union. The real power of his holiness, however, is here put to the test. He is successful in delivering the king from the censures of the church, and his offspring from the civil consequences of illegitimacy; but the Creator yields not one jot or tittle of His law. The union is either altogether unfruitful, or children miserably constituted in body and imbecile in mind are produced; and this is the form in which the divine displeasure is announced. The Creator, however, is not recognized by his holiness, nor by priests in general, nor by ignorant kings, as governing, by fixed laws, in the organic world. They proceed as if their own power were supreme. Even when they have tasted the bitter consequences of their folly, they are far from recognizing the cause of their sufferings. With much self-complacency, they resign themselves to the events, and seek consolation in religion. 'The Lord giveth,' say they, 'and the Lord taketh away; blessed be the name of the Lord:' as if the Lord did not give men understanding, and impose on them the obligation of using it, to discover his laws and obey them; and, as if there were no impiety in shutting their eyes against His laws, in pretending to dispense with them; and, finally, when they are undergoing the punishment of such transgressions, in appealing to Him for consolation.

"It is curious to observe the enactments of legislators on this subject. According to the Levitical law, which we have adopted, 'marriage is prohibited between relations, within *three* degrees of kindred,' computing the generations through the common ancestor, and accounting affinity the same as consanguinity. Among the Athenians, brothers and sisters of the half-blood, if related by the fathers' side, might marry; if by the mothers' side, they were prohibited from marrying. 'The same custom,' says Paley, 'prevailed in Chaldea; for Sarah was Abraham's half-sister.' 'She is the daughter of my father,' says Abraham, 'but not of my mother; and she became my wife.'—Gen., xx., 12. The Roman law continued the prohibition, without limits, to the descendants of brothers and sisters."

"Here we observe Athenian, Chaldean, and Roman legislators prohibiting or permitting the same act, apparently accord ing to the degree of light which had penetrated into their own understandings concerning its natural consequences. The real divine law is written in the structure and modes of action of our bodily and mental constitutions, and it prohibits the marriage of all blood relations—diminishing the punishment, however, according as the remoteness from the common ancestor increases, but allowing marriages among relations by affinity, without any prohibition whatever. According to the law of Scotland, a man may marry his cousin-german, or his great-niece, both of which connections the law of nature declares to be inexpedient; but he may not marry his deceased wife's sister, against which connection nature declares no penalty whatever. He might have married either sister at first, without impropriety, and there is no reason in nature why he may not marry them in succession, the one after the other has died. There may be reasons of expediency for prohibiting this connection, but I mean to say that the organic laws contain no denunciations against it.

"In Scotland, the practice of full cousins marrying is not uncommon; and you will meet with examples of healthy families born of such unions, and from these an argument is maintained against the existence of the natural law which we are considering. But it is only when the parents have both had excellent constitutions that the children do not attract attention by their imperfections. The first alliance against the natural laws brings down the tone of the organs and functions, say one degree; the second, two degrees; and the third, three; and perseverance in transgression ends in glaring imperfections, or in extinction of the race. This is undeniable, and it proves the reality of the law. The children of healthy cousins are not so favorably organized as the children of the same parents, if married to equally healthy partners, not at all related in blood, would have been. If the cousins have themselves inherited indifferent constitutions, the degeneracy is striking, even in their children. We may err in interpreting nature's laws, but if we do discover them in their full import and consequences, we never find exceptions to them.

"Another natural law relative to marriage is, that the parties should possess sound constitutions. The punishment for neglecting this law is, that the parties suffer pain and misery in their own persons, from bad health, perhaps become disagreeable companions to each other, feel themselves unfit to discharge the duties of their condition, and transmit feeble constitutions to their children. They are also exposed to premature death; and, of consequence, their children are liable to all the melancholy consequences of being left unprotected and unguided by parental experience and affection, at a time when these are most needed. The natural law is, that a weak and imperfectly-organized frame transmits one of a similar description to offspring; and the children, inheriting weakness, are prone to fall into disease and die. Indeed, the transmission of various diseases founded in physical imperfections from parents to children, is a matter of universal notoriety: thus consumption, gout, scrofula, hydrocephalus, rheumatism, and insanity, are well known to descend from generation to generation. Strictly speaking, it is not *disease* which is transmitted, but organs of such imperfect structure that they are unable to perform their functions properly, and so weak that they are easily put into a morbid condition by causes which sound organs could easily resist."—(*Combe's Moral Philosophy, p.* 114.)

(*d*) Hitherto the general opinion has been that the determination of the sex of offspring was a mere matter of chance, dependent on no law of nature, therefore beyond human control.

Dr. Ryan, in his "Philosophy of Marriage," regrets the obscurity in which this subject is involved, and remarks that, in a country where the laws of primogeniture exist, any knowledge which would insure the birth of male heirs, would be of the first importance; but that no such knowledge does, at present, exist. Yet, more recent observation, and the statistical tables of births, show that the laws which govern this subject are as certain in their operations as those of any other portion of organized nature; and closer observers of human nature have also discovered that the sex of offspring is determined by the comparative strength of constitution, temperament, age, and habits of the parents.

The following remarks of Mr. Combe respecting the laws of polygamy, throw much light on this subject:

"It is generally admitted by physiologists, that the proportion of the sexes born is thirteen males to twelve females. From the greater hazards to which the male sex is exposed, this disparity is, in adult life, reduced to equality; indeed, with our present manners, habits, and pursuits, the balance among adults, in almost all Europe, is turned the other way—the females, of any given age above puberty, preponderating over the males. In some eastern countries more females than males are born; and it is said that this indicates a design in nature that *there* each male should have several wives; but there is reason to believe that the variation from the proportions of thirteen to twelve is the consequence of departures from the natural laws. In the appendix to the Constitution of Man, I have published some curious observations in regard to the determination of the sexes in the lower animals, from which it appears that inequality is the result of unequal strength and age in the parents. In our own country and race it is observed, that when old men marry young females the progeny are generally daughters; and I infer that, in the eastern countries alluded to, in which an excess of females exists, the cause may be found in the superior vigor and youth of the females;* the practice of polygamy being confined to rich men, who enervate themselves by every form of disobedience to the natural laws, and thereby become physically inferior to the females."

Dr. Ryan also suggests the importance of continence on the part of the husband desirous of male heirs, and illustrates his hypothesis by several examples.† Accordingly, it may be

* When we reflect upon the degraded condition of the females of those eastern countries, the little intellectual culture which they receive, their indolent, luxurious, and sensual habits, another very palpable inference may be arrived at, which is, that the habits of those women are more favorable for producing female, than male offspring.

† The reasoning of this author is so exceedingly conclusive, that the writer regrets the book is not at hand to quote from.

observed that the first child of many young married people is generally of the male sex, while those that immediately follow are females.

The influence which the comparative age of the parents has in determining the sex of offspring, is shown by the following table of Professor Hofacker. This table coincides perfectly with those referred to by Mr. Combe.

AGE OF THE HUSBAND.	AGE OF THE WIFE.	Number of Boys born for every 100 Girls.
Husband is younger	than the wife	90 6
Husband is the same age . . .	as the wife	90 0
Husband is older	by from 3 to 6 years	103 4
do. do.	by from 6 to 9 years	124 7
do. do.	by from 9 to 18 years . . .	143 7
do. do.	by from 18 years and upwards	200 0
Husband's age between 24 and 36	wife's between 16 and 26 . .	116 6
do. do. do. .	wife's between 36 and 46 . .	95 4
Husband's age between 36 and 48	wife is younger	176 9
do. do. do. .	wife is of middle age	114 3
do. do. do. .	wife is older	109 2
Husband's age between 48 and 60	wife of middle age	190 0

According to the preceding table, it may be inferred that the majority of the first children of very young parents would be females; and observation shows this to be the fact. There are, however, many apparent exceptions to this law; but if all the circumstances under which those exceptions occur were known, they would, doubtless, tend to prove the law.

Strength of constitution and age having been considered, it only remains to notice the effect which the temperament and habits of the parents have in determining the sex of offspring. The effect which a powerful vital or sanguineous temperament has, when possessed by the female, is shown by the following observation and fact. In speaking of the Empress Maria Theresa, Mr. Swinborn remarks, "She has such an internal fever and heat of the blood, that she cannot bear to have the windows closed at any season of the year." Maria Theresa was married at the age of eighteen: her first children were twin girls, and in twenty years she had *twelve* daughters and four sons.

"The lymphatic temperament," says Mr. Combe, "gives

the greatest activity to the animal organs;" and it may be observed, that women in whom this temperament obtains, generally have more daughters than sons.

The nervous temperament, on the contrary, is more favorable to greater intellectual activity; and women of this temperament have most sons, and are generally *less prolific* than either of the former temperaments. The cause of this appears to be the greater expenditure of nervous energy through the brain, induced by the superior activity which the nervous temperament gives to that organ. When, however, the husband is of a lymphatic temperament, and the wife bilious and nervous, the progeny will generally be daughters; for, although, to the superficial observer, appearances may indicate the contrary, superior strength of constitution is possessed by the wife. And when we reflect that the temperament and habits can be very materially modified and changed, the inference is, that the sex of offspring may, in some degree, be controlled by the will of the parent.

A very pious lady, of a lymphatic temperament, indolent and luxurious habits, married young, and had a large family of daughters; at the birth of each of whom she experienced a severe disappointment, so great was her desire for a son. "That the Lord would be pleased to grant her a son," she constantly and devoutly prayed, but without effect, until the preceding views were explained to her; and it was suggested, that if she fasted as well as prayed she would be much more likely to attain her object. For, as the laws of the Creator were unalterable, it became her duty to ascertain those laws, and conform to them; and, instead of blindly supplicating the Almighty to grant her request, to change her habits of life, and endeavor to live in accordance with His physical as well as spiritual laws. Being a woman of some original force of character, until spoiled by prosperity, and seeing the truth of this reasoning illustrated in the families of her own acquaintances, she immediately commenced a course of physical and mental training, which, in effect, has made her a wiser, happier, healthier woman, and the mother of a fine, promising boy.

Mothers generally prefer the greater number of their children to be sons, knowing that the chances of happiness for women are much less than for men. If, in the present condition of society, the proportion of males to females born were two to one, there would be much less suffering in the world, and married women, being more tenderly cherished, would attain to greater age. For, that more of this class die prematurely, from the effects of unkindness and neglect, than are set down in the bills of mortality, there can be but little doubt.

In connection with the preceding observations, a few remarks respecting the causes of sterility may be useful.

There is, probably, no subject on which there is so little general knowledge, as that of barrenness, or sterility. The principal cause of this want of information is, that the subject has usually been considered of so delicate a nature, that it could not be treated of, with propriety, except in medical works. When, however, we reflect upon the importance of such knowledge to the happiness of a vast number of the most amiable and worthy of our sex, the great and natural desire they have for offspring, the distress and perplexity of mind which they experience by not being able to discover the causes of sterility, any light on this subject must be most welcome. Those, therefore, who possess this light, but withhold it from mere motives of false delicacy, must be, in the estimation of all truly philosophical minds, exceedingly reprehensible.

The authoress does not propose treating this subject at the length of which it will admit, but merely to give a few conclusions, arrived at by much study and observation. She would suggest, that there may be much error in the popular opinion that sterility is more commonly the fault of the female than of the male. For, when we contrast the temperate and chaste habits of the former with the too frequently intemperate, luxurious, and dissipated lives of the latter, the most superficial knowledge of physiology might point out the error. When, however, knowledge becomes more generally diffused, and parents perceive the necessity and importance of enlightening their children on the vital subject of the laws of health, sterility, from this cause, will be less frequent.*

There is another cause of sterility, more common, perhaps,

* Many of our miseries, misfortunes, and even crimes, are to be attributed to the misplaced indulgence, or culpable neglect of our parents; and however startling and unpalatable to the unintentional offenders this maxim of the venerable author of the "Economy of Health" may be, its truth cannot be gainsayed. The censure contained in this remark, so deeply important to the human race, should open the eyes of the thoughtless to a sense of their duty, and to the adoption of every available means, aided by precept and example, to obviate such disastrous results.

Too many of the guardians of youth, using ignorance as a shield, aim to conceal from their charge all knowledge of the vicious and impure tendencies in our nature. Vain and impotent defence! What is to supply the warning voice, the lessons which could be inculcated by one experienced in the world's ways—who could tear from the front of vice the smiling mask, and point to the haggard features, distorted by pain and misery, as the too sure result of unhallowed indulgences? a sight that would surround the votary with an armor "thrice mailed in proof," which no accidental change of circumstances could endanger, or moment of temptation assail with success. "An admonition from the experienced physician," says the author just quoted, "frequently makes a deeper impression on the mind of headstrong youth, in this respect, than a sermon from the priest." Speaking in regard to the passion of love, Dr. Johnson continues: "Cupid is represented by the ancients as a winged infant, amusing himself with catching butterflies, trundling a hoop, or playing with a nymph. These representations are not inappropriate to the character of LOVE in the third septemnied. It is then guileless, innocent, ardent, and devoted! Would that it always maintained this character! But, alas! like every thing in this world, LOVE itself changes with time, and assumes such a different aspect and temperament, that the poets were forced to imagine two Cupids—one, heaven-born, the other, the offspring of Nox and Erebus, distinguished for riot, debauchery, falsehood, and in constancy! Instead of the bundle of golden arrows, designed to pierce, but not to wound the susceptible heart, we too often see the sable quiver surcharged with darts and daggers, dipped in poisons more potent than the UPAS, and destined to scatter sickness and sorrow through every ramification of society—poisonous, both moral and physical—unknown to Greek or Roman, whether philosopher, satirist, or physician; but fearfully calculated to taint the springs of life, and involve the innocent and guilty in one common ruin! From the quivered son of Jupiter they have little to fear, but oh! let them beware of that other deity, sprung from Nox and Erebus!" The following examples are in support of this view.

Alfred B——, son of the strong-minded and sensible Colonel E——

than the preceding, and more difficult to comprehend; as it occurs with those of the soundest constitutions, who have always led the purest and most exemplary lives. These

passed through college with distinguished honor; and it was determined to send him, for a season, to the medical school of the gay city of temptations—the capital of France. Previous to his departure he had formed an attachment and became engaged to a young lady of superior talents. accomplishments, and beauty. This circumstance was very gratifying to his father, who thought that a virtuous attachment would serve to guard him from forming any improper connections abroad. He, however, did not depend entirely upon this, but enlightened him thoroughly with regard to all the dangers, temptations, and snares to which an enthusiastic and impetuous youth is exposed in spending a winter in Paris. Fearful that his injunctions might be forgotten, and being desirous of making an indelible impression on the mind of his son, his father requested him, immediately on his arrival at the French metropolis, to visit an exhibition in wax, representing, with the most perfect truth, the effects of vice in all its stages, in the most horrible and disgusting forms.* A view of that revolting exhibition had the desired effect. The youth passed unscathed, surrounded by as many snares as were spread by Calypso and her nymphs, and returned to his country pure in person and mind as he left it, and is at present the happy husband of an adoring and adorable wife, and the proud and affectionate father of a talented, beautiful, and healthy offspring.

Mr. L—— was the son of an opulent merchant, who had devoted his life, from early youth, to acquiring wealth. Gratified with success, his next ambition was, that his only son should make a splendid figure in society, and become a distinguished man. With this view, he bestowed upon him the best education that money could procure; that accomplished, he sent him to travel in foreign countries to attain a knowledge of the world, and the highly polished manners of good society. Before leaving the parental roof, the youth received a general injunction to avoid low company, the gaming table, and sharpers, and to associate only with his superiors. These, judging from his own experience, the father thought included all the evils to which his son would be exposed. Thus, with suddenly-acquired liberty and a splendid allowance, without any practical knowledge of the world, nor any noble aim in view, was this inexperienced youth exposed to temptations, requiring the firmest principles of virtue to withstand. The result was, as might be apprehended. After a

* "Let the most thoughtless and dissipated youth," says a young medical writer, "frequently visit the ward of our City Hospital appropriated to the disease induced by sensual excesses, and he must be deficient, indeed, in reflective powers, if the scenes of suffering and death there witnessed do not prove a sufficient warning to deter him from the practice of conduct incurring such a dreadful penalty."

cases, doubtless, may be explained when we shall have obtained a sufficient knowledge of the laws which constitute the different temperaments, and the rules by which they should

few years' absence, he returned to his home with the loss of health, character, and peace of mind. Could those misfortunes have been confined to the culpable in this case, the evil would have been less; but, unfortunately, the innocent and the virtuous shared the penalty of the guilty. Hoping to retrieve his character and standing in society, after a few months' apparent reformation, Mr. L—— made proposals of marriage to an amiable, gentle being, who accepted him upon the supposed truth of the maxim, "that a reformed rake makes the best husband." Like many others of her sex, she proved the fallacy of this maxim by a life of suffering and sorrow. Five children died in infancy, from the dreadful effects of a virulent disease inherited from their father.* One bright bud of promise, however, lived long enough to entwine itself around the heart

* That the dreadful disease here alluded to is one of the forms by which the "sins of the fathers are visited upon the children unto the third and fourth generation," there is but little doubt. The following extract from a lecture delivered by a distinguished professor in one of our medical colleges, may serve as a warning to inexperienced youth; for how should they know if the fatal penalty of sin, descending through many generations, has not tainted their constitution, and rendered it susceptible to the condition therein referred to.

"It is my firm impression—and one, too, that I have not failed to impress on the minds of my students ever since I have been a teacher—one that I have not hesitated to promulgate in writing and in debate—that most of the constitutional symptoms of syphilis depend on the inoculation of this disease in a scrofulous constitution. For many years I have had this subject impressed on my mind. I have examined with care every case of this disease that has occurred in a laborious practice. I have inquired into the previous history and circumstances of the unfortunate beings who have fallen victims to the fell destroyer. I have looked at every case of this disease transplanted into a strumous diathesis, with peculiar attention, and I do not hesitate to assert, that when a scrofulous patient presents himself before me, with even a common chancre, I consider his death-warrant signed and sealed. He may, it is true, linger on a miserable life, disgusting to himself, and loathed by his friends; but, even if his life be spared, what is he but a miserable, emaciated, deformed, wretched being, beyond the power of medicine, capable of indulging in no hope but that of a speedy death? And the early death of such an unfortunate being is a relief from misery and despair. And who are the victims to this unenviable conjunction? Who are the young men that fall victims to the union of this disease and scrofula? Alas! it is among the young, the talented, the manly.

"Too often have I seen young gentlemen whose early mental developments, whose just and fair proportions, whose general character for scholarship and accomplishments have rendered them the delight of their friends, the hope of their parents and of their country, cut off by their own imprudence. And those, too, are the very men that are most easily led away—young, ardent, and enthusiastic.

"It is for the scrofulous, for the young, for the talented, for the beautiful, that the snare is laid; and many a physician can testify how often they have followed to the grave the blighted hopes of parents, in the persons of those who have, by imprudence and dissipation, wrought out their own destruction."

be united in the opposite sexes. It is a well-known law of nature, that issue follows the union of contrarieties. These contrarieties, it is found, must not only be male and female, but, in the human species, there should also be a difference in the temperaments. And hence it has been noticed, by one who has given considerable attention to the subject, that those wives who are of the same temperament as their husbands, are either sterile, or, if they have issue, their children are feeble, and, generally, very short-lived. When, on the contrary, there is the most marked difference in the temperament of the husband and wife, other things being equal, we usually find the most numerous and healthy offspring.

From this view of the temperaments, we are enabled to understand that well-established law of nature which produces sterility and feeble offspring from the union of blood relations ; and, also, the reason why a severe fit of illness, a sea-voyage, change of air, habits, and diet, or, in fact, any circumstance which would produce a change of temperament, should result in offspring, to those who had been united many years previous to that event.

It is also generally believed, that a stimulating, luxurious diet is conducive to fecundity. That the converse is, however, true, can be shown by the concurrent testimony of both the physiologist and the naturalist. It is a well-ascertained fact, that nature, both in the animal and vegetable kingdoms, when threatened with causes of danger or decay, makes the greatest effort to propagate itself, in order to preserve the species. The prolific powers of the starving peasantry of Ireland, and the no less rapidly multiplying inhabitants of Eastern Asia, who subsist upon a handful of rice daily, bear witness to the truth of this law. Hence, the conclusion arrived at is, that a simple and abstemious diet, and temperate and chaste habits, are more conducive to fecundity than the reverse.

Another frequent cause of sterility, is functional derange-

of its mother, when its frail constitution was shattered by a simple disease of childhood, and one grave received the innocent sufferer and the heart-broken mother.

ment of the uterus, caused by an irritation of the spinal nerves, connected with the ganglia distributed to that organ. This cause, fortunately, is completely within the power of medical skill to remove. There are, doubtless, many cases of sterility from this cause, in which the sufferer thinks that it is the will of the Almighty that she should not have offspring, therefore takes no further thought on the subject. Whereas, if a wise and experienced physician were consulted, the physical derangement might be corrected, and nature assisted to perform her natural function.

"There is no question," says Dr. Elliotson, "that the cultivation of any organ or power of the parent will dispose to the production of offspring improved in the same particular."

"It is well known," says Mr. Walker, "that the whelps of well-trained dogs are, almost at birth, more fitted for sporting purposes than others. The most extraordinary and curious observations of this kind have been made by Mr. Knight, who, in a paper read to the Royal Society, showed that the communicated powers were not of a vague or general kind, but that any particular art or trick acquired by the animals was readily practiced by their progeny without the slightest instruction.

"It was impossible to hear that interesting paper without being deeply impressed by it. Accordingly, in taking a long walk afterward, for the purpose of reflecting upon the subject, it forcibly struck me, that the better education of women was of much greater importance to their progeny than is imagined; and in calling on Sir Anthony Carlisle, on my return, to speak of the paper and its suggestions, he mentioned to me a very striking corroboration of this conclusion.

"He observed, that many years since, an old schoolmaster had told him, that in the course of his personal experience, he had observed a remarkable difference in the capacities of children for learning, which was connected with the education and aptitude of their parents; that the children of people accustomed to arithmetic, learned figures quicker than those of differently educated persons; while the children of classical scholars more easily learned Latin and Greek; and that, notwithstanding a few striking exceptions, the natural dullness of children born of uneducated parents was proverbial."

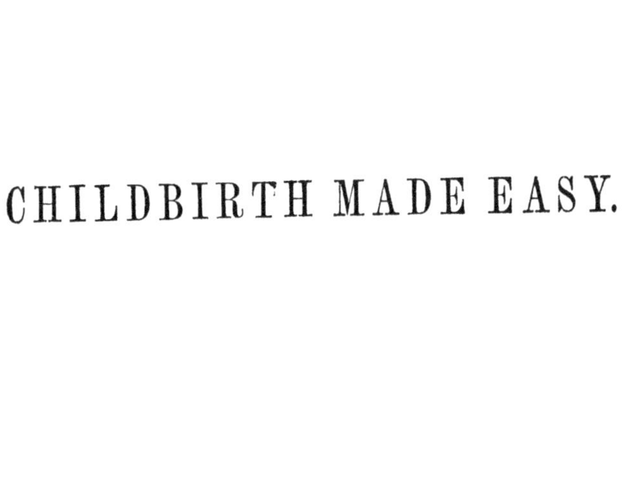

CHILDBIRTH MADE EASY.

CHILDBIRTH

PRESUMPTUOUS and unnatural as the assertion contained in the title of this work may appear, it is, nevertheless, sustained by the highest medical authority. Dr. Dewees, Professor of Obstetrics in the Medical School of Pennsylvania, in an elaborate Thesis on Childbirth, took the broad ground, that pain in childbirth was a morbid symptom, the consequence of artificial modes of life and treatment, and could be avoided by appropriate habits and treatment.

It is a well established fact, that women are to be found in almost every country who suffer no pain in childbirth.

Now, as a natural law never admits of an exception, this exemption from pain could not occur in any individual, unless it were fairly within the capabilities of the race.

"If the public mind," says Dr. Combe, "were only sufficiently enlightened to act on the perception, that no effect can take place without some cause, known or unknown, preceding it, to which its existence is really due, many evils to which we are now subject might easily be avoided. If, for example, women in childbed could be convinced, from previous knowledge, that, as a general rule, the danger attending that state is proportioned to the previous sound or unsound condition of the system, and to its good or bad management at the time, and is not the mere effect of chance, they would be much more anxious to find out, and successful in observing, the laws of health, both for their own sakes and for the sake of the future infant, than they now are, while ignorant of the influence of their own conduct. Accordingly, I entirely agree with Dr. Eberle, when he says that "the pregnant female, who observes a suitable regimen, will, *caeteris paribus*, always enjoy more tranquillity both of mind and body, and incur much less risk of injury to herself and child, than she who, giving a free reign to her appetite, indulges to excess, or in the use of improper articles of food."

"In sorrow shalt thou bring forth," says the text, alluding to woman and her offspring. This sentence has resulted in a general belief that the pains of childbirth, in their present aggravated intensity, are unavoidable. That this is, to a certain extent, a popular error, we think, is conclusively shown in the following paragraph from "Combe's Constitution of Man," a work of undeniable authority:*

---

* The following remarks of Mr. Combe, "On the Relation between Science and Scripture," apply to the present subject:

"If the views of human nature expounded in this work be untrue, the proper answer to them is a demonstration of their falsity. If they be true, they are mere enunciations of the insti-

"The sufferings of women in child bed have been cited as evidence that the Creator has not intended the human

---

tutions of the Creator; and it argues superstitious, and not religious feelings, to fear evil consequences from the knowledge of what divine wisdom has appointed. The argument that the *results* of the doctrine are obviously at variance with *scripture*, and that *therefore* the doctrines *cannot be true*, is not admissible; 'for,' in the words of Dr. Whately, 'if we really are convinced of the truth of scripture, and consequently of the falsity of any theory, (of the earth for instance,) which is really at variance with it, we must next believe that the theory is also at variance with observable phenomena; and we ought not, therefore, to shrink from trying the question by these:'

"Galileo was told, from high authority in the church, that his doctrine of the revolution of the globe was obviously at variance with scripture, and that therefore it *could not be true*: but as his opinions were founded on palpable facts, which could be neither concealed nor denied, they necessarily prevailed. If there had been a real opposition between scripture and nature, the only result would have been a demonstration that scripture, in this particular instance, was erroneously interpreted; because the evidence of physical nature is imperishable and insuperable, and cannot give way to any authority whatever. The same consequences will evidently happen in regard to phrenology. If any fact in physiology does actually and directly contradict any interpretation of scripture, it is not difficult to perceive which must yield. The human understanding cannot resist evidence founded on observation; and even if it did resist, nature would not bend, but continue to operate in her own way in spite of the resistance, and a new and more correct interpretation of scripture would ultimately become inevitable. Opposition between science and revelation I sincerely believe to be impossible, when the facts in nature are correctly observed, and divine truth is correctly interpreted; but I put the case thus strongly to call the serious attention of religious persons to the mischievous consequences to religion of rashly denouncing, as adverse to revelation, any doctrine professing to be founded on natural facts. Every instance in which the charge is made falsely, is a gross outrage upon revelation itself, and tends to lead men to regard scripture as an obstacle to the progress of science and civilization, instead of being a system of divine wisdom, in harmony with all natural truth."

being, under any circumstances, to execute all its functions free from pain. But, besides the obvious answer that the objection applies only to one sex, and is therefore not to be too readily presumed to have its origin in nature, there is good reason to deny the assertion, and to ascribe the suffering in question to departures from the natural laws, in either the structure or the habits of the individuals who experience it."

We might multiply authority to any extent, to prove the correctness of this opinion. Reasoning from analogy with the animal kingdom—the book of nature, the handwriting of God, which bears on every page evidence of His wisdom and goodness, amply testifies to its correctness. Comparative anatomy, also, which shows the difference of capacity between the male and female pelvis, sustains the opinion that nature has made ample provision for the performance of the function of parturition unattended by danger or suffering.

The following extract from "Mrs. Gove's Lectures to Ladies," supports the view last quoted, as to the effects of wrong habits, in aggravating the pains and perils of child bearing.

"Many lovely young women enter the married state frail as the gossamer, from wrong physical training, unable to bear the slightest hardship, when it is their right, by God's intendment, to be hardy and robust. They fall victims immediately, and often the grave covers them and their first born, and 'mysterious Providence' heads their obituary. Parent of wisdom! shall such ignorance forever shroud our world?

"The functions of gestation and parturition are as natural as digestion; and were mankind brought into a natural and healthy state, we have reason to believe that these functions would be attended with little, if any pain. But the healthy tone of the nervous system is destroyed, and diseased, convulsed, and erratic action established, by the various abuses of civic life; and the most tender and endearing of all relations becomes a horror and a curse.

"I know many mothers who, with their husbands, have adopted the 'Graham System,' or in other words, those correct habits recommended in these lectures; (that is, attention to diet, exercise, and bathing freely and constantly with pure cold water,) and these mothers have abridged their sufferings in parturition from forty hours to *one hour*, and have escaped altogether the deathly sickness of the three first months of gestation. But they avoided all excesses as far as possible. We know that the Indians, the lower orders of Irish, and the slaves at the South, suffer very little in childbearing. Why is this? God made us all of one blood. Is it not that these, living in a less artificial manner, taking much exercise in the open air, and living temperately, have obeyed more of the laws of their being, and consequently do not suffer the penalty of violated laws, as do our victims of civilization?"

A manuscript, containing an account of the progress and successful termination of an experiment for securing childbirth with safety, and almost without pain, published in London, 1841, by S. Rowbotham, author of an "Essay on Human Parturition, &c." was sent to the writer, requesting her to add her views on the subject, and to prepare it for publication.

The request was cheerfully complied with, in view of improving the opportunity of collecting and arranging in a popular form, information of such vital importance to the health and happiness, not only of the present, but also future generation of her own sex. For, however well-informed and intelligent our countrywomen may be on other subjects, the one under consideration is, to the majority of them, shrouded in more than Egyptian darkness. This state of things, however, cannot long remain. A spirit of inquiry is abroad ; and in the present age of progress, ignorance and prejudice must yield to more liberal and enlightened views. The time cannot be far distant when a knowledge of the functions of gestation and parturition will be considered as necessary as those of digestion, circulation, or any other natural law of the human system.

A former copy of this work, which had been prepared with much attention, research and labor, together with the original manuscript, containing an account of the experiment, were destroyed by the late fire in the Tribune Buildings. Not being able to procure another copy, without much loss of time, the writer will be obliged to give a synopsis of the experiment from recollection. Fortunately, however, two of the first pages of the manuscript had been copied, and were thus preserved.

"While reading the article *Age*," (says Mr. Rowbotham,) "in the 'Penny Cyclopædia, published by the Society for the Diffusion of Useful Knowledge,' I was forcibly impressed by this paragraph : 'When first the human embryo becomes distinctly visible, it is almost wholly fluid, consisting only of a soft gelatinous pulp. In this gelatinous pulp solid substances are formed, which gradually increase and are fashioned into organs. These organs, in their rudimental state, are soft and tender, but, in progress of their developement, constantly acquiring a greater number of solid particles, the cohesion of which progressively increases, the organs at length become dense and firm. As the soft solids augment in bulk and density, *bony particles* are deposited, sparingly at first, and in detached masses, but accumulating by degrees; these, too, are at length fashioned into distinct oseous structures, which, extending in every direction, until they unite at every point, ultimately form the connected bony framework of the system. This bony fabric, like the soft solids, tender and yielding at first, becomes by degrees firm and resisting.'

"Mr. Rowbotham reasoned from this, that the firmness and density of a fœtus depends upon the amount of *bony matter* deposited, or entering into its constitution; and as the fœtus is built up, nourished and supported by the mother's blood, the mother's blood must be the source of *bony matter* which hardens and consolidates the fœtus. But blood is derived from food and drink—consequently, if different kinds of food and drink contain different proportions of this bony matter, it follows, that according to the kind of food which the mother subsists upon during pregnancy, that is to say, according to the amount of earthy or *bony matter* existing in it, will be the amount existing in, or entering into combination with, her blood; and consequently, the fœtus will be more or less firm and resisting.

"Diet, then, is the principal thing. Exercise has a favorable effect no doubt, but nothing more: it is not a primary cause of either difficult or easy parturition.

"Many midwifes and experienced matrons admit, that not to indulge in eating and drinking more than is barely necessary, retards the growth of the fœtus, and thus contributes to the safety of childbirth.

"Every mother knows," continued Mr. Rowbotham, "that the cause of the extreme pain in the birth of a child, is the consolidation of its bones while yet in the womb. Some persons may suppose that this consolidation is desirable. But this is a mistake. For the free expansion, beauty and grace of its form, it is, on the contrary, desirable, that the bones of the child should be in the state of gristle, soft, elastic, yielding; no less than to save suffering to the mother. Many children are so much injured at birth that they suffer through life in various ways; while it is often observed, that seven months' children are remarkable for their size, grace, and general fine form."

Mr. Rowbotham, having thus come to the conclusion that no injury would result to the child by this de-ossifying system, endeavored to persuade his wife to enter into his views, and test his favorite theory.

Although Mrs. Rowbotham had suffered severely in two previous labors, she could not be induced to practice the self-denial necessary to insure a safe and easy labor, until six weeks, as it proved, previous to the expiration of her time. At the period in which she commenced this depleting system, she was suffering under all the evils of pregnancy, which resulted principally from a plethoric habit; as nausea, varicose-veins, vertigo or dizziness, accompanied by a disagreeable sensation of lassitude and dullness, both of body and mind. These painful symptoms, however, were soon relieved by abstemiousness, a simple diet, bathing, fresh air, exercise, and attention to the healthy action of all the organs; a regimen, in the opinion of the writer, sufficient to account for the easy labor that followed, independently of the theory of her husband, in regard to the softening of the fœtal-bones.

In order fully to carry out her husband's views, Mrs. Rowbotham abstained as far as possible from all articles of food containing the phosphate of lime and magnesia.

Wheat, barley, beans, peas, rice, and all farinaceous substances, Mr. Rowbotham stated, contained a much greater amount of earthy phosphates, than fruits, vegetables, or even animal food. Fine wheaten flour, whether used in the form of bread, cakes, pastry, or puddings, was particularly objectionable, on account of the large portion of earthy matter it contained. Milk, butter, and cheese, were, for the same reason, to be avoided. All kinds of fruits, on the contrary, were highly recommended; more particularly acid fruits, such as lemons, oranges, currants, grapes, &c. These, when used with sugar, were not only highly nutritious and grateful to the stomach, but served the important purpose of dissolving and carrying off much of the earthy matter, unavoidably taken with the food.

Water, and the different kinds of drink in which it enters, as tea, coffee, beer, &c., were also put under interdict by Mr. Rowbotham, as containing the constituents of bone. In answer to the question that might be asked, as to the means of allaying thirst, he stated that his wife experienced no thirst after she had entered upon the temperance system, except such as could be readily allayed by juicy fruits; and that this system agreed well with her health; she felt cheerful, strong, and active, attended to her domestic duties, and performed active household labor, up to the very hour of her accouchement.

Certificates from the attendant physician and nurse accompanied these statements, showing the remarkable easy labor, and rapid convalescence, of Mrs. Rowbotham. Nor was the child a sufferer by this experiment; for although small and soft when born, it soon grew to be a large, finely-formed, and perfectly healthy child. Thus proving, to the entire satisfaction of Mr. Rowbotham, the truth of the principle on which his theory was founded.

This experiment has terminated with equal success in several cases in this country, although the writer is not at liberty to mention names.

The investigations of modern chemistry have shed a brilliant light upon many subjects hitherto considered obscure and incomprehensible. The vital principle of animal heat is no longer a speculation—agriculture no longer an experiment; while the advantages which many of the arts have derived from this science are almost invaluable; by its light order is evolved out of chaos, and all the laws of matter discovered to be invariable and harmonious.

With all its splendid discoveries, however, modern chemistry has added little to our knowledge of physiology previous to the investigations of Liebig: to whose invaluable work, on "Animal Chemistry," we must now look to elucidate the present subject:

"The combinations of the chemist relate to the change of matter, forward and backward, to the conversion of food into the various tissues and secretions, and to their metamorphosis into lifeless compounds; his investigations ought to tell us what has taken place, and what can take place, in the body."

Accordingly, from these investigations we learn, that the phosphate of lime and magnesia contained in the food and from thence conveyed into the blood, cannot be converted into cellular tissue, neither can these be consumed by the respiratory organs, but that a portion of them is deposited in the form of bone, and the residue, after performing the important purpose of keeping up the peristaltic motion, is thrown out of the system. Hence, it appears probable, that if only those articles of food containing the least amount of the phosphate of lime or magnesia were taken by pregnant women, the ossification of the *fœtus in-utero* might be retarded in such a degree as to obviate the imminent danger at the period of parturition, so frequently fatal to either mother or child. The writer is perfectly aware that all reasoning *apriora* is without value, and that carefully conducted and well observed experiments only, can test the truth and utility of this principle.

Meanwhile, the important question arises as to the effect which this abnormal condition of the bones may have on the constitution of the offspring; as no mother would be justified in guarding herself against pain at the expense of the health of her child; for what are a few hours, or even days suffering to her, in comparison to a life of disease, debility, and pain to her offspring.

It is well known that many of the most fatal diseases of infancy originate from a want of earthy matter in the bones; as rickets, mollities-ossiana, or softening of the bones, and spina-biffida, a want of one or more of the arches of the vertebre, thereby allowing the contents of the spinal column to exude in the form of a tumor, which is almost always fatal. A knowledge of such facts should render every mother particularly careful of transmitting even a tendency to those diseases to her offspring. This un-ossifying system, therefore, may prove in the hands of the timid and ignorant a source of infinite mischief, in transmitting a weakly organized constitution, and thereby enfeebling and deteriorating the race. There are, however, many cases in which this system might prove highly beneficial; it should at all events be resorted to, where there has been a succession of stillborn births, caused *only* by the large size of the fœtus.

There is, perhaps, no department of medical science which can boast of more excellent treatises than Midwifery. It is, therefore, much to be regretted that the many valuable popular works, intended expressly for females, should meet with so little attention. The time, however, cannot be far distant, when a knowledge of the laws which govern the human system under *all* circumstances, will be considered an indispensible branch of female education. Hitherto palliatives and curatives have been the principal means sought after and relied on ; but when more liberal and enlightened views obtain—when the cobwebs of false delicacy have been swept from society—when women are taught the importance of a knowledge of the organic laws, preventive and first principle will take their place.

"The physical and organic laws," says Mr. Combe, "when truly discovered, appear to the mind as institutions of the Creator ; wise and salutary in themselves, unbending in their operation, and universal in their application. They interest our intellectual faculties, and strongly impress our sentiments. The necessity of obeying them comes to us with all the authority of a mandate from God. While we confine ourselves to mere recommendations to beware of damp, to observe temperance, or to take exercise, without explaining the *principle*, the injunction carries only the weight due to *the authority of the individual* who gives it, and is addressed to only two or three faculties—veneration and cautiousness, for instance, or self-love, in him who receives it. But if we be made acquainted with the elements of the physicial world, and with those of our organized system—with the uses of the different parts of the human body, and the conditions necessary to their healthy action—with the causes of their derangement, and the pains consequent thereon ; and if the obligation to attend to these conditions be enforced on our moral sentiments and intellect, as a duty which is imposed by the Creator, and which we cannot neglect without suffering punishment ; then the motives to observe the physical and organic laws, as well as *the power of doing so*, will be prodigiously increased. It is only by being taught the *principle* on which consequences depend, that we become capable of perceiving the *invariableness* of the results of the physical and organic laws, acquire confidence in, and respect for, the laws themselves, and fairly endeavor to accommodate our conduct to their operation."

The important principles which govern the health of both mother and child during the period of gestation, are fully explained in that most useful and excellent work, "Combe on Infancy."

This author, also, explains the effect of the mother's imagination and sentiments, on the mental constitution of her offspring—a subject of the deepest interest to mankind; as on obedience or disregard to this important law of nature, depend the happiness or misery of the domestic circle; the birthplace of the affections, the shrine of the heart. Prosperity may shower its brightest gifts on man—wealth and art may combine to beautify and embellish his habitation—science and literature may elevate his understanding and refine his taste—the good and the wise may court his society—he may be exalted to the highest place in the gift of his countrymen: of what avail are all these advantages, if his home presents a scene of corroding anxiety, or humiliating mortification, caused by feeble, sickly, or inefficient and badly organized children? Not until the public mind is fully awakened to the importance of the laws which govern a healthy action of mind and body, and also the hereditary descent of intellectual and moral qualities, can domestic happiness be predicated to a moral certainty, or approximate to a more perfect state. That order and law govern all matter, animate and inanimate, is too well established to admit of a doubt. Shall it then be said, that so important a subject as the physical and mental constitution of our children, is a mere matter of chance, the only department of creation not subject to fixed and invariable laws? Forbid it, every just appreciation of the wisdom and goodness of a beneficent Creator!

For the benefit of those who cannot procure the work just alluded to, (it being nearly out of print) the writer will extract from its pages much valuable counsel in regard to the subject under consideration.

"The only circumstance which can explain or excuse the indiffence shown by many mothers to the state of their own health during pregnancy, is their *entire ignorance* of the injury which they thereby inflict on their future offspring. Many a mother, who will not deny herself the temporary gratification of a simple desire or appetite on her own account, would be the first and firmest in resisting the temptation, if her reason was fully convinced, that every transgression which she commits diminishes, in so far, the chances of health of the being whom she carries in her bosom. And such is unquestionably the fact."

"A notion is very prevalent, that an unusual supply of nourishing food is required during pregnancy, on account of the rapid development of the new being in the maternal womb. In some instances in which the general health, digestive powers, and appetite improve during gestation, an increased allowance of food becomes necessary, and is productive of much advantage. But in the great majority of cases, when no such improvement takes place, and the appetite is already more vigorous than the powers of digestion, nothing but mischief can follow from increased eating.

"It is true that substance is expended on the development of the infant being in the mother's womb, but Nature herself has provided for that demand, by the suppression of the periodical discharge to which they are at other times subject, and which ceases altogether when the age of child-bearing is past; and, therefore, when during pregnancy the health is good and the appetite is natural, there is no need whatever of increasing the quantity or altering the quality of the food which is found by experience to agree with the constitution, and nothing but harm can result from attempting to "support the strength" by too nutritious a diet.

"When, from mistaken views, a change is made from a plain and nourishing diet to full and generous living, and especially when the usual exercise is at the same time diminished, a state of fulness not less dangerous to the mother than injurious to the embryo, is apt to be induced, or is prevented onlv by the digestive powers giving way, which leads to much suffering from nausea, heartburn, flatulence, inordinate craving, disagreeable breath and perspiration, and other symptoms well known to mothers as incapable of cure until gestation is at an end. Where digestion continues unimpaired, and the superfluity of nourishment is taken into the system, a fulness and sense of oppression ensue, which infallibly lead to mischief, when not timely relieved either by nature or by art. Occasionally, bleeding from the nose or lungs, or from piles, removes the impending danger. At other times blood is purposely drawn from a vein to avert it; but now and then it happens, that nature seeks relief by attempting to re-establish the customary discharge from the womb, and if she is aided in her efforts by any accidental imprudence on the part of the parent, the attempt will be successful, and accompanied probably by a miscarriage and a risk of life. In short, the fulness of system thus imprudently induced, must have vent somewhere, and it will depend upon the existence of any local weakness or other accident, in what organ or in what way the vent shall be effected, and with what extent of danger it shall be accompanied. To the child, not less than to the parent, its consequences are injurious, not only as endangering premature birth, but as effecting the *future soundness of its organization*: and it therefore becomes a solemn moral duty of the mother, not to place herself voluntarily in circumstances which may not only defeat her fondest hopes of happiness, and leave her a prey to broken health and endearing regret, but permanently diminish the happiness of the offspring.

"But, while avoiding one error, we must be careful not to run headlong into the other extreme, and sanction an insufficient diet. Many of the lower orders suffer grievously in this way, and from absolute inability to procure nourishing food in due quantity, give birth to feeble and unhealthy children, whose whole life is a scene of suffering, although, fortunately, they do not survive long. This is, in truth, one cause of the physical inferiority of, and greater mortality among the working classes; and as it almost necessarily leads to moral inferiority as its result, it is one of the points which eminently deserve the attention of the philanthropist and enlightened statesman.* As well may we expect fine fruit and rich harvests from an impoverished soil, as well-constituted children from parents exhausted by physical exertion and insufficient food. It is in work-houses that the evil is seen in its most glaring form. These are peopled by the children of the lowest, most sickly, or most improvident parents. From birth they are the worst fed, and the most miserably clothed, and in consequence, their bodies are stunted and weak, and their minds and morals impaired and degraded. If the children in any work-house are contrasted

* ["In this country, happily, the working classes do not suffer in the manner described in the text. They are in more danger of excess, than deficiency of food."—B.

with the children of even any common country school, their physical and moral inferiority is seen to be very marked, and in the expression of innate heartiness and enjoyment peculiar to early youth, the difference is still more striking.

"It is naturally the children of the poor who suffer most from the inadequate nourishment of the parent during pregnancy; but those of the higher classes also suffer, though in a different way. The system is duly nourished only *when the proper food in itself is also properly digested:* if the digestion be imperfect, no food, however nutritious, will afford a healthy sustenance. Many mothers in the higher classes, give birth to feeble and badly developed children, from inattention to this fact. Fond of indulging in every luxury, they eat unseasonably and largely, till the powers of the stomach are utterly exhausted, and digestion becomes so much impaired that the food ceases to be nutritious. As regards the infant, the result is the same, whether the want of nourishment arises from want of food or want of digestion; and hence the duty so strongly incumbent upon the mother, of acting like a rational being, for her infant's sake, if not for her own. Morally considered, it is as culpable on her part, to starve the infant before birth, by voluntarily impairing her own power of nourishing it, as by directly refusing it food after it is born.

"In all instances, the great aim ought to be, to act according to the laws of the human constitution, and, consequently, adopt the kind and quantity of nourishment to the wants of the individual. Following this rule, we shall find that while, *in general*, no increase is required during pregnancy, there are, nevertheless, many females who enjoy a higher degree of health in the married state, and especially during pregnancy, than they did before, and in whom the appetite becomes more acute, only because digestion and the other organic functions are carried on with greater vigor. In such cases, an improved diet is not only safe, but natural and necessary ; and all that is required is, not to push it so far as to impair the amended tone, or oppress the system. The proper limit can, in general, be easily determined by a little attention. So long as healthy activity of mind and body, aptitude for exercise, and regularity in all the animal functions, continue unimpaired, there will be nothing to fear; but if oppression, languor, or other indications of constitutional disorder, begin to show themselves, no time should be lost in taking the hint, and adopting the necessary restrictions.*

"There is no period of life at which it is of so much consequence to observe moderation and *simplicity* of diet, and avoid the use of heating food and stimulants, as during pregnancy. Not only is the general system then unusually susceptible of impressions and disordered by the slightest causes, but, in nervous constitutions, the stomach is the seat of a peculiar irritability, accompanied by a craving and capricious appetite, to which it requires much good sense and self-denial on the part of the parent, to refrain from giving way. Dr. Eberle notices

* [Doctor Dewees, in his valuable "*Treatises on the Physical and Medicinal Treatment of Children,*" expresses himself on this point in the following language: He had just mentioned the subject of nausea and vomiting being such common symptoms in the early period of pregnancy. "Now do these not most emphatically declare that the svstem requires reduction, rather than an increase of fluids? or why should this subduing process be instituted? It certainly cannot be intended for any other purpose, since it is not only almost universal, but highly important when it occurs, as it would seem to add much to the security of the fœtus; for it is a remark, as familiar as it is well grounded, that very sick women rarely miscarry ; while, on the contrary, women of very full habits are disposed to abortion, if exempt from this severe, but it would seem, important process."—B.]

several remarkable instances in which indulgence in indigestible articles of diet produced excruciating colic, followed by abortion, even so early as the fourth month. During the latter stages of pregnancy, the risk from this cause is greatly increased; and, to long-existing intestinal derangement, produced by a redundant, mixed, heterogeneous diet, the same author justly ascribes the appearance of a peculiar and highly dangerous affection, resembling puerperal fever, which comes on soon after delivery, and is characterized by a remarkable sinking of the vital energies. In cases of this kind, the disorder of health, previous to parturition, is not so striking as to arrest attention, although perfectly obvious to experienced eyes; and when, after delivery, danger declares itself, it is viewed with all the surprise and alarm of an unexpected event, although, in reality, it might have been foreseen, and, to a considerable extent, guarded against by a well-conducted regimen, and due attention to the action of the bowels.

"If the public mind were only sufficiently enlightened to act on the perception, that no effect can take place without some cause, known or unknown, preceding it, to which its existence is really due, many evils to which we are now subject, might easily be avoided. If, for example, women in childbed could be convinced from previous knowledge, that, as a general rule, the danger attending that state is proportioned to the previous sound or unsound condition of the system, and to its good or bad management at the time, and is not the mere effect of chance, they would be much more anxious to find out, and successful in observing the laws of health, both for their own sakes, and for the sake of the future infant, than they now are, while ignorant of the influence of their own conduct. Accordingly, I entirely agree with Dr. Eberle, when he says that "the pregnant female, who observes a suitable regimen, will, *caeteris paribus*, always enjoy more tranquillity, both of mind and body and incur much less risk of injury to herself and child, than she, who giving a free rein to her appetite, indulges it to excess, or in the use of improper articles of food."

On the subject of *longings* for extraordinary kinds of food, much caution ought to be exercised. Longings rarely occur in a healthy woman of a well-constituted mind. Indeed, they are almost peculiar to delicate, nervous, irritable, and above all, *unemployed* women, who have been accustomed to much indulgence, and have no wholesome subject of thought or occupation to fill up their time. If they are indulged from the first, they gain strength by what they feed on; the whole mind becomes centered on their contemplation, and the fancy is incessantly excited to produce new whims for their gratification, to the infallible disturbance of the health of both mother and child. Longing is a disease of the brain and mind, much more than of the stomach; and the way to cure it is to provide the mind with wholesome occupation, and the feelings with objects of higher interest, and to give the stomach the plain and mild food, which alone, in its weakened state, it is able to digest. In very capricious and confirmed cases, it is sometimes better to yield temporarily; but, even then, the main object, the means of cure, ought never to be lost sight of.

"During pregnancy, the great aim, for the sake of both parent and child, ought to be to sustain the general health in its highest state of efficiency; and in order to attain this, the mother ought to pursue her usual avocations and mode of life, provided these be compatible with the laws of health. Regular daily exercise, cheerful occupation and society, moderate diet, pure air, early hours, clothing suitable to the season, and healthy activity of the skin, are all more essential than ever, because now the permanent welfare of another being is at stake, in addition to that of the mother. But any of these, carried to excess, may become a source of danger to both mother and child. Dancing, riding, travelling over rough roads, and vivid exertions of mind, have often brought on abortion.*

" For many years past, common sense and science have combined to wage war against custom and fashion on the subject of female dress, and particularly tight-lacing, and the use of stiff unyielding corsets ; but hitherto with only partial success. Of late, however, a glimmering perception has begun to prevail, that the subject for which the restraint is undergone may be more certainly attained by following the dictates of reason, than by physical compression ; and if this great truth shall make way, fashion will ultimately be enlisted on the right side, and the beautiful forms of nature be preferred to the painful distortions of art. Already sounder views of the nature of the human frame, added to the lamentable lessons of experience, have convinced many mothers that the surest way to deform the figure and prevent gracefulness of carriage, is to enforce the use of stiff and tight stays ; and the most effectual way to improve both, is to obey the dictates of nature in preference to the inspirations of ignorance. It was not by the use

* [Most practitioners of extended experience have met with cases of delicate women, who have only been able to avoid a miscarriage by taking regular exercise and attending to their domestic avocations, in place of confining themselves to the house, or even to their chamber, as they had been in the practice of doing before, but without its protecting them from the misfortune they so much dreaded.

More harm is done by sudden efforts, as in lifting, pulling, pushing, stepping with a bound, so as to light only on the fore part of the foot, or by jumping, than by prolonged exercise, or even labor, though neither of these is proper for persons unaccustomed to them.—B.]

of tight bands and stays the classic forms of Greece and Rome were fashioned; and if we wish to see these produced, we must secure freedom of action for both body and mind, as an indispensable preliminary. If the bodily organization be allowed fair play, the spine will grow up straight and firm, but, at the same time, graceful and pliant to the will, and the rest of the figure will develope itself with a freedom and elegance unattainable by any artificial means; while the additional advantage will be gained, of the highest degree of health and vigor compatible with the nature of the original constitution.

"If, then, perfect freedom ought at all times to be provided for in the construction of female dress, it is plain that during pregnancy it must be doubly imperative. And, accordingly it is well remarked by Dr. Eberle, 'the custom of wearing tightly-laced corsets during gestation cannot be too severely censured. It must be evident to the plainest understanding, that serious injury to the health of both mother and child must result from a continued and forcible compression of the abdomen, while nature is at work in gradually enlarging it for the accommodation and development of the fœtus. By this unnatural practice, the circulation of the blood throughout the abdomen is impeded—a circumstance which, together with the mechanical compression of the abdominal organs, is peculiarly calculated to give rise to functional disorder of the stomach and liver, as well as to hemorrhoids, uterine hemorrhage, and abortion. The regular nourishment of the fœtus, also, is generally impeded in this way; a fact which is frequently verified in the remarkably delicate and emaciated infants born of mothers who have practised this fashionable folly during gestation. It may be observed, that since the custom of wearing tightly-laced corsets has become general among females, certain forms of uterine disease are much more frequent than they were sixteen or eighteen years ago.'*

"Hence it ought to be the first duty of the young wife, who has reason to believe pregnancy has commenced, to take special care so to arrange her dress as to admit of the utmost freedom of respiration, and to prevent even the slightest compression of the chest or abdomen.

"After these most judicious and forcible observations, I need only add, that the evils of tight-lacing do not end with the birth of the child. The compression further prevents the proper development of the breasts and nipples, and renders them unfit to furnish that nourishment on which the life of the infant may entirely depend; and yet it is only when absolutely compelled to give way, that many mothers, as pregnancy advances, loosen their corsets sufficiently to admit of common breathing space, and remove the unnatural obstacles of steel or whalebone, which Dr. Eberle has shown to be so injurious.

"But although I strongly advocate the propriety of bringing up young girls without the use of such ill-judged support, I by no means recommend that those mothers, to whom long custom has rendered corsets necessary, should at once lay them aside. They ought, however, to be very careful to wear them sufficiently loose to admit of the free enlargement of the womb in an upward direction, and to substitute thin whalebone blades for the stiff steel in common use. If this precaution be neglected, both mother and infant may be seriously injured, and ruptures or other local ailments induced. To afford the necessary support, a broad elastic bandage worn round the body, but not too tight, will be of great service; but every approach to absolute pressure should be scrupu-

* Eberle on the Diseases and Physical Education of Children. Cincinnati, 1833, p. 9.

lously avoided. The Romans were so well aware of the mischief caused by compression of the waist during gestation, that they enacted a positive law against it; and Lycurgus, with the same view, is said to have ordained a law compelling pregnant women to wear very wide and loose clothing.*

"In regard to regular exercise in the open air, the greatest attention is requisite on the part of the mother. Nothing contributes more essentially than this to a sound state of health during gestation, and to a safe and easy recovery after delivery. With ordinary care walking may be continued almost to the last hour, and with excellent effect upon all the functions. Hard riding on horseback, dancing, and every kind of violent exertion, ought, however, to be scrupulously avoided; as also fatigue, damp, cold, and late hours. The early part of the day ought to be selected in preference, especially in winter, as there is always a degree of dampness at sunset which is unfavorable to health. Riding in an open carriage is a very useful addition to walking, but ought never to supercede it. I have seen even delicate women pass through the whole period of pregnancy and delivery without a single bad symptom, merely from scrupulous but cheerful observance of the laws of exercise and health; and it cannot be doubted that the degree of danger attending it depends very much upon the mother herself. *Child-bearing is a natural and not a morbid process; and in the facility with which healthy and regular-living women*

[* Beauty, grace, cheerfulness, a good temper itself, are all sufferers from this practice of lacing and wearing corsets. The editor may be excused from referring on this occasion to his work, entitled "*Health and Beauty*," in which this subject is examined, together with all the other causes which influence the form and carriage. —BELL.]

pass through it, we have abundant evidence that the Creator did not design it to be necessarily a time of suffering and danger. Where the mode of life and the habitual occupations of the mother are rational, the more nearly she can adhere to them during pregnancy, the better for herself, and consequently the better also for her infant.

"Cleanliness and fresh air are important aids to health at all times, and doubly necessary during gestation. Hence the propriety of having recourse to a tepid bath every few days, especially in the case of females of the middling and higher classes, in whom the nervous system is unusually excitable. It promotes the healthy action of the skin, soothes the nervous excitement, prevents internal congestion, and is in every way conducive to health. But it must not be either too warm, too long continued, or taken too soon after meals. For the cautions which its use requires, I must refer the reader to my former work, as it would be out of place to repeat them here.*

"Other circumstances might be mentioned as influencing the mother's health, and indirectly that of the child; but as they have reference to her only, in common with other individuals, and therefore come under the head of general laws of health, I need not now enlarge upon them. Many sensible people, who have not thought on the subject, may be surprised at the earnestness with which I have thus recommended attention to the mother's state as the surest way of influencing the health of the child; but let them observe and reflect upon what is passing around them, and they will meet with many proofs of the principle which I have been enforcing, and soon be induced to admit its importance."

All the authors, in this department of medical science,

* Principles of Physiology applied to Health and Education chap. III.—[Also, Bell on Baths and Mineral Waters.]

of the present age, concur in opinion, as to the importance of regimen during the period of gestation. The following remarks coincide perfectly with the preceding, and are worthy of high consideration, as eminating from the best possible authority—Dr. GILMAN, Professor of Obstetrics in the New-York College of Physicians and Surgeons:

"*Regimen of Pregnant Women.*—This is a most important subject, but physicians are not as frequently consulted about it, as they might be with advantage, perhaps —because, *when consulted they make light of it.*

"*Diet.*—This should be light, not very nutritious, and rather laxative. Nature in most cases points out this course; the appetite is for fruits, vegetables, and the lighter meats, while gross food, such as goose, pork, fat, &c. are loathsome. Follow here the dictates of nature, let the patient take vegetables, and especially fruits, freely, and abstain from gross articles, from highly seasoned meats, and from stimulating drinks. These rules are most appropriate for the first four months; after quickening, when the digestion improves, a rather more nutritious diet may be allowed, but as the patient approaches the term of her gestation, the diet should again be light. Dr. Delafield, my predecessor in the professorship of obstetrics, gives it as the result of his experience, that women generally do best, when, before they fall into labor, the system is reduced to a little below par; for this purpose he lowers the diet, and gives occasional laxatives during the ninth month. This, as has been said, is an excellent practice. Articles likely to produce flatulency are to be avoided at this time.

"*Influence of Atmosphere in Pregnancy.*—This is well established; cold, rainy weather, and low, damp miasmatic localities, have been recognized since the time of

Hippocrates, as disturbing pregnancy and causing abortion. To the influence of the atmosphere is to be attributed the frequency of abortion, miscarriage, or rather mishap in pregnancy, by which some years are signalized. Miasma is, probably, the unsuspected cause of many abortions, and when this unpleasant accident recurs frequently to a woman residing in a low, damp, or miasmatic district, she should remove during pregnancy.

"*Exercise.*—This should be strongly insisted; none ot the means of preserving the health of pregnant women are more valuable than this. It should always be taken in the open air, and carried so far as to produce fatigue, but not absolute exhaustion. As to the kind of exercise, walking is best, riding in an open carriage will do well; horseback exercise is not to be permitted, unless the patient be very well accustomed to it, ride well, and have a gentle horse.

"Nothing is so likely to overcome the persistent insomnia,* with which some women are troubled towards the close of pregnancy, as to exercise in the open air, carried to fatigue; this, with warm-bath, will do more than all the anodynes you can give.

"*Dress.*—The great thing to be avoided is tightness. Anything that compresses the body, and obstructs circulation, does harm. Inflammation of the mammae is sometimes excited by the exposure of the parts to cold, in consequence of the dress being too low. This should be avoided, and the patient induced to dress *decently*.

"Pregnant women should never be allowed to witness any scene that will be likely, very powerfully to excite, alarm, or distress them—the evil influence of rash impres

* Sleeplessness.

sions is well established. Even the more exciting pleasures of life, they should partake of sparingly, as balls, parties, theatrica exhibitions, &c."

While thus showing the physical causes and external circumstances which affect the health of pregnant women, we must not overlook the moral causes of evil to which this condition is peculiarly susceptible. During the first months of gestation, and immediately after parturition, (owing in the latter case to the severe depletion of the vascular system,) the nervous temperament predominates, and the mind is thus rendered susceptible in the highest degree to impressions from moral causes. An unkind word, a cold or severe look, or even apparent neglect, will frequently, in this state of health, derange the whole physical system, prostrate the most promising state of convalescence, and set medical skill at defiance. Nor does the evil end here. A deep sense of injury and wrong is engendered, and the hitherto sweet sources of domestic happiness, affection and confidence, are embittered for life. If, however, in this morbid condition of the system, unkindness and neglect are more keenly felt, so, also, the kind offices of affection are doubly appreciated.

The injurious effects of moral impressions on the health, are thus forcibly described by Dr. James Johnson:

"The moral impressions on the brain and nerves are infinitely more injurious than the physical impressions ot food and drink, however improper, on the stomach. The multifarious relations of MAN with the world around him, in the present era of social life, are such as must inevitably keep up a constant source of perturbation, if not irritation; and this trouble of mind is not solely, or even chiefly, expended on the organ of the mind, viz: the brain, and its appendages, the nerves, but upon the organs of the body most intimately connected with the brain—namely, the DIGESTIVE ORGANS, including the stomach, liver, and bowels.

"Let us exemplify this. A man receives a letter communicating a piece of astounding intelligence—great loss of property, or death of a child, wife, or parent. The mind, the brain, the nervous system, are all agitated and disturbed. But the evil does not rest here. The organs not immediately under the will, or directly connected with the intellectual portion of our frame—the organs of digestion, circulation, nutrition, &c., are all consequently disturbed, and their functions disordered; the tongue turns white, the appetite fails, and the complexion grows sallow. These corporeal maladies are those which naturally attract most the sufferer's attention. He seldom comprehends, or even suspects, the nature and agency of the MORAL cause. He flies to physic; and it may very easily be conceived that he generally flies to it in vain!"

The following letter from Mrs. P. S. Wright was not received in time for the work for which it was intended; but as the facts and observations apply equally to the present work, the writer takes the liberty of giving it entire; although perfectly aware that some of the opinions, being in advance of the age, may prove unpopular:

JULY 3, 1844.

DEAR MADAM: It was with sincere pleasure that I learned from yourself that you were to republish and enlarge your valuable work, on the transmission of parental qualities. That the circulation of that work should be greatly extended is my sincere desire, and in compliance with your request, I send you a few facts which have come within the range of my own observation.

That the subject of which your work treats is one of immense importance to the rising generation, no one can dispute; but that the child takes more in its mental constitution and temperament of the father than the mother, I am somewhat inclined to think. That the physical constitution is derived or controlled almost exclusively by the mother, appears to me self-evident.

Physiologists reason from analogy; and the facts established with regard to some animals, such as in their physical organization most resemble man, may be considered as finger-marks pointing to some similar law which governs the human family. Combe (I think it is, although I have not the author here to refer to) says that in the generation of the horse, in order to produce vigorous and sprightly offspring, the sire should be actively exercised. Hence we may properly reason, that if a father is dull, heavy, and stupid habitually, or even at the time of generation, the child will partake of his mental temperament to a greater or less degree. I will here cite one or two facts in elucidation of my position. A mother of my acquaintance, now somewhat advanced in years, gave me the following relation:

"I was," said she, "married at the age of twenty-five, inheriting from both my parents a most vigorous constitution. My husband was four years my senior, and alike blessed with most perfect health. But we started wrong after all, for we both determined to be rich, let what would come. We occupied a large farm, and I, in my eagerness to amass wealth, which has been as a canker to my happiness, would never employ help for a day, frequently doing all the labor for a family of twenty during the period of gestation. My first children were twins. My living at the time was what is commonly called the plain living of farmers, but what I now consider as much too luxurious for health.

"Previous to my accouchement a cutaneous eruption appeared on my face, neck, and hands, together with swelling of the joints. This I looked upon as the effect of heat, which would soon pass off; but what was my disappointment, at the birth of my babes, to have presented to me two emaciated little beings, covered with the same eruption, which proved to be scrofula induced by heating my blood with wrong living. I had most ardently desired children, and my love of riches gave way to my maternal feelings; but in less than four months both the little sufferers were carried to their resting-place. I regarded myself as stricken of God; I sought to submit to my trying fate as a Christian, for I did not regard myself as having had anything to do with my affliction. A third, fourth, and fifth child followed, diseased in the same way, and only lingered for a short period. At length my desires were gratified in everything except living children. I wept and prayed much for a child that might bless our old age.

At length the illness of a beloved parent called me to a different scene, and during almost the entire period of pregnancy with my sixth child, I was occupied in her care. Being no longer actively engaged, having scarcely sufficient exercise for my health, my mind turned naturally to investigating the causes that had co-operated to produce such painful results, if causes there were. Does God, I asked, arbitrarily punish us in this world for infringements of his moral law? if so, of what use is the atonement or death of Christ? Then first dawned upon my mind the belief that there were natural as well as moral laws given to govern us, and that an infringement of them would be followed by a just punishment. The period of parturition arrived. Conceive, if you can, the joy and gratitude of my heart to find myself the mother of a fair and beautiful boy, which still lives to bless and comfort me; but although he lives, and the three daughters which followed him, yet they too partake of the feeble constitution which I have entailed upon them, for my own health had become greatly impaired during my struggle after riches."

I will here give my own observations of the family in question. The mother was a woman of fine mental and moral organization, with the exception of her large acquisitiveness, and of an active nervous temperament. Her superior mental endowments are proven by her having thought so correctly, more than twenty years since. The father had retained his fine natural constitution, but he was an exceeding dull heavy man of the lymphatic temperament. The children, particularly the daughters, were much like the father in mind, and it was often remarked, that were it not for the broad fields, and accumulating interest money, they would be a very dull family.

Another illustration proving the almost unlimited control of a mother over the physical organization of her child, I will here cite : Mrs. B. a lady moving in a fashionable circle in one of our large cities, possessing a fine natural constitution and good mental organization, became *enciente* soon after marriage. Wishing to enjoy society as long as possible, she habitually laced herself so tight as to conceal her situation for six or seven months.

Her three first children were sickly and weak, weighing not more than three or four pounds at birth. In the first period of gestation with her fourth child, an accident occurred which prevented her desiring to enter society, consequently her corsets were abandoned, and as she was cut off from the brilliant festivities of the winter, she resorted to reading. I should have mentioned that she had suffered exceedingly in parturition. Her husband, a man of excellent sense, placed in her hands physiological works, and she, seeing her gross neglects of duty, resolved to fit herself for the high sphere of a mother. She followed the light as she received it, and the result was a great diminution of suffering in giving birth to a fine boy, weighing nine pounds.

She often remarks that it would be less trouble to train half a dozen such than one like her first children. Oh, said she, (for she had the tender feelings of a mother) I have done to those little ones, an injury that a whole life can never repair! * * * That the world is to be regenerated, physically, mentally, morally, is a theory that has ever appeared most delightful to my mind; not that I have ever expected any miracles wrought to bring it about, but that it would be done by natural means, and that the investigation of subjects treated of in this work are to do much towards accomplishing this object, I have not a doubt.

But there is one exceedingly delicate point which, in the first edition, is not alluded to, and as it has so strong an influence upon the purity of unborn generations, I feel myself constrained to give it least a passing notice:

The father can have no influence directly over the fœtus after its formation; it is then the mother's exclusive prerogative to nourish and cherish the being she carries. What character then, should the father desire to fix upon his child? Should it be that of gross licentiousness? Nay! Then let the father as well as the mother be pure-hearted. Let both utterly repudiate the almost unlimited married licentiousness that now prevails. Let them never come together, but for the great purpose for which marriage was at first instituted.

Let these principles be adopted and carried out, together with a course of living, and the great work of purifying the world is accomplished. Hitherto reformers have been dabbling with effects, while the great cause or causes have been left untouched. In proof of the last principle advanced, let me cite a case just in point:

J. P. finished early his college course, and with a rapidity surpassing even the most sanguine hopes of nis friends, acquired the profession of law. The evening that he was admitted to the bar saw him the husband of a lovely and pure-hearted woman. He rose in his profession with a rapidity unequalled, but his wife drooped in spirits and health, her happiness had been evanescent as the dew, for she had too late learned that her husband, like his father, was a profligate, licentious man. A few months previous to the birth of their son he had abandoned the young and tender wife. That son, at the age of nineteen, when I first knew him, was the most briliant young man in mind, the most noble in form and feature of any person I had ever known, but he was pursuing a reckless licentious course, and was self-indulgent in all his appetites, to a degree almost unparalleled. This child was trained, with the exception of proper physical training, (and that was the great point which ruined him) with great care. Often after receiving a letter from his mother, in which she gave excellent advice, and much religious council and exhortation, have I known him to shut himself up for days, and fast and pray, and weep like an infant over his transgressions. I have heard him make the most solemn promises before God of entire reformation. Again and again, I have seen this strong man bowed for days to the very earth under a sense of his transgressions.

But when he went forth it was to eat and drink, and again to go out and commit the same sins, perhaps to a more fearful extent.

Now, did not that father stamp his character upon his child most perfectly. The mother was a noble, highly-gifted woman, but the baser passions of the father were stronger than the moral ones of both. But had one-half of the study of the mother been directed to acquiring a knowledge of the laws of nature, she might have saved him much suffering; she might have given to his consti.

tution a shield that would have protected him from temptations to which he was exposed. For she would have taught him, that by living on a mild unstimulating diet, together with bathing, air, and exercise, those baser passions might be controlled, and brought into due subjection to his higher nature. But ignorantly she fed the volcanic fires in him, which in after life she vainly sought to quench.

She loved, when her fair boy came home from school, to have something prepared to please and pamper his vitiated appetite. Thus she, like thousands of others, took the most sure means to prevent an answer to her daily, nay, almost hourly prayer, that God would keep pure her son. Would that parents, when they surrounded their luxurious boards, furnished with tea, coffee, flesh, meats, condiments, &c. and lift up their voices, and ask of God to bless that food to the strengthening of their bodies, and then rise with those bodies stimulated and unnaturally excited, and their spirits grovelling and fleshly, could but see their inconsistency. To a mind truly enlightened, such scenes are most revolting. It savors strongly of pagan idolatry. It is at least mocking God with lip-service, while the heart is so debased, low, and sensual, that the higher natures are dormant, their religion sensualism. Their God is like themselves.

I have no hope for the purifying of the world, but through those who have learned to look at these subjects in their true light.

Yours, with sincere respect,

P. S. W.

In the treatment of so important a subject as that of alleviating human suffering, it were inexcusable to overlook any system, however new or unpopular, which has in view this important object. Hydropathy, or the water cure, therefore, claims our particular attention.

This system, however, merits consideration not only on account of its inherent principles of truth and practical utility, but also on account of the high character and talent enlisted in its dissemination throughout Europe and our own country

The following cases, taken from the "Water-Cure Journal," show the favorable influence which this treatment exerts in pregnancy and child-bearing:

WATER-CURE IN CHILD-BEARING.

The following remarkable case might by many be reckoned as one forming an exception to the general rule, as to what would be the general result under similar circumstances. In reality, striking as the case is, it is only an exemplification of what has frequently been proved, that it is possible for women of ordinary health so to live that childbirth and the period of pregnancy can be rendered comparatively free from pain and suffering.

A lady of this city, whose name from motives of delicacy, we are not at liberty to mention, of 17 years of age, small form, with very good constitution, was lately with child, and passed through the whole period as follows: She took regularly a shower bath every morning, exercised every day, wet or dry, in the open air, and when by any means, the amount of exercise was considerably less than common, a quick bath was taken before dinner, and regularly a sponge or rubbing bath was used before going to rest. Sitz baths were taken daily and the body bandage worn much of the time. No permanent chill was allowed to take place. The evening sitz bath seemed to have a decided effect in causing sound rest. The bowels were kept free by clysters of cold water whenever these were necessary. Very plain vegetable and farinaceous food and fruits constituted the sole diet. The meals were light, and for three months previous to confinement, the supper was always omitted, so that only two light meals were taken daily and no food between times. Drinking of water is a powerful means to reduce the inordinate craving appetite with which many are afflicted in childbearing. In the case of this lady no other drink than pure soft Croton water was taken during the whole time.

As the expected time drew near, one morning while in the sitting bath labor commenced. The pains were prompt, and in about twenty minutes a fine healthy child was born. In about ten minutes more the after-birth came away, followed with but little flowing of blood. The patient was allowed to rest a short time, after which the body was sponged over and quickly made dry and comfortable. Wet cloths were laid upon the breasts to prevent inflammation or undue swelling of the parts. A wet bandage was also placed about the abdomen covered with a dry one, so as to be of comfortable temperature. The sponging, rubbing and bandages were the means of reducing the feverish excitement caused by labor, and of soothing the body in a remarkable degree, so that sweet and quiet sleep soon followed. On the third day, water having been used as the case seemed to require in the mean time, the woman walked in the open air without injury, but on the contrary with benefit. Daily exercise, however, was previously taken, in the sick room, which was at all times kept well aired.

In this remarkable case there was not a single scar left upon the body, it being the first child, and the amount of suffering was by far less than is often experienced in mere menstruation, by women who do not bathe regularly and adopt a generally correct hygenic course. Physiology cally as well as morally, "wisdom's ways are ways of pleasantness," and happy is that mother who understands Nature's laws, and who has in them a confidence sufficient to live accordingly.

It may be objected in reference to the above case, that it would be unsafe for most females to attempt to carry out a similar course to the one described. This is not true. Every individual, old or young, sick or well, and of either sex, should have at least, a daily bath. Who would think of leaving for a single day the face and hands unwashed? Those who have adopted daily bathing, know well the comfort and advantages arising from it. Nor is a rigid vegetable, farinaceous and fruit diet, as was used in the above case, a dangerous one as many suppose. On the contrary, such a diet judiciously selected, is highly conducive to bodily vigor and comfort, and renders one in all cases far less liable to disease of every kind. All who will in every respect take a judicious course, similar to the one described, will, as certainly as the sun shines, render their sufferings in child-bearing very much less than by any other possible means that can be adopted, and in most cases, so great will be the benefit derived that, comparatively speaking, child-bearing will be unattended with suffering—be without pain.

The condition of the child in this case, was not less remarkable than that of the mother. It was healthy and vigorous, and as a natural result was far less liable to disease than children generally are. It is not at all natural for one-half of the race to die under five years of age. If mothers and children were universally managed as in the case above, mortality of infants and children would be comparatively unknown.

CHILD-BEARING.

"Of no one thing relating to physiology and medical treatment, have those particularly interested, been so ignorant as that indicated in the above caption. Woman may study and know all the fashions and frivolities of the day, and the art of perverting everything furnished us for daily sustenance, by the All Good; but to know *why* and wherefore she suffers sorrow and pain and anguish, and often death, in the advent of a new being upon our earth, is not to be thought of by any but a *man* making a *profession* of physiological knowledge, which the Indian woman of the forest would cause him to blush and hang his head in shame for. Every woman ought to know enough of the laws of her own physical being and of generation, to avoid and prevent the cause of the evils so generally attendant upon child-bearing. And to show that it is possible to avoid these evils, just to the extent that she conforms to the physiological law of purity and health, I will give you a fact.

"Mrs. ——, about eight years since, had her attention directed to the subject of physiological truth and reform, and from that time has followed a generally correct course with regard to diet and general regimen. During this time she has bathed daily. Becoming with child the past year, she continued daily bathing the whole period of gestation to the day of her confinement; and the result was most happy. That which is to most women an hour of unutterable torture, was passed by her with comparatively no pain or suffering. Her husband's knowledge of anatomy and physiology was all-sufficient, and the presence of a physician was not required; neither were all the *old ladies* in the house and neighborhood called in to embarrass the patient with their presence and officious interference. It being early in the morning, no one in the house was aroused or disturbed, and quietude in the room, with no one present but the husband, proved very favorable. Instead of castor oil or drugs, cold water was the only thing given to mother and child, and both were thoroughly bathed in tepid water. The mother was not *confined* to her bed even a whole day, and on the second day arose and bathed herself. In less than two weeks from the birth of the child, the mother and infant rode thirty-six miles; and in three weeks went a journey of four hundred miles, with no inconvenience. As the mother did not inherit constitutional health adapted to produce so favorable a result, what but a strict regard to bathing and conformity to the physiological law in diet and dress could have produced such a result? She has lived for the last eight years on a farinaceous and fruit diet exclusively, abjuring tea, coffee and flesh-meat. And she is confident that the use of water as a beverage exclusively, and daily bathing, were the most efficient means used. Its soothing and invigorating power, after confinement, was very great."

INFLAMMATION AND SWELLING OF BREASTS.

"On the evening of the third day after my wife's first accouchement, I came home from Guy's Hospital, where I had been detained since morning, and found her groaning and weeping with intense pain, the breasts red and enormously enlarged, which the frightened nurse was vehemently rubbing with brandy and oil. The skin was excessively hot and dry, and the pulse was leaping along at the rate of 120. It was in the month of January—so I walked into the street with a pail, which I filled with snow, and bringing it into the sick room, I piled a heap of it over both breasts, continually adding fresh snow as it melted. In a very few minutes the milk spun out in streams, to the distance of more than a foot, and the tears of torture were at once changed for those of pleasure, accompanied by that hysterical sobbing, which is the common result of a sudden transition from intense suffering to perfect ease. The mere absence of pain in these cases takes all the characters of the most delicious and positive pleasurable sensations. In half an hour the inflamation had subsided, the breasts had become *comparatively* flaccid, the fever had entirely subsided, and not only all danger, but all inconvenience, had utterly vanished. But for this timely succor, suppuration must have supervened in both breasts, and large abscesses would have been the inevitable consequence."—Dr. Ed. Johnson.

Dr. Shew of this city informs the writer that he has never known of an instance in which this painful affection, swelling, or caking as it is called, of the breasts, could not be wholly prevented; that is, so that no troublesome effects of the kind would follow childbirth. Dr. Shew's mode is to direct females, some days before labor is expected, to make the application of wet bandages to the breasts, these cloths to be of a temperature suited to the feeling of comfort in the case, and to be applied as frequently and continuously as is necessary to keep down inflammation. He always in every case directs these bandages to be applied immediately after labor, whether there is any undue inflammation or not. To prevent evaporation, the bandages are to be covered with dry flannel. They not only have a soothing effect upon the breasts, and act to prevent inflammation, but aid also in causing a healthy and natural secretion of milk. In cases of sore nipples, it may at times, be necessary to use some mechanical means to shield the effected or painful parts, and perhaps some adhesive substance or plaster to keep the cracked surfaces in a favorable situation for healing; yet nothing is so good for healing as pure clean water rightly applied; and in any case where the cracked parts naturally remain in a good situation for becoming healed, and are not subject by motion to have the cracked surfaces re-exposed to the atmosphere, clean wet cloths are alone sufficient, and also the best.

To prevent that extreme and troublesome nervousness with which child-bearing females are sometimes troubled, Dr. Shew recommends that wet bandages be worn frequently, and especially at night. He relates the following case: A lady of extremely irritable nerves, having unfortunately a variety of moral causes acting to increase that nervous irritability, as well as too much and irregular physical exertion while pregnant, found it exceedingly difficult to obtain anything like sound and refreshing sleep. A persistent nervous headache was also at times present. The lady had been in the daily habit of shower-bathing, but this headache had at one time become so severe, that the bathing increased it, as is sometimes the case in such instances. To prevent this severe headache, and to cause sleep, the patient was directed to have a heavy night-dress well wrung out of cold water, together with cold bandages applied to the head, and the body warmly wrapped in flannel blankets, with warm applications to the feet, as indicated by the feelings of comfort. In a very short time after being enveloped, she declared that the headache wholly left her, and, as is common in such applications, a sound night's rest was enjoyed. In the morning the shower-bath was taken as usual; and by wearing wet bandages over the whole body each night, well bound on with woollen shawls, the headache and nervousness were prevented, notwithstanding the unfavorable causes mostly remained.

The daily shower-bath and sitting-bath are highly recommended in cases of pregnancy, as producing a most excellent effect. Clysters of water, either warm or cold, are also to be frequently taken, to keep up a natural action of the bowels. The following directions for their application are taken from "Dr. Shew's Water-Cure."

CLYSTERS.

"Cold or tepid water injections constitute an important part of the treatment of pregnancy. The bowels can at any time be easily kept free, and the evils and unpleasantness of constipation thus be at once removed. This application is also of great service in all bowel complaints. Severe diarrhœa, dysentery, cholera morbus and cholic, can often be speedily arrested by this application alone. In inflammation of the bowels it is of most signal benefit. The author has, in different instances, given immediate relief in this disease, when the bowels had been for days obstinately closed, resisting the action of the most powerful medicines.

"This application should be made with an instrument, by which no air will be introduced into the parts. Air often causes pain. It should always be carefully expelled by pouring the water through the instrument a few times before it is inserted.

" The quantity of water to be used will vary. As much as can be retained, be it more or less, can be taken. The temperature is to be made according to the feelings of comfort, never too warm or too cold. Many take cold water.

" Some have a prejudice against this application, thinking that it will weaken the bowels like cathartic medicine or cathartic clysters, but this is not true. Pure water, rightly used in this way, strengthens. When constipation proceeds from too great a degree of internal heat, cold water injections are the safest and most efficient remedy."

SITTING BATH.

" Pregnant women receive much benefit from a constant use of this bath. A small tub of sufficient size, set upon a very low stool, or anything by which it may be raised a few inches, is quite sufficient. Unpainted wood is the best material, metal being unpleasant and cold. The water is used from one to five or six inches deep. The length of time this bath is used, varies from a few minutes to two hours or more. To avoid exposure to cold, it is best to uncover only the part of the person to be exposed to the water. This bath is to Priestnitz of so much importance, that it is prescribed to nearly or quite every patient. It has the effect of strengthening the nerves, of drawing the blood and humors from the head, chest, and abdomen, and of relieving pain and flatulency, and is of the utmost value to those of sedentary habits. It is sometimes well to take a foot bath, tepid or cold, at the same time. If a large quantity of cold water were used in this bath, it would remain cold too long, and thus drive the blood to the head and upper parts of the body, which might be very injurious; but the small quantity of water used at once becomes warm, and thus admits of speedy re-action. In some local diseases of the lower parts, where there is inflammation, and the cold water feels most agreeable, the water is frequently changed. If there is any inclination to head-ache, or too much heat in the head, a cold bandage upon the forehead or temples is good. It is often well to rub the abdomen briskly during this bath.

"The sitz bath may be used by any person, whether in health or otherwise, without the slightest fear of taking cold. Let those subject to giddiness, head-aches, or congestion of blood in the upper regions, try this, and they will at once perceive its utility."

In endeavoring to unfold useful truths in the language of reason, the writer has felt no apprehension of offending the natural delicacy of any well constituted mind. Actuated, also, by a deep sense of the misery arising from the prevailing ignorance on this subject, she has not permitted any false notions of delicacy to prevent her from directing attention to the calm and deliberate examination of the bearing which the present ignorance has on the health and happiness of the sex.

The reader who has followed the writer thus far, will have become convinced, not only from the opinions and high authority of the medical writers quoted, but also from the facts and arguments which have been aduced, that no truth is more apparent than this: *That the degree of suffering and danger at the period of parturition is entirely dependent on the previous mode of life and habits of the mother;* and also, that the sound or defective constitution transmitted to her offspring will be the result of her attention or inattention to the laws of health during the period of gestation.

When habits of indolence and luxury have been indulged in, the appetite pampered to excess, and as a natural consequence, the vascular system overcharged, to the imminent danger of convulsions, or congestion of the brain—it is vain for the imprudent sufferer to call in the aid of science; it is *then* too late to avert the fatal errors of ignorance or self-indulgence. No human power can save both mother and child!

The necessity for the use of the numerous instruments of torture and death, so common in the practice of Midwifery, has arisen in a great measure from the habits referred to in the preceding paragraph. Yet we might hope that every woman possessing the common feelings of humanity, would inform herself of, and avoid the causes which lead to the necessity of using implements so destructive to infant life. A knowledge of the well-known expedients resorted to in such cases of extremity—as the breaking up of the infant skull, or the dismembering of its tender limbs while quivering with life, should arm every mother with sufficient resolution to practice self-denial to any extent, in view of averting such fearful consequences, and preserving the life of her child.

It is deeply painful to reflect upon the amount of infant life sacrificed in such cases; more particularly when we consider in which class of society it generally occurs. Not in that of the indigent, uneducated, and laborious; on the contrary, in that of the educated, refined, and affluent, who, with these advantages, possess the power of transmitting an improved organization to their offspring, and thereby promoting an evident design of the Creator—the progress and improvement of the race. A subject not yielding in interest and importance to any to which the human mind can be directed.

Fortunately, this opinion is not new; nor is it limited as respects the number and intelligence of those who entertain it. That it is taking deep root in the public mind, with the most gratifying rapidity, and promises to be productive of invaluable fruit, appears from an abundance of concurrent testimony, not only in the writings of our own talented and philanthropic countryman, Dr. Caldwell, but also in those of George and Andrew Combe; and, in fact, all the observing and inquiring minds of the present age, whose attention has been directed to the subject.

The following case is from the Water-Cure Manual:

Possibly some may doubt the propriety of giving cases of the following kind in a popular work. Do we not all buy our Bibles, circulate them among all readers, and make them tokens of friendship to those we hold most dear on earth? And yet, with all its allusions to delicate subjects, who would think of objecting to the Bible on this account? "To the pure, all things are pure;" so, also, to the impure are all things impure. There is, then, no need of an apology for introducing matters of this kind.

Out of numbers of cases of the most marvellous kind, I select here only one. I will take the liberty, however, of referring the reader who may be interested, to a work now in preparation by myself, designed more especially for the perusal and study of females, on the water treatment, as applicable in pregnancy, childbirth, and the rearing of infants and children. A work of this kind is, I believe, needed not less than any other at the present day. Water-cure is destined yet to accomplish untold, unheard-of wonders, in childbirth, and the rearing of children.

Case of Mrs. Shew.—On the 16th of September, 1845, Mrs. Shew gave birth, under peculiar circumstances, to a child. Her ancestry on both sides are consumptive, so that she inherits a strong predisposition to that disease, and has, in fact, for years had much to contend with, in reference to the condition of the chest. Pleurisies, inflammation of the lungs, cough, and hemorrhages, she had at different times, and is constantly liable to affections of this kind. She is likewise naturally of very delicate frame and extreme nervous sensibility, and it has been only by exercising great care in everything that pertains to health, that she has now for a number of years, with two or three exceptions, kept free from the outbreaks of disease, and has enjoyed, what would ordinarily be termed, good health.

The summer of 1845, it will be recollected, was very tedious and hot. The whole season the drought was severe, and there was scarcely a single shower to refresh the earth. It was, therefore, very depressing to the health. However, by daily bathing and being much in the shade in the open air, wearing usually a part of each day the wet girdle, to refresh the system, using the cooling hip bath and injections now and then, as occasion required, and partaking lightly of food but twice a day, Mrs. S. passed through the summer remarkably well; but more than once during the season, certain things transpired that were very much against the quietude, peace of mind, and mental repose so necessary in the condition she was then in.

At length her expected time drew near. By the exercise of great prudence and care, she was enabled, up to the very last, to discharge the ordinary duties of overseeing the household affairs of her family, and to walk and ride daily and frequently for exercise, or as business called, in the open air.

I must here mention, that one of my respected preceptors in medicine, and a man who is scarcely second to any other in his thorough acquaintance with medical lore, gave it as his decided opinion, that from the extreme smallness of the pelvis, Mrs. Shew could never give birth to a full-formed living child. The expedient of causing premature birth, or the still more horrible one, of destroying the child, seemed to him inevitable, either of which Mrs. S. could not for an instant listen to. That the labor must be exceedingly severe, was evident enough to all. But she was resolved to let nature take her own course, whatever it might be.

Labor came on at evening, of the 15th of September, the weather being yet hot and sultry. Mrs. S. would not listen to the proposal to have medical aid besides myself; nor would she consent to have any nurse or female attendant of any kind. Ordinary servants only were to bring water, and do whatever of like service was necessary.

The labor-pains went on, becoming exceedingly severe, and continued until three o'clock in the morning, at which time she gave birth to a large, healthy, and well-formed female child. Almost immediately the after-birth was expelled, followed by most frightful flooding. The night was, I confess, a long, dark, and dismal one to me. There was, I knew, in my wife's system, and always had been, as well as in her family, a strong tendency to hemorrhages. I understood perfectly well the different modes resorted to in these dangerous extremes. Cold applications are, the world over, the means relied upon. As to the mode of applying the cold, I had resolved, in this case, to take a different course from any I had ever heard of. I had procured a large hip bath, with a good back, in which a person could be placed in a sort of half-reclining position, with the head supported upon pillows. Instead of applying the cold water by the stream from a pitcher, by wet cloths, and the like, I had resolved, that if flooding came on, I would take Mrs. S. in my arms, and instantly place her in this hip bath; and thus, as I believed, I could more quickly chill the whole of the pelvic viscera, than by any other means. Be it remembered, that wherever there is hemorrhage, whether from the lungs, stomach, bowels or womb, there is great heat in and about the part from which the blood issues; and the quicker and more effectually this heat can be abstracted and the parts chilled, the more certain are we to arrest the flow, by the constringing effect of cold upon the open vessels. As for the *shock* of the douche, or pouring of water from a height, so much in vogue, I believe that, so far as the shock is concerned, it is better avoided. If I am not mistaken, *that* only tends to keep up the flooding. The cooling should be passive, and not violent.

Having everything in readiness, I took Mrs. S. in my arms, and before she had time to faint entirely, I placed her in this hip bath of cold water. The water covered from near the knees over the whole abdomen, and no sooner had these parts come in contact with the water, than it seemed, as if by magic, the flooding ceased The water revived her, and in a few minutes before she had become much chilled, I raised her carefully and laid her in bed, put wet cloths about the abdomen, and wrapped her warmly in blankets. The feet were cold, as they generally are in severe hemorrhage. These parts, and from the knees down, I rubbed briskly, with the warm hand, to restore the natural warmth. I kept good watch that she should not become too warm, as in that case flooding would be apt to return. It was not long before Mrs. S. fell into a sound sleep, in which she rested for some time.

I have regretted much that I did not, at the time, write down notes of this case ; that is, of the remaining part of the treatment to be spoken of. From the severity of the labor and the loss of a large amount of blood, Mrs. S. said she felt a greater degree of weakness than she had ever before experienced, a sense of sinking of the vital powers, and an oppression at the heart, with which she was before wholly unacquainted. The sleep I have spoken of did her much good, and was, of all things, the most desirable. Still, she was very weak, and after-pains set in, growing more and more severe. Her *system being so highly sensitive, I expected this, and resolved* upon the use of the hip bath. I would here remark, that the objection that would be raised by almost any practitioner to this procedure, here as well as in the flooding before spoken of, would be, that the position, the raising up a person in this weak state, and placing the trunk of the body in an upright position, would be likely to cause a return of the flooding. This objection, I admit, would have great weight, were it not for the fact that the water acts so powerfully to check that symptom Still, there is nothing like the danger feared, even without the use of the water, that there is supposed to be. And persons are found everywhere, in fact, it is almost a universal thing in childbirth, that females are required to lie, day after day, in too warm beds, thus debilitating the body by the heat caused by the fatigue of remaining much in one position, and by the unnatural position of the brain. Females thus become debilitated, nervous, restless, and are kept back day after day, and often for weeks, and all for the want of what may well be called good nursing; and then in this debilitated state, when they do begin to get about after the ninth day, as superstition has it, the opposite extreme is practiced; too much is done at once, a cold is taken, inflammation of the breasts occurs, or falling of the womb takes place, or perhaps a powerful hemorrhage. I repeat, that in my practice, as a rule to which there can seldom be any exception, my patients of this kind sit up, even if it be but one or five minutes at a time, the first day of the confinement and onward. This sitting up to *rest* the patient, that is, to rest from the fatigue of the lying position, is one of the best means that can be adopted. The bed is at the same time aired and becomes cool, so that when she returns to it, the change back again is salutary, and the reclining position becomes one of rest. The patient should be taught not to overdo in this matter, for every good thing has its abuse as well as use. I had now, in Mrs. Shew's case, a good opportunity to test fully the powers of water and good nursing. There were in her mind no prejudices to overcome—no lack of confidence, no superstitious, yet good-meaning, old women about us, to whisper their fears and prognosticate evil. There was nothing in the way, and what was better than all the rest, Mrs. S. had herself a good knowledge of the principles that should guide us in the management of such cases.

After Mrs. Shew had slept, as before mentioned, and the after-pains had commenced, I administered the hip-bath. These pains, as well as hemorrhages, are attended with internal heat; but, as regarded the general system, Mrs. S. had now a feeling of dread of *cold* water. The objects in view in the use of the hip bath and frictions, were to lull the pain, and to invigorate the system by the tonic effect of the water and friction. I laid a folded blanket in the bottom of the bath, in which was put a small quantity of tepid water, of such temperature as would produce no unpleasant sensation. Blankets were also used to wrap about the feet and limbs, and the whole surface, except the parts exposed to the water. Reaching my hand under these blankets, I commenced rubbing the spine, abdomen, and other parts; and as the surface became accustomed to the water, I dipped the hand into that which was of a little lower temperature, and at length lowered the temperature of the water in a bath gradually, by adding to it cold water. In a short time the pains ceased. The bath was continued some fifteen or twenty minutes, possibly a little longer, and then Mrs. S. was placed comfortably in bed. It was indeed truly wonderful to behold the change produced by this bath. Besides the removal of all pain, it seemed as if the strength was increased ten-fold, all in the space of less than half an hour.

The after-pains returned frequently during the day, and as frequently they were combated with the hip bath and frictions. At least as many as ten times, and I think more, through the day and evening, I administered these baths, every one of which appeared to do an astonishing amount of good. Besides the removing of after-pains and the tonic effect of the baths, there was another palpable one: at times, sharp, cutting pains were experienced in the bowels, caused by flatulency. The bath removed them like a charm. The urine was found to pass freely, in consequence of the bathing and drinking; and the soreness so much felt in these cases was all removed.

As Mrs. S. grew stronger, the water was used somewhat colder, but all the time of moderate temperature. She slept very well during the night, having little or no more of the after-pains. In the evening, she sat up, bore her weight, and walked a little about the room.

In consequence of more than usual fatigue, I did not awake the next morning until between six and seven o'clock. I confess I was not a little surprised, on awaking, that Mrs. Shew had left the room. This was only twenty-six hours from the birth; and she had taken her child in her arms, and gone down to the kitchen. She felt that she was perfectly able to do this, and acted accordingly, on her own responsibility. She was, however, very careful this day; took but little nourishment; and in three days time, we moved to the large house, 56 Bond street, Mrs. S. walking up and down stairs numbers of times during the day, overseeing things as they were moved and so every day onward. Bathing was kept up as usual, daily, and she partook now, as was her usual habit, of the plainest food, and but twice per day, using no other animal food, except a trifling quantity of milk, and no other drink except pure water.

The second day after the birth of our child, a worthy old gentleman, one of our patients, from New England, called upon us. He inquired, kindly, respecting Mrs. S.'s health, he having seen her much in the summer, and in a few minutes she met him in the parlor. He raised his hands, and, in astonishment, exclaimed, "This is indeed bringing things back to nature!"

In conversation with one of the first medical men of our city, or of the world, I described this case of Mrs. Shew's, and also others of like results. He said that he could not conceive it possible for a woman to get up and go about, with any thing like safety, in twenty-four, or even forty-eight, hours after childbirth. I admit, that as a rule, women could not, under ordinary modes of treatment; but, at the same time, asked him how it was that the Indian women were so little troubled with these matters. I then said, our patients practice bathing daily bathing continually; drink no tea or coffee, to weaken the powers of digestion, constipate the bowels, destroy the relish for food, shatter the nervous system, and impair the soundness of natural and refreshing sleep; their modes of dress do not distort and debilitate their frames, and, instead of remaining mostly within doors, according to the foolish customs of civil life, they go regularly and often in the open air, thus gaining strength upon strength, by means of these natural and powerful tonics, exercise, pure air, and light. He admitted that such modes persevered in, must produce powerful effects of some kind, and added, that he intended always to sustain good health by means of the shower bath, the daily use of which he had adopted with the greatest benefit.

I hold that, strong and enduring as are the Indian women, the generality of females of the present generation even, may, if they commence in early life, become more hardy and strong than are those daughters of the forest, whose habits are, in many respects, unnatural and detrimental to health. But all this requires an amount of knowledge that few yet possess.

I could add numbers of cases of childbirth scarcely less

striking than that of Mrs. Shew; and if the reader has any doubts of the authenticity of such narrations, I ask him to take the names and residences of my patients, and hear their stories for himself. Persons who have experienced the invaluable, untold, and apparently miraculous effects of cold water, will not hesitate to make known the blessing of the new system.

Before closing this little volume, the writer is impelled by a sense of duty to add a few remarks on a subject of the highest importance, both in a moral and physical point of view, to the well-being of society. The practice of procuring abortion, or, to use a less offensive expression, inducing a miscarriage, has of late become so common, that it requires to be placed before the public in all its naked atrocity. From the increasing number of unprincipled persons who publicly advertise this destructive practice, it is evident that it is extending to a fearful degree throughout our country: some knowledge, therefore of the dreadful consequences attending such utter violations of nature's laws, may be useful. That the act of procuring abortion is a crime of the deepest dye, on a par with that of murder, no argument can controvert; nor can any, except the weak-minded or the vicious, be persuaded to the contrary. Is it possible that any woman of sane mind can look upon her living child, and admit for a moment that it would be a greater crime to deprive it of life by violent means then, than it would have been while in a state of embryo? Many early married, unreflecting females, to avoid the cares and responsibilities of a large family, allow themselves to be deluded by the miserable sophistry, that there is no harm, previous to quickening, in taking the most deadly drugs, or in making use of the most violent means to procure abortion. Let them not, however, thus deceive themselves, for whatever apparent success may, for a time, attend these atrocious practices, retribution is sure to follow such gross violations of nature's laws. The moral and physical institutions of a wise and just Creator cannot be thus outraged with impunity—effect follows cause as unceasingly here as in any other department of organic life.

Scarcely any misfortune to which humanity is liable, is more to be dreaded than a natural tendency to miscarriage. How often has it been the bane of an otherwise happy existence? Its uniform evil effect, upon the general health of the sufferer, is well-known and admitted: and yet, strange perversity, an incredible number of females, in all ranks and conditions of life, are found, who in their pitiable ignorance are willing, often for slight personal considerations, to risk a constant liability to this constitutional evil, and thereby commit, in an indirect manner, the crime of self-murder. Among several cases fresh in the memory of the writer is that of Mrs. W——, a woman highly respected for her piety, and in some respects good sense, having borne four healthy children, and thereby acquired a priceless treasure. Some plausible demon incited her to the use of these unhallowed means, to avoid, in the cant phrase of the day, a too numerous family. After five years of success, she is now a helpless ruin, totally prostrated in her nervous system, and entirely blind. And again, these days of modern refinement have given rise to another baneful practice. The newly-married, youthful couple, must for a season enjoy the butterfly-life of gayety proper to their condition in the present improved scale of existence, to do which, it is absolutely necessary to avoid the inconvenience and cares of offspring. This can only be accomplished by encouraging—harmlessly and for the present only, mind you—a miscarriage, forgetting that this outrage upon nature can only be inflicted by incurring the heavy liability to the mother of permanent and irreparable injury, or perhaps laying the train for a premature death.

Thus it is with the family of R.—or, more properly speaking, thus it is with that lonely, unhappy, because childless couple, who, in their early marriage day, long years ago, threw away, like the unbelieving Jew, the pearls that would have enriched his tribe.

"In England," lately remarked a native of that country, "every mother feels proud of having reared a large family of healthy, joyous children—ten or fifteen being no unusual number. While the American mothers, I observe, generally have small families, particularly in the higher classes of society." An old and experienced physician present significantly referred the speaker to the advertisements of professed female physicians, remarking, that these fiends in human form escaped unwhipped of justice, because the patronage they received enabled them, when prosecuted, to employ the best legal defence in the country; and that their practice being principally confined to the wealthy portion of the community, many a dark deed of iniquity has been concealed—the patients in such cases preferring any amount of suffering, or even death, to the public exposure which must ensue in bringing the criminal to justice.

In a subsequent conversation, this physician stated to the writer, that many distressing cases of this kind had fallen under his observation—cases in which it was clear to the experienced eye of the physician, that the patient had most ignorantly tampered with her constitution, interfered with, and interrupted the natural functions of her system. For after giving birth, at regular intervals, to healthy children, the young and vigorous mother suddenly becomes sterile. Years pass, during which frequent indispositions occur, leaving behind them a constitution strangely shattered, and a nervous system in ruins. The misguided sufferer at length perceives the dreadful results of her practices, and desists—pregnancy ensues, but the whole term of gestation is one of painful debility, and at its close, in the effort for relief, outraged nature denies the necessary energy: the patient sinks to the tomb, another victim to the Moloch of selfishness, leaving a family of young children motherless, to grow up in ignorance and tread the same path of error which led to her destruction.

Oh, Justice! where is thy whip of scorpions to lash the vile Charlatan, who thus makes a trade of death, naked through the world?

The very painful and dangerous consequences which attended an unsuccessful attempt at abortion, is thus given by an eminent practitioner of this city:

"*December* 19*th*, 1843.—Drs. Vermeule and Holden requested me to meet them in consultation, in the case of Mrs. M——, who had been in labor for twenty-four hours. On arriving at the house I learned the following particulars from the medical gentlemen:

"Mrs. M—— was the mother of two children, and had been suffering severely, for the last fourteen hours, from strong expulsive pains, which, however, had not caused the slightest progress in the delivery. I was likewise informed that, about four hours before I saw the case, Dr. Miner, an experienced physician, had been sent for, and, after instituting a vaginal examination, remarked to the attending physicians, that, "in all his practice, he had never met with a similar case." Dr. Miner suggested the administration of an anodyne, and, having other professional engagements, left the house. Mrs. M—— was taken in labor Monday, Dec. 18th, at 7 o'clock, P. M., and on Sunday, at 7 o clock, P. M., I first saw her. Her pains were then almost constant, and such had been the severity of her suffering, that her cries for relief, as her medical attendants informed me, had attracted crowds of people about the door. As soon as I entered her room she exclaimed, "For God's sake, doctor, cut me open, or I shall die; I never can be delivered without you cut me open!" I was struck with this language, especially as I had already been informed that she had previously borne two children.

"At the request of the medical gentlemen, I proceeded to make an examination per vaginam, and I must confess that I was startled at what I discovered, expecting every instant, from the intensity of the contraction of the uterus, that this organ would be ruptured in some portion of its extent. I could distinctly feel a solid, resisting tumor, at the superior strait, through the walls of the uterus—*but I could detect no os tincæ.* In carrying my finger upward and backward towards the *cul de sac* of the vagina, I could trace two bridles, extending from this portion of the vagina to a point of the uterus which was quite rough and slightly elevated. This roughness was transverse in shape, but with all the caution and nicety of manipulation I could bring to bear, I found it impossible to detect any opening in the womb. In passing my finger, with great care, from the bridles to the rough surface, and exploring the condition of the parts with an anxious desire to afford the distressed patient prompt and effectual relief, I distinctly felt cicatrices, of which the rough surface was one. Here, then, was a condition of things produced by injury done to the soft parts at some previous period, resulting in the formation of cicatrices and bridles, and likewise in the *closure of the womb.* At this stage of the examination, I knew nothing of the previous history of the patient more than I have already stated, and the first question I addressed to her was this: Have you ever had any difficulty in your previous confinements? Have you ever been delivered with instruments? &c. She distinctly replied that her previous labors had been of short duration, and that she had never been delivered with instruments ; nor had she ever sustained any injury in consequence of her confinements. Dr. Vermeule informed me that this was literally true, for he had attended her on those occasions. This information somewhat puzzled me, for it was not in keeping with what any one might have conjectured, taking into view her actual condition, which was undoubtedly *the result of direct injury done to the parts.*

"I then suggested to Drs. Vermeule and Holden the propriety of questioning the patient still more closely, with the hope of eliciting something satisfactory as to the cause of her present difficulty ; repeating, at the same time, that it would be absolutely necessary to have recourse to an operation for the purpose of delivering her. On assuring her that she was in a most perilous situation, and, at the same time, promising that we would do all in our power to rescue her, she voluntarily made the following confession :

"'About six weeks after becoming pregnant, she called on one of these infamous female physicians, who, hearing her situation, gave her some powders, with directions for use; these powders, it appears, did not produce the desired effect. She returned again to this woman, and asked her if there were no other way to make her miscarry. 'Yes,' says this physician, '*I can probe you ; but I must have my price for this operation.*' 'What do you probe with?' '*A piece of Whalebone.*' 'Well,' observed the patient, 'I cannot afford to pay your price, and I will probe myself.' She returned home and used the whalebone several times, it produced considerable pain, followed by a discharge of blood. The whole secret was now disclosed. Injuries inflicted on the mouth of the womb, by other violent attempts, had resulted in the circumstances as detailed above. It was evident, from the nature of this poor woman's sufferings and the expulsive character of her pains, that prompt artificial delivery was indicated. As the result of the case was doubtful, and it was important to have the concurrent testimony of other medical gentlemen, and as it embodied great professional interest, I requested my friends, Drs. Detmold, Washington and Doane, to see it. They reached the house without delay, and, after examining minutely into all the facts, it was agreed that a bi-lateral section of the mouth of the womb should be made.

Accordingly, without loss of time, I performed the operation in the following manner: The patient was brought to the edge of the bed and placed upon her back. The index finger of my left hand was introduced into the vagina as far as the roughness, which I supposed to be the seat of the *os tincæ*. Then a probe-pointed bistoury, the blade of which had been previously covered with a band of linen to within about four lines of its extremity, was carried along my finger, until the point reached the rough surface. I succeeded in introducing the point of the instrument into a very slight opening which I found in the centre of this surface, and then made an incision of the left lateral portion of the mouth, and before withdrawing the bistoury, I made the same kind of incision on the right side. I then withdrew the instrument, and in about five minutes it was evident that the head of the child made progress. The mouth of the womb dilated almost immediately, and the contractions were of the most expulsive character. There seemed, however, to be some ground for apprehension that the mouth of the uterus would not yield with sufficient readiness, and I made an incision of the posterior lip, through its centre, extending the incision to within a line of the peritorial cavity. In ten minutes from this time, Mrs. M—— was delivered of a strong full-grown child, whose boisterous cries were heard with astonishment by the mother, and with sincere gratification by her medical friends. The expression of that woman's gratitude, in thus being preserved from what she and her friends supposed to be inevitable death, was an ample compensation for the anxiety experienced by those who were the humble instruments of affording her relief. This patient recovered rapidly, and did not, during the whole of her convalesence, present one unpleasant symptom. It is now ten weeks since the operation, and she and her infant are in the enjoyment of excellent health.

"At my last visit to this patient, with Dr. Forry, she made some additional revelations, which I think should be given, not only to the profession, but to the public, in order that it may be known, that in our very midst there is a monster who speculates with human life, with as much coolness as if she were engaged in a game of chance.

"This patient, with unaffected sincerity, and apparently ignorant of the moral turpitude of the act, stated most unequivocally to both Dr. Forry and myself, '*that this physician, on previous occasions, had caused her to miscarry five times*, and that these miscarriages had, in every instance, been brought about by drugs administered by this trafficer in human life. The only case in which the medicines failed was the last pregnancy, when, at the suggestion of this physician, she probed herself, and induced the condition of things described, and which most seriously involved her own safety, as well as that of her child.' In the course of conversation, this woman mentioned that she knew a great number of persons who were in the habit of applying to this physician for the purpose of miscarrying, and that she scarcely ever failed in affording the desired relief; and, among others, she cited the case of a female residing in Houston-street, who was five months pregnant; this physician probed her, and she was delivered of a child, to use her own expression, '*that kicked several times after it was put into the bowl.*'

"It indeed seems too monstrous for belief that such gross violations of the laws of both God and man should be suffered in the very heart of a community professing to be Christian, and to be governed by law and good order. Yet these facts are known to all who can read. This creature's advertisements are to be seen in most of our daily papers. Thus she invites the base and the guilty, the innocent and the unwary, to apply to her. She tells publicly what she can do, and without the slightest scruple urges all to call on her who may be anxious to avoid having children. Here, then, is a premium offered for vice, to say nothing of the prodigal destruction of human life that must necessarily result from the abominations of this mercenary and heartless woman.

"With all the vigilance of the police of our city, and with every disposition, I am sure, on the part of the authorities to protect public morals, and to bring to merited punishment those who violate the sanctity of the law, this *physician*, as she styles herself, has as yet escaped with impunity.

"Occupying the position I do, and fully appreciating the important trust confided to my care, in connection with the department over which I have the honor to preside in the University, I have felt it to be a duty I owe to the community, to the profession, and to myself, publicly to expose the facts of this case ; and I fervently hope that the disclosures here made may tend to the arrest of this woman, and the infliction of the severest penalty of the law."

THE END.

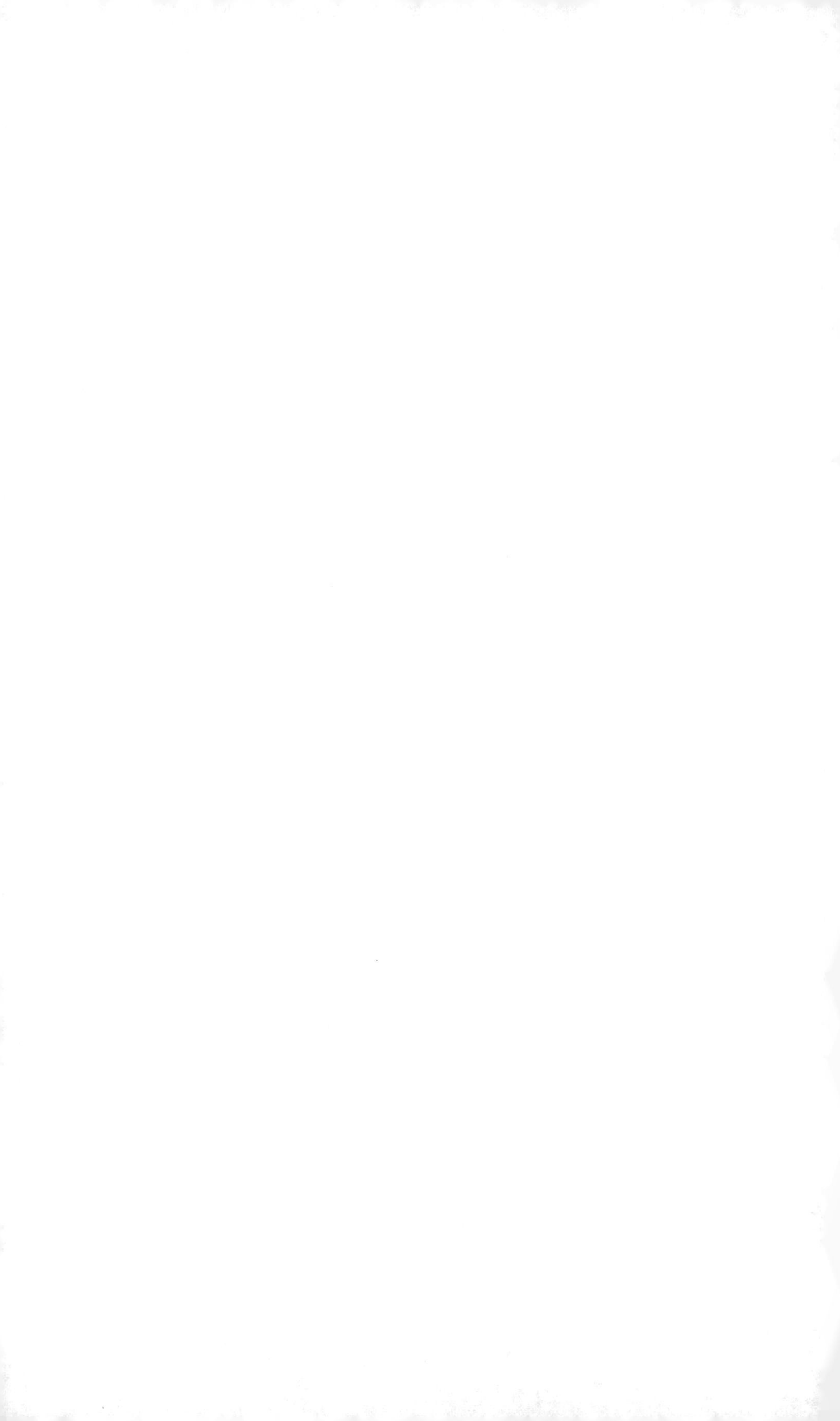

www.ingramcontent.com/pod-product-compliance
Lightning Source LLC
LaVergne TN
LVHW010144110826
845151LV00002B/424